Extraordinary Healthcare

To Leslie

Best of Health

Sarvasri

Extraordinary Healthcare

Low-Cost, No-Cost Natural Healthcare
For Physical, Mental, and Emotional Health

Sri Ananda Sarvasri

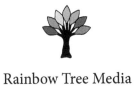

Rainbow Tree Media

Disclaimer
This book is designed to reduce suffering and healthcare costs by 90-95%. It is a new multi-disciplinary approach to healthcare beyond what doctors, hospitals, the pharmaceutical industry, and healthcare specialists currently offer. Allopathic healthcare is remarkable in the case of accidents, emergencies, and reconstructive surgery. For virtually all degenerative and lifestyle diseases, it has proven ineffective, because doctors are being asked to do the impossible. They cannot make your decisions about what you eat, think, feel, do, believe, or know. This book is intended to help you make the best decisions for your healthcare. But the truth is, no one can assume responsibility for your well being except you. Take advantage of all options available to you including the services of health care professionals if your intuition guides you in that direction. Neither the author nor the publisher is responsible for any consequences incurred by those employing the remedies or treatments reported herein. It's simply not possible. Even doctors and hospitals will not guarantee that you will survive a visit to any hospital or medical institution. No one can or will take responsibility for your health, whether allopathic or otherwise. You are the only one who can take responsibility for your well being. Therefore, any application of the material set forth in the following pages is at the reader's discretion and is his or her sole responsibility.
Extraordinary Healthcare: Low-Cost, No-Cost Natural Healthcare For Physical, Mental, and Emotional Health is published by Rainbow Tree Media, a subdivision of a developing non-profit educational/spiritual trust dedicated to the welfare of the people of the world regardless of race, culture, or faith. Its primary goal is to create new innovations to uplift humanity into a new era of peace, understanding, and well-being, and to create and distribute literature and media that make it easy to put knowledge into practice.

Rainbow Tree Media
1060 Tyler Rd.,
Walnut Cove, North Carolina, 27052
http://RainbowTreeMedia.com
Manufactured in the United States of America

Publisher's Cataloging-in-Publication Data
Ananda, Sri Sarvasri 1946 –
    Extraordinary Healthcare : low-cost, no-cost natural healthcare for physical, mental, and emotional health / by Sri Ananda Sarvasri
    p. cm.
    ISBN 978-0-9915067-0-5
1. Holistic health 2. Self-care, Health. 3. Naturopathy 4. Complementary therapies 5. Mental health   I. Ananda, Sri Sarvasri II. Title
R733.A53   2014
615.53   2014902653

First Edition - February, 2014
10 9 8 7 6 5 4 3 2 1

Dedication

I dedicate this book to the youth of the world. They have not yet suffered so much pain and heartache as we adults have. It is my hope that by learning and utilizing this knowledge, they can be spared as much pain and suffering as possible.

In the future, all healthcare will be easier and more effective as we learn to utilize our innate wisdom and intuition and learn to understand the laws of nature and apply them. My intent is that this book will give our youth a head start.

I gratefully dedicate this book and thank my many teachers who have unselfishly shared their knowledge, especially, Paramahamsa Sri Nithyananda

— Sri Ananda Sarvasri

The pain which has not yet come is avoidable.
— Yoga Sutras of Patanjali, 2:16 —

Contents

Introduction

The Journey Begins

Over forty-two years ago, I began to research whether it is possible to heal the human body, mind, and heart through knowledge alone. No medical procedures, no surgery, no drugs, no expensive supplements, no exotic foods or herbs, no expert intervention, no costs whatsoever. Just knowledge. Could we stimulate the body's own inner pharmacology to create a superior form of healthcare beyond anything the medical industry can offer, all for free? I searched the world's healing traditions to discover if, by making different choices in our daily activities, we could create an immune system capable of rapidly healing virtually any disease and every psychological condition – even add decades to human life in perfect health. Could simple exercises, changes in the foods we choose to eat, what we drink, the thoughts we think, what we visualize, the emotions we feel, allow us to eliminate the need for medicines, drugs, and surgery altogether, except in cases of traumatic injury? The answer is a resounding "YES!"

Your body has an amazing pharmacy built in – far superior to any pharmaceutical industry. Your body can do surgery one cell at a time, far superior to any surgeon. Your mind and emotions have self-healing properties. You are actually self sufficient in your capacity to heal virtually every condition. You just need knowledge.

This book introduces a new natural multidisciplinary approach to healthcare, a non-medical approach that can be practiced by individuals, families, businesses, nurses, doctors, and hospitals. It is a realistic solution to the healthcare crisis in America and elsewhere. The premise is that humans are designed to be self healing. We heal easily when the right resources are provided and destructive practices are avoided. This manual of natural healthcare should be taught around the world in every country, city, town, village, and family. These low-cost, no-cost solutions are just what the world needs in these times of exorbitant healthcare costs.

Natural healthcare has been used to prevent and cure cancer, diabetes, heart disease, and virtually all chronic and degenerative diseases and conditions. Companies and organizations use it to reduce healthcare costs by over 80% and keep their employees alive and productive. It makes bottom-line economic sense to care for employees through natural healthcare and maintain a healthy work environment. Benefits to industry include lower turnover, lower absenteeism, higher quality workplace, improved performance, and lower healthcare costs (5:1 ROI).

Our healthcare system cannot be fixed with a new insurance program or any other superficial fixes. It is fundamentally broken because it has not addressed the ultimate cause of disease – a depleted immune system. In the U.S., over half of the population uses prescription drugs regularly. Non-prescription and illegal drugs are widely used. Prescription psychotropic drugs for depression are pervasive. Yet, we are not healthier or happier. In fact, medical intervention itself is the third leading cause of death. Statistics vary from a few hundred thousand to over a million deaths per year due to medical negligence and mistakes, wrong prescriptions, botched surgeries, hospital and doctor induced infections (35-40% of all disease), wrong diagnosis, and toxic therapies. This is happening because we have been asking doctors to do the impossible. No matter what skills doctors may have, they cannot make our decisions for us. Most doctors, including former Surgeon Generals, understand that over 3/4 of all deaths are actually due to poor diet and lifestyle choices. This is where we need to put our focus if we desire to be healthy. With this book, you should be able to eliminate 90-95% of healthcare costs and drastically reduce premature deaths in your family or organization. Natural healthcare can produce remarkable effects in stimulating the immune system to regenerate your body. Let's look at a few healing stories.

Healing Stories

An 82 year old woman suffered from multiple conditions: Hypertension (180/140), diabetes (requiring insulin injections), heart disease, rheumatoid arthritis, nephritis, gallbladder inflammation, bronchitis, and cataracts. She was on many medications. Several times a day she took at least 17 pills. She began a simple regimen of self-administered natural healthcare that consisted of percussive acupressure on GV-14, and a few other locations for 30 minutes each – basically, an hour and a half of self therapy, twice a day. Being an invalid, she didn't have much else to do.

She also did a stretching exercise, starting with 5 minutes, gradually increasing to 30. In one month, symptoms of hypertension, rheumatoid arthritis, nephritis, cholecystitis, and bronchitis gradually disappeared. She was able to stop related medications, except for anti-hypertensive drugs and insulin. Soon, her blood pressure returned to normal, and she was able to discontinue the drugs for hypertension that she had been taking for 20 years.

She was still taking insulin injections, 16 units twice a day. As her diabetes responded to her healthcare regimen, she reduced to 12, then 10, then 7 units, until finally, she was able to discontinue insulin altogether.

Her eyesight was poor, she had cataracts, vitreous opacity, muscae volitantes (floaters), a very dark view from one eye, and blurry vision in the other. She began a technique of percussive acupressure for her eyes. Within a month, she had clear, bright eyes and normal vision. Her cataracts disappeared. She is now healthy, has stopped all medications and no longer suffers from any of her previous conditions, or side effects from her medications.

She can now go up and down stairs carrying a heavy load with no symptoms of arthritis. In her advanced age, she was humpbacked, with flabby facial skin, many wrinkles and age spots. Her body is now straight, she has firm facial skin, significantly fewer wrinkles, and her color spots are almost gone. Her skin is much smoother. She can lift both arms overhead and bend to touch her hands to the floor. She now looks a dozen years younger, without any signs or symptoms of a woman over 80 years old. All this transformation happened within one year.

—

A man comes to my office having received a diagnosis of prostate cancer. His PSA is over 120. He is a prominent man in the community, one of the county commissioners. He wants to try a natural healthcare approach since his prognosis is not good. I describe to him a simple regimen of two alternative therapies that people have used in the past. He decides to try it. Within a few weeks, he returns to the office with stories to tell. As he tried his self-administered natural healthcare, he continued to visit his doctor. Each time he visited his doctor, his doctor would grill him and ask him what he was doing, but he would never tell. He didn't want anyone to know what he was doing because of his prominent position in the community.

Finally, after a few visits, his doctor was insistent to know more. He asked his patient if he would join him for dinner, after all, he was also a friend. When he attended the dinner, his doctor friend again brought up the question of what he had been doing. Still he would not tell. Finally the doctor became even more insistent and demanded to know. The patient finally ask, "Why are you so insistent about what I've been doing?" The doctor said he had never seen this before, the PSA dropped from 120 to 0.1 and according to his training, this was impossible. He wanted to know what was responsible for it, how he was able to get rid of the prostate cancer so rapidly and so completely. Still the patient would not tell. He had healed his cancer and that was enough. He wanted to put that part of his life behind him and didn't want to make waves because of his prominent position.

—

A friend of a friend calls me from Florida. He has a woman friend who is in the hospital. She is in a coma. She's been in a coma for a long time and her prognosis is not good. He asks if I can do a healing session on her. He knows that I know how to do bio-energetic, life-force healing and that I can do it at any distance. I agree to do the healing and proceed to do a one-hour distance healing session on her from where I live in North Carolina. Within three days, the woman is out of the coma and out of the hospital.

—

A medical doctor, a woman, finds that there is a lump growing in the center of her chest. It's growing extremely rapidly. Within the short timespan of a few weeks this small lump turns into a tumor the size of a grapefruit. It's cancer, of course. Being a medical doctor, she consults with an oncologist, to see what can be done. The tumor is rapidly growing larger. When the oncologist does his assessment, the only recommendation he gives is that she should immediately make out her will. The cancer has already spread throughout her chest cavity and there is no hope. He recommends the usual chemotherapy, which he says could perhaps extend her life for a while. Being a doctor herself, she knows the medical odds with conventional intervention. She recognizes that there is no hope through the established medical protocols and methods. The woman doctor decides against all medical intervention, with the exception of surgery to remove the external tumor. She then adopts a radical high enzyme, high life-force, natural, vegetarian diet. Within a few months of her self-administered natural healthcare, she is completely cancer free and returns to a normal life.

—

I'm teaching a seminar on bio-energy healing. On the second day, one of the participants doesn't show up. I ask her roommate about her and she says that her friend won't be able to make the workshop today because she has a terrible migraine headache. She says that when she gets a headache like this, she is usually bedridden for at least two days. She can hardly see, she's in tremendous pain, she can't really walk, she's in a really bad way. I told her that this is a healing workshop and that she should go upstairs and lead her friend down here for me to help her. She does.

When she comes into the room, she's in a really bad way – in tremendous pain and completely dysfunctional. I place my hands on her head and began streaming bio-energy into her from her forehead to the back of her skull. Within eight minutes she is completely out of pain. Within 13 minutes she is completely normal. She attends the second day of the workshop and everybody is happy. She could not believe that her migraine headache could be completely eliminated in less than 15 minutes. It was a real awakening for her.

—

I'm working in my yard, in my front garden. I hear a noise and look up. One of the neighborhood kids has fallen on his bicycle and hurt himself. He's crying. I run over to see him and find that he is in pain from some pretty intense scrapes and bruises from falling on the asphalt. Immediately, I examine his hand, which is bleeding slightly and in substantial pain. I begin streaming life-force, bio-energy into his hand. Within about a minute his hand is pain-free. Next, I move to his knee and stream healing energy into his knee. Again, within a minute or so his knee is also pain-free. He is smiling. The next step is to clean the injuries and apply some bandages. He is without pain and goes to rest at home. After a few days, I see him playing in the neighborhood. He comes over to show me how his wounds have healed so well that he can return to his bicycle riding.

—

Several patients are having heart trouble. Upon medical examination it's discovered that their arteries are 80 to 90% blocked and that they are going to need either triple or quadruple bypass surgery. They cannot afford such expensive healthcare. They began a self-administered natural healthcare program using two simple therapies – drinking slightly mineralized water in sufficient quantities, combined with gentle, daily walks. Within 3 to 6 months their arteries are completely free of obstructions. They no longer need surgery and return to a normal life.

—

My wife and I are driving back from Atlanta to North Carolina, traveling through a rural part of the country. In front of us there is an accident. A family just totaled their car. The husband and son are able to get out, but the wife is trapped behind the wheel. She cannot get out and she is going into shock. She is a very large woman with multiple medical problems, including diabetes. She is still conscious enough to talk. I climb in on the passenger's side and tell her that I am a healer and I'm going to do some energy healing for her. I began streaming life-force, bio-energy into her. Within a short time, normal color returns to her face. She is not going unconscious and avoids going into shock. I continue to stream bio-energy into her – into her head, her heart, and anywhere she has pain.

EMS, emergency medical services, arrives on the scene. They assess the situation and realize that she cannot be freed from the vehicle through any ordinary means. They asked me what I am doing, and I tell them that I am a healer and that I'm doing bio-energy healing on her. To my surprise, they tell me to keep doing what I'm doing, because there is nothing they can do for her until the Jaws of Life, a powerful pneumatic demolition tool, arrives on the scene. They are going to have to cut her out of the car using the Jaws of Life to break her free.

I continue to stream energy into her until the equipment arrives. By this time her transformation from the bio-energy is substantial. She is laughing and carrying on as if nothing has happened, as if she has not just totaled her car and been pinned behind the wheel – trapped. She is out of shock and her spirits are high, she is calm. The EMS people are taking her medical history, and she is totally clear and conscious as she gives them the exact details of her extensive medical problems.

The Jaws of Life show up and they proceed to cut and pry her out of the car. As they do so, I leave the vehicle to avoid the potential of flying glass, but I continue to stream energy from a distance and the woman sails through the experience of being extricated from the car. They put her on a gurney and take her to the hospital for examination.

There is no doubt in my mind that had we not arrived on the scene and kept her from going into shock, the outcome could have been totally different – with her medical history, perhaps deadly.

—

A woman calls me about her shoulder. She's been told that she needs to have a shoulder replacement because there is hardly anything left. She is in severe pain, her shoulder muscles have atrophied, and mobility is limited. We schedule a couple of bio-energy healing sessions. After the second session she is out of pain. A few weeks go by and she decides to attend one of my seminars on bio-energy healing. On the last day of the class, she demonstrates the extraordinary level of healing that has taken place since I first worked with her. She has been completely out of pain, her shoulder mobility is completely restored, and she no longer needs a shoulder replacement operation.

—

My wife gets a call from a couple she met at a trade fair. Their little dog is not doing well, in fact, it is at the vet hospital with congestive heart failure and is not expected to live through the night. There's a lot of water around the heart, and for such a little dog, the prognosis is not good. They call in a panic to see if there's anything we can do. My wife has an affinity for animals, and has been trained in bio-energy healing as well. She is accomplished in her own right.

My wife begins a session of streaming bio-energy, long distance, to the little dog. It's after hours at the vet hospital and no one is there. Everyone expects that they may have to bury the dog the next day.

The next morning, we get an excited call from the couple. They went to pick up their dog with the idea of taking it to a specialist and found the dog alive and alert. She had done her morning business, and is friskily running around the place. The vet is amazed. She says the animal is totally normal and the blood work shows near-perfect scores, the best she has ever seen, considering the prior situation. The couple picks up their dog and returns to normal life. Bio-energy healing is not a placebo. Even an animal, which of course cannot respond to psychological placebo effects, gets healed.

—

A woman shows up with severe psychological problems. She has been seeing a psychiatrist and the psychiatrist had prescribed Xanax, a psychotropic drug. The psychiatrist kept increasing the dosage because she was continuing to have psychotic episodes. She had reached the maximum dosage, but she was still having psychosis, hallucinations, and could not function well in society. She was unable to hold a job.

The woman tells the psychiatrist that the drug is not working and that she would like to get off drugs altogether if possible, that she needs some other help. The psychiatrist then has her sign an affidavit that he is no longer responsible for her and he abandons her. She leaves his office. She had reached the limit of what psychiatric drugs could do for her. She arrives at my door.

She had taken it upon herself to stop taking the drugs altogether. I am aware that this is a dangerous thing to do, to stop taking such drugs cold turkey, but she had already done it, and now she is here in front of me, coming loose at the seams. When she enters my office she is in a terrible state. She starts screaming that Hitler is trying to kill her. She is having an intense psychotic episode, as if her life is being threatened this moment. She is having a horrible hallucination. It's impossible to reason with a person during a psychotic episode. I give her some simple straightforward instructions that she can do. Within five minutes she begins to return to normal. I began working on her with various acupressure methods. Within 30 to 40 minutes, she is stable and somewhat functional.

She has nowhere to go and no money for medical help. She asked me to help her so I continue to educate her regarding natural approaches to mental health. She learns and applies the principles of natural mental healthcare. Within a few weeks she has improved substantially. Within a few months she is able to function in society, hold a job, and live a normal life. She is completely drug-free and continues to develop into a balanced human being.

—

Hundreds and thousands of such stories of natural healing exist for physical, mental, and emotional health. I could go on and on, but I think you get the idea. *Extraordinary Healthcare* is possible and very real. It's practically free and you are going to learn how to accomplish it for yourself, your family, and your organization by reading this book. I've included the best of what I've learned over the past 40+ years. Armed with this information, you may never need to see a medical specialist again, except for accidents or true emergencies. For the most part, conventional "healthcare," as we know it, should be refined and upgraded to natural methods wherever possible. We need to realize that true healthcare can never be achieved through a medical industrial complex based upon injecting us with exotic chemicals, pumping us full of pills, slicing up our tissues, and disfiguring our bodies. Current practices in allopathic medicine have proven to be a misguided attempt at "healthcare," mostly because they lack knowledge of effective alternatives. There is a better approach. Achieving extraordinary health doesn't have to be difficult. It is simple. It is rational. It is straightforward. You just need the right knowledge.

A New Era of Healthcare

Healthcare is ultimately about your journey, your quest to become all that you can be – to be happy, to live well, to live a long and successful life. Yet, how long will you live? How much happiness will you find? How much pain can you avoid? How do you pursue this quest? What are the methods, the techniques you can use to create a whole and complete life – a life of health, happiness, and purpose? That's what I present in this book. I am introducing you to a new era of healthcare. My goal is to reduce healthcare costs and restore natural healthcare worldwide. I'm going to give you the knowledge and teach you practical methods of natural healthcare, to heal yourself, to heal others, to revitalize your company or organization, and help awaken everyone to their highest health potential.

This is the knowledge I wish I had known 50 years ago, when I was a youth just starting out. I could have avoided so much pain and heartache. You don't need to learn everything the hard way. It takes too much time and it's painful. Why not make it easy on yourself? It doesn't matter what your age, it's never too late to learn something new. In this book, you'll discover how to eliminate your current pain and suffering, and how to avoid future pain and suffering. Ultimately, you'll discover an easier way to live the fulfilling life you really want.

I'll provide insights into health that are known only to a very small community of people – insights that may help you choose a path for your own healthcare, or the healing of a friend or loved one. How you use this information is totally up to you. Personally, I believe everything can be healed. I prefer to believe there are no limits to healing, except the limits we impose on ourselves.

The reason I believe in such extraordinary possibilities is because of my experience. I've experienced miraculous healing thousands of times. We've all read stories or heard about people who were given up for dead and then suddenly were healed. They resumed a normal life. In case after case, there are people who should have died, but didn't. It's referred to as "spontaneous remission." I believe it isn't spontaneous at all, that is, it is never random or accidental. There's always a cause for every effect. There are definite reasons why health returns and there are rational methods that promote healing.

I believe that your body has miraculous healing powers when it has the resources it needs. These resources are physical, bio-energetic, emotional, mental, and spiritual (consciousness), which you'll discover throughout this book.

9

Healing vs Medical

I have a great respect for medical doctors. They go through arduous training and often work under difficult conditions. The problem is, they are being asked to do a job they cannot do. With the tools and training doctors are given, it's impossible to create a healthy society. The reason we have a healthcare crisis today is because our medical model is totally inadequate. No new insurance program, no state run access to medical care is going to make any difference. The problem is with the medical model itself, both in methods and administration.

There are many compassionate doctors who want to see substantial changes in the medical system. They know it's not working. It's unfortunate that our healthcare system developed the way it did. I believe that healthcare should never have become a profit-making industry. It should be universally available and free. It should have developed as a spiritual profession, like the practice of religion or spirituality. When it became a profit-making industry, several things happened:

1) The medical educational system became dominated by industry in order to promote expensive pharmaceutical and surgical solutions.

2) Simple and inexpensive solutions are no longer taught or practiced.

3) The healthcare system as a whole lost its heart and became corrupt and greedy.

4) Science became politicized, honest science is rarely practiced.

5) Simple and effective solutions used for centuries were forgotten.

6) People enter the profession with the goal of making lots of money, which is the wrong motivation for the healing arts.

The result is that medical care became both prohibitively expensive and ineffective. One of the biggest problems with the healthcare system today is that it is based on inherently dangerous practices. Drugs and surgery both have high costs and dangers. That's why doctors and nurses need to be licensed to begin with. In many cases, medical practitioners often cause death or permanent disability. Statistics vary, but in the USA alone, medically-caused deaths range between 250,000 to over 1,000,000 every year – inadvertently, but directly caused by medical doctors and staff. These deaths are caused by botched surgeries, wrong prescriptions, wrong diagnosis, introduction of new infections that did not previously exist, and many other factors I will cover later. Debilitating injury could be 10 times this amount. We need a much gentler, noninvasive approach to healthcare. Doctors are well aware of the problems, but they are not given solutions.

Patients aren't the only ones who are suffering. Doctors themselves are often deeply frustrated with their profession. Through their education, they were led to believe that they have the best knowledge of healthcare. But when the methods they were taught fail to work, they become frustrated and blame themselves, when in fact, it's the system. This failure is particularly apparent with degenerative diseases like diabetes, cancer, heart disease, and mental disorders. The body is already weakened, and the introduction of harsh methods of treatment often causes further degradation of health. It's a difficult profession because of the way doctors have been trained. Among professions, doctors have the highest rates of alcoholism and suicide.

From a business or administrative point of view, the medical system depends upon an endless stream of very sick people to continue to support its huge infrastructure. What would happen if we all became healthy? This would be great for people, but intolerable to our vast medical industrial complex and vast insurance complex. More than 20% of the economy would disappear. Vast expenditures for medical expenses does not produce a better real economy any more than war does. The only real solution that benefits people is an economy based on health, not disease. It's essential for us all to become healthy naturally. That's the purpose of this book. Worldwide, it doesn't make sense to fund a huge medical complex any more than it makes sense to fund continuous war. It's a losing proposition for people.

Let's compare the profession of natural healthcare with conventional medicine. Natural healthcare is a completely different approach to health. Medicine is concerned with diagnosis, powerful drugs to alter body chemistry, and surgery to remove damaged or diseased tissues. It is actually derived from battlefield necessities. On the other hand, natural healthcare is a regenerative approach. It empowers the body to heal itself. The basic philosophy is that our body can never be healthier than our cells. If our cells are healthy, then our body will be healthy. From this positive health approach, it's difficult to imagine how powerful drugs or surgery could make better cells, and without better cells, how can we have a healthier body?

The art of natural healthcare doesn't require that we diagnose or treat diseases with specific cures. Your body doesn't care what you name a disease. Also, there are virtually no diseases with only a single cause. The quest for a magic bullet that will heal any disease like cancer is a myth. All diseases are caused by multiple weaknesses. With natural healthcare, the main purpose is to empower the body to heal itself in multiple ways. The body has more wisdom, more ability to heal than you can possibly imagine. This is very important. Unlike a machine, the body is designed to be self healing. If we provide sufficient resources, and restore harmony and balance to mind and body in a profound enough way, then the body uses its incredible wisdom to heal itself. We don't even have to know the nature of the condition or the disease.

Even conventional, allopathic medicine ultimately relies on the body to heal itself. The difference is that with natural healthcare, we start there. We empower the body to heal itself from the beginning. It resolves the problem without much external intervention. True healing is ultimately self healing – easily self-administered natural healthcare.

This is not to say that there is no place for allopathic medicine. There are times when surgery is necessary, 1) in case of accidents, 2) when abnormal growths in the body have become too large, and 3) in emergency situations. In these situations, allopathic medical intervention is necessary. Medical discoveries have benefited all of us greatly. Who can imagine surgery or dentistry without painkillers? Antibiotics have saved countless lives. Yet, with all the medical technologies at our disposal, we see mental and physical health deteriorating rapidly around the world. It's because we're asking the medical profession to do the impossible. Medicine can never substitute or compensate for bad diets, high stress, emotional turmoil, destructive thinking, or our disconnection from our inner self and nature. To reverse this downward spiral, we must return to natural, regenerative ways of caring for ourselves and our families. This is something only we can do for ourselves.

In this book, I make no medical claims. I don't approach healthcare as a medical discipline. If you think about it, even the medical world makes no guarantees. Doctors can't and won't guarantee that you'll survive even the simplest medical procedure – that you'll leave the hospital alive. When you enter a hospital you sign papers to that effect. Fortunately, the methods in this book are non-destructive by nature. But even water is lethal – people drown in it. People choke on ordinary food. Your common sense and intuition are what save you. These methods, practiced sensibly, are safe and powerful, but nothing in life is guaranteed. The only real guarantees you have in life are the ones you create for yourself. Ultimately, you are the one who is responsible for your life and your health. No one can assume that responsibility for you. The methods in this book come from various sources

– the ancient Vedic tradition, enlightened masters, master healers, naturopathic studies, and my own experiences.

Two Approaches, Two Choices

A century ago, the medical system had a choice of two basic approaches to healthcare. One approach was promoted by Louis Pasteur, who you may have learned about in school. The other approach was developed by Antoine Beauchamp (you probably never heard of him). At that time, the world had endured plagues of infectious diseases, and the hunt was on to stop these devastating threats to health. Louis Pasteur, you may remember, is credited with the discovery of microorganisms. He claimed that germs were the cause of disease. The medical world took that approach, followed his lead, and began the search for chemicals that could destroy germs. They're still looking for more powerful drugs, because over time, germs became more powerful, more resistant. Now we have super pathogens, super strains of diseases like strep and tuberculosis, that we can't destroy with any existing medical antibiotics. These resistant microorganisms resulted from the choice that medical science made years ago.

Antoine Beauchamp, a contemporary of Pasteur, noticed that not everybody contracted diseases even though they were exposed. He even proved that disease was not caused by single organisms, but was a complex process of environmental opportunity. Basically, the health of the immune system, the ability of the body to resist infection, was more important than germs.

Pasteur wasn't entirely wrong, germs are a factor in many diseases, but the environment of the body is much more important. This is especially true today, since most diseases like cancer, heart disease, and diabetes, are degenerative in nature, and not caused by single pathogens. At the end of his life, Pasteur withdrew support for his own theory and supported Beauchamp. But the medical world had already committed to the path of destroying germs, looking for and finding powerful drugs. In spite of evidence to the contrary, medicine chose the path of destruction of microorganisms as the primary path to health. Kill the germs, surgically remove bad tissues, force powerful chemical changes in the body through drugs. These have become the fundamental approaches of modern medicine.

This combative approach not only influenced the medical profession, it colored every aspect of our society. Everything became a battle. Agriculture, for instance, found poisons to destroy insects. But just like the germs, insects became immune, so more powerful poisons were needed. Now we've poisoned virtually all life in our soils. We keep "needing" more types of poisons and more powerful poisons. Just as we created super germs, we created super pests on our crops.

Society attempts to stamp out what it doesn't want by destroying the opposition. We see it today in politics, religion, law and justice, education, in business, and of course, in the war machine that pervades the news. Everywhere, we see competition, battles. Good against bad. It's an approach with a proven record of failure. The bugs, the opposition, only get stronger, more sophisticated, more cunning.

It seems clear that to be successful, we must examine the environments that cause the original problems. We must understand whole systems. This is the new approach to healthcare, just as it's also the new approach in organic agriculture. Repair the environment. This is the approach that conventional medicine left behind. We need to create environments which foster health and positive values, rather than trying to destroy what we don't want. When we look at environments, healing becomes much easier. This concept applies to all our institutions.

Healing Is Easy

It turns out that healing the human body can be surprisingly easy! This may seem to be a farfetched idea, especially considering the vast medical problems that exist today, and the extreme difficulty of conventional medicine to find cures. The reason this new approach is so much easier, is because the body and mind want to heal more than anything else. Plus, the body KNOWS HOW to heal. The body knows more chemistry than any scientist has ever known. It has a better pharmacy than any pharmaceutical company. It can do microscopic surgery at the cellular level, one cell at a time. No surgeon could ever possibly do that. The body is a miraculous system, but it has not been empowered with a favorable environment. When we change the environment, the body heals itself, using its own powerful systems of regeneration.

As a result, our job really becomes simple. Create a new internal environment: physically, energetically, emotionally, mentally, and consciously, and, if possible, improve the external environment as well. Since natural healthcare is so easy, every parent should learn it. It will prevent high stress, help avoid feeling powerless with your family, and save a fortune in medical costs. For organizations, it will greatly increase productivity and job satisfaction, because people won't be overwhelmed or in pain at work.

How Natural Healthcare Works

In a nutshell, here's how natural healthcare works. We're all subject to two kinds of forces, destructive forces and constructive forces. Destructive, degenerative forces are the forces that tear us down: high stress, toxic exposures, congestion, depression, poor nutrition, and so on. Constructive, regenerative forces are the forces that lift us up: high quality nutrition, clean internal environment, deep rest, a boost in energetic life forces, a positive self image, and increased conscious awareness.

When degenerative forces predominate, 1) the harder it is to heal, 2) the fewer things we can heal, and 3) the slower we heal. We're simply dragged down. When regenerative forces predominate, 1) the easier it is to heal, 2) the more things we can heal, and 3) the faster we heal. Therefore, in order to heal any condition, all we have to do is minimize destructive forces and increase regenerative forces. The body then heals itself. Doesn't this make sense? Regenerative forces must outweigh degenerative forces. It's simple, and it always works. Create a regenerative environment, and if conditions haven't deteriorated too much, it's virtually impossible NOT to heal. The only question is, can we minimize degenerative forces and maximize regenerative forces fast enough to undo existing damage?

Five Levels of Natural Healthcare

Regenerative and degenerative influences operate on five levels. The five levels are: 1) physical, 2) bio-energetic, 3) emotional, 4) mental, and 5) conscious awareness. These are the five basic pathways or approaches we can take to minimize degenerative forces and increase regenerative forces. By approaching every human condition on all five levels, we can bring about a transformation in the field of healthcare. For the ultimate in healthcare, we must create new environments on all five levels.

In this book, I'll share with you how people used this approach to transform their life to one that no longer supported disease. This is what we all want. The first step is to set your intention, set goals for the kind of life you want.

Setting Goals on Five Levels

It's important to set goals for yourself. When you set goals you take your attention away from problems and put it on solutions. You can set goals on all five levels: Physical, Bio-Energetic, Emotional, Mental, and Conscious Awareness. You can also set goals for other areas of your life according to the commitments you have made. In the upcoming section on organizing, you'll dive deeper into goal setting when you have your organizing system set up.

We are going to go far beyond ordinary healthcare to create a profound level of life, beyond suffering of any kind. This is what I call Extraordinary Healthcare. This is not only possible, it is our birthright. Reversing diseases is just the beginning. There is an incredible transformation and adventure awaiting you.

If you have a serious condition, you should know that this kind of healthcare is extremely practical. Many people have reversed the most devastating, life threatening conditions, long after the medical world gave up and left them to die. I'll explore the methods they used to create the conditions that empowered their body to heal itself. The powers of your body are amazing. Your body can do surgery, pharmacology, it can repair DNA, it can create new cells, new tissues, and repair organs. The goal is to create an extraordinary, regenerative environment. Then powerful healing responses happen in both mind and body. The innate, vastly intelligent resources within you produce the transformative healing that you desire.

Our extraordinary healthcare approach is also preventive. It begins before any health concern ever arises. It is restorative, it applies powerfully when we need it most, and it continues long after you're healed. It's not just for sick people. It's for everyone to create a new super quality of health.

How long and how happily you live depends on *you*. You must learn how your living system works, how to create supportive inner environments, and apply the basic laws of nature for your own benefit. Then you can help those around you.

Getting the Most From *Extraordinary Healthcare*

First of all, you're in control: Whenever you don't understand something, STOP, back up and re-read again. Keep your focus. If you begin to lose focus because you're tired, then stop and come back after a short rest. Every few months, you'll want to review the text, or at least sections of it, until you really understand. You probably won't understand every aspect of what's presented here the first or second time through. Some learning depends on *experience* with the concepts and methods. You'll understand the methods more deeply with experience.

You don't have to agree with everything presented. If something doesn't appeal to you right now, let it go for a while. Concentrate on what you find most useful and acceptable. To get a deeper understanding, maybe you'll need to research the concepts on your own. Sometimes, it's just semantics. You may need to hear it a different way. Some concepts might take awhile to assimilate. Take your time.

This is actually a workshop, not just a book to read. After I cover a method or technique, pause and do the exercises. Work your way through the book doing the exercises. When you're finished with an exercise, move to the next section.

Taking Responsibility

Remember to use your intuition. I can't be there to guide your every step. No one can guarantee success but you. No one can assume responsibility for your well-being. You have to do that. I do not diagnose diseases nor prescribe "cures." I only describe how to empower your mind and body through natural, time-tested methods, to heal itself. You have to be responsible for yourself and know when and how much to utilize any method or concept. Sometimes you may need to go easy. Sometimes you may need to "pour on the coals." You are your own responsibility and no one can take that away from you. So be wise and listen to your body, listen to your intuition to gauge how far to take each exercise or suggestion. One of the first topics I'll cover is how to develop and use your intuition so you can get answers for yourself. If you need or want expert advice, whether medical or otherwise, then get it. This knowledge is not a substitute for common sense or expert advise when it's warranted. As you heal, often the need for prescription drugs drops drastically, often within days or weeks. This means you could overdose on the drugs you've been taking if the dosage is not reduced. If you are taking any drugs, you should consult with your doctor about how to respond accordingly. If you take both herbs and medications, learn about any conflicts. Constantly monitor medications until you no longer need them. Be aware of the effects of overdose. Look up every drug you take and be aware of all its characteristics. One resource is http://www.rxlist.com

In this book, I'm not going to focus on all the scientific data behind the recommendations. That would take several more books. If you're curious about any of the suggestions, then study the subject on the Internet and read books that target your specific interests. Learn Internet searching skills. Today, the ability to use Internet search engines effectively is one of your most powerful allies. But remember that most sources usually have an agenda to convince you to buy (or not buy) various products and services. You have to use your intuition and discernment wisely. Don't believe everything you read on the Internet, especially if products are being sold. You must be wise and intuitive. Creating extraordinary health is not expensive. It will probably cost far less than what you are spending now.

Enjoy this book and take your time working through it. It's not a race, but spend at least some time every day working through it. Devote extra time on weekends when you can. This information was developed over a period of over 40 years, with lots of investigations and trials. It's designed to get you up to speed very quickly, but it could still take a few weeks to really develop a thorough understanding. I wish you the best of health and an exciting journey into the future.

Chapter 1
Create Your Own Healthcare Plan
Deciding What to Do and How to Do It

Use Your Intuition for Healthcare

Most of us are just muddling through. Many of us never think about the important questions in life or consciously plan to achieve worthwhile goals. When we do attempt it, we constantly wonder whether we are doing the right things. Usually, we choose to do what our educational systems, parents, friends, or so-called authorities recommend, or else we rebel and oppose everything. There is a better way. You can consciously learn about your purpose for being here and consciously plan your life through the use of intuition. Intuition is superior to guessing or logical analysis.

Accessing Your Intuition

Everybody has perfect intuition, but most of us were never taught how to access it. Intuition is a deeper level of knowing that is beyond the mind. The mind is not a good tool to access intuition because it is so cluttered with prior conditioning and expectations. For most of us, our mind is a chaotic space, filled with anxieties, worries, concerns, confusions, and prejudices. Until our inner space is purified, the mind won't be a very reliable tool to get information. In a later chapter you will work with your mind more intensively, but right now you need to be able to get answers. You need to know how to proceed with your own healthcare. There are easy tools to access intuition.

Your body is a better guide than your mind for accessing your intuition. There are many ways to get answers from those deeper parts of you that have access to perfect intuition.

The Body Strength Method

When you ask yourself a question, your body immediately responds with either weakness or strength. This is the method used with the art and science called kinesiology. It's a very simple method and very effective. All you do is ask a question and then test the strength of your body. If your body is strong, then the answer is "yes." If your body is weak, the answer is "no." There are different ways to test body strength. One way is to work with a partner. You extend your arm out to the side, and your partner presses down on your arm with two fingers. It's not a battle of strength. Your partner is just going to use enough downward force to see whether you're holding your strength (or even stronger) or not. Here's the procedure:

1) If you're right handed, extend your left (non-dominant) arm, horizontally. If left handed, use your right arm.

2) Before asking the question, your partner says, "Hold" and presses to test your initial strength. You also can sense your initial strength.

3) Then you or your partner asks any question that can be answered with a yes or no answer.

4) Again, your partner says "Hold" and then presses gently on your outstretched arm to test whether you are stronger or weaker.

5) If you're stronger the answer is yes, if weaker, the answer is no. If your arm is kind of wobbly, giving an uncertain response, rephrase the question.

Asking the Right Questions

The secret to getting good answers is to ask good questions. Your body is literal and doesn't have a sense of humor. It simply answers the questions. If you formulate the questions poorly, you can get misleading answers. You may want to formulate your questions ahead of time, carefully and thoughtfully, and then go through them one by one. As you get answers to each question, you may want to pursue a deeper question, based upon the response. In this way, you can probe deeply into any area of your life and get the answers you need.

You can ask any question and get answers. You can ask what parts of your body are weak. You can ask about different approaches to healing your body. You can ask if a particular food is good for you, or not, at this time. Perhaps the food is tainted or for some reason is not agreeable to your system. Food choices are a very good thing to test frequently. You can ask about relationships, employment options, anything about any area of your life. Because everything is connected, you have access to all knowledge regarding everything that exists. If you are uncertain about an answer, ask the question a different way. You don't need to live your life with nagging uncertainties. When faced with a problem, just ask!

Whenever you ask a question, let your mind be inactive, passive. Take the attitude that you have no idea what the answer may be. Just be completely open. If you get too attached to wanting a particular answer, you can influence the result. Take the attitude that you don't care what the answer is. If the answer turns out to be something you don't want, you can always ask and determine how you can set things right. So don't be afraid of any kind of answer.

Other Body Strength Options

For long question and answer sessions, holding your arm out can become tedious. Also, this method requires a partner, which may not be available. There's another way to test your strength by yourself. Here's the method:

1) If you're right-handed, use your left hand (non-dominant hand) for the test. Press the tip of your left thumb against the tip of your ring finger (or your little finger). You are making a circle or ring using your left-hand finger and thumb. Press them together with modest strength. If you're left-handed, use your right hand to make this loop. As with the arm resistance test, this is not a battle of strength, just a way to gauge relative strength. Don't strain to do this.

2) With your other hand, make a similar ring with your thumb and longest (middle) finger, which is naturally stronger.

3) Now, interlock the two rings, one inside the other.

4) As you pull your hands apart, it will be easier to break the ring made with your non-dominant hand, which is also using a weaker finger.

5) First test your initial strength. How easy is it to break the ring? Gauge the strength.

6) Now ask a question. As before, if you're stronger, then the answer is yes. If it's easy to break the ring, then you are weaker and the answer is no.

Accessing Intuition Using A Pendulum

Another way to get answers is to use a pendulum. You can get four kinds of answers with a pendulum. 1) Yes, 2) No, 3) Maybe, and 4) Better not to know. Here's how it works:

1) First make a pendulum using a piece of string and any kind of weight. The string can be 8 to 12 inches long, but you will only use about 3-5 inches of the string. The weight can be anything from a paperclip to a small stone.

2) Hold the string between your thumb and first finger with just 2-3 inches of string between your fingers and the weight. Hold your hand still. The pendulum's movement, when it happens, does so without any obvious movement of your hand. It does not move by your conscious control or will. It moves from the deep connection with your body and your body's connection to everything. It is a subtle and wondrous process. Now, ask to be shown what a "yes" is. The general convention is for the pendulum to rotate clockwise to express a "yes" answer.

3) Now ask to be shown what a "no" answer is. Generally, a "no" answer is given when the pendulum rotates counterclockwise. Although these are the conventions for a "yes" and "no" answer, you may be given something else. You can set it up any way you want to, as long as you are consistent. You can decide how the "yes" and "no" answers come to you. Just get comfortable with how you get your "yes" and "no" answers. Test your system using known questions with known answers. Such as, "My first name is…" Yes or no?

4) You can get two other kinds of answers, a "maybe" and "better not to know." You get a "maybe" answer when the question is not defined very well. In other words, the answer is dependent upon circumstances that you have not properly defined in your question. So the answer could be "yes" or "no" depending upon something not clearly defined. The solution is to define your question more precisely. A "maybe" answer is often indicated by the pendulum swinging side to side.

5) A "better not to know" answer is an answer that comes when knowing the answer would influence your behavior in such a way as to alter the answer. In other words, knowing the answer is not necessary or desirable. In this case, pursue another line of questioning to get a resolution to the deeper question that you are after. A "better not to know" answer is often indicated when the pendulum swings to and fro, toward you and away from you.

Now you have a system for getting more detailed answers. Practice your system with easy and simple concerns at first. It's better not to start with life-changing questions unless there is no choice. Essentially, you want to get comfortable with the system so that you can put your trust in it. As you practice, you may start to get intuitive answers before you even test. This leads to a quicker system of getting intuitive answers.

Using Physical and Emotional Feelings To Access Intuition

Once you get some experience with accessing your intuition, you realize that the answers are coming even before you can finish asking the question. There is a kind of certainty and immediacy of knowing exactly what the answer is. As this intimacy with your intuition develops, you will begin to get emotional and physical responses to your questions. Both emotionally and physically, you feel a kind of lightness when the answer is "yes." Similarly, when the answer is "no" you feel a kind of heaviness. The reactions are immediate, before you can even think about them. There may even be a slight physical movement such as the up or down movement of your head. This kind of response is not coming from your head (your mind), but is coming from your heart and your body.

Once you recognize this ability – an immediate physical and emotional response – you can access your intuition very quickly for "yes" and "no" answers. Everyone has this ability built in. It's just a matter of getting comfortable with it. Once you have it available, use it for everything important. Don't let your mind guide you. Your mind, with all of its embedded patterns, projections, prejudices, investments, and confusions, will often mislead you.

Logic and analysis are also not the best ways to get answers. There are so many possible options for any possible choice in life, there's not enough time to logically analyze all the combinations and permutations of any direction you might take. Intuition is the shortcut that can compute everything at once. Live your life by intuition, not mental analysis. It's easier, more accurate, and more fulfilling.

As your intuition develops further, your inner guidance will include more detail. Intuition can come as a complete package that includes 1) certainty of knowingness, 2) complete concepts with enough detail, and 3) moving or still images. It's unfortunate that most adults were never taught how to access intuition at an early age. If you work with children or young adults, share this information with them. It can prevent so many hardships and misguided actions.

Getting Organized

Healing doesn't happen by accident. In order to heal, you have to take certain steps, certain actions. You have to change the way you live. This means forming new habits, new ways of living, new choices. Ultimately, the problem boils down to remembering to do things!

Everyone has made resolutions at one time or another only to drop those resolutions within a few days. We usually don't *decide* to drop a resolution, we just forget - very conveniently. The ego part of us doesn't want to change and often gets its own way - usually, by just forgetting about it. The truth is, you can't count on your memory. When you want to develop a new lifestyle or develop a new habit, it's easy to get distracted. You may have good intentions, but for most people, life gets pretty hectic and you forget to do the things you want to do. Also, there are many negative programs buried in your forgotten memory. These buried negative programs cause self sabotage. You need a system to overcome these limitations.

What you really need is a personal assistant to remind you of what things to do and when to do them. The best personal assistant is one that never complains, is always around, and never fails - a digital personal assistant.

these high-tech times, it's so much easier to get organized using the multitude of devices and apps that are available. Practically every smartphone, every computer, every tablet, and even many music players have basic apps. You are looking for these eight apps: 1) *Calendar* (with color-coded sub-calendars), 2) *Reminder List*, 3) *Checklist*, 4) *To Do List* (for more extensive planning), 5) *Timer* (count down timers can be used to set your meditation time), 6) *Alarms* can be set to go off many times a day at certain intervals, 7) *Note Taking* and/or audio recording apps, and 8) *Contacts/Address Book*. Find something to start with in each of these eight categories. You can refine your system as you go along. For people not plugged into the high-tech world, there are paper organizer systems at any office supply. A simple kitchen timer at the dollar store works for timing activities. Here are the basics:

Contacts, Calendars, Reminders, Checklists, ToDo's, Timers, Alarms, Notes

Probably everyone already has a contacts list or an address book. People are the most important aspect of your life. Everything happens by virtue of your relationships with people. Keep your list updated. Your list will include both people and organizations. Set up categories for work, home, relatives, friends, shopping, volunteering, etc. as you see fit.

Calendars are an essential part of life. Whether you use a paper system or an electronic system, you need to have some system that you look at every morning. With electronic calendars, you can create multiple calendars for greater clarity and ease of use. Each calendar can be color-coded. Create calendars for your daily schedule, work schedules, work appointments, family, home, social events, holidays, and various projects. It wouldn't be unusual to have 10 or 12 calendars. In this case, the most important calendar to create is your healing calendar. If you have some kind of device or access to Google Calendar, create one now. Learn how to keep your calendars in sync on your portable devices.

The same is true with reminders and checklists. Create multiple reminder categories and checklists categories according to your needs, the major categories of your life.

Reminders are used to help you remember to do things you commit to do. They are great for creating new habits. It usually takes 21 days to create a new habit. You can create a reminder to jog your memory every day to: read a book, meditate, do exercise, learn a language, master a new computer application, or do affirmations. Reminders can be assigned to a project category to provide a list of the next few steps for a project. Another great use of reminders is to note down new ideas, inspirations, or other things to go into your to-do list (or you might use a note taking app for such activities). When inspiration strikes, you want to capture it while it's still fresh in your mind. Don't think you will remember it later. Inspirations are fleeting. If I am near WiFi, I often use Siri to quickly speak such items into a reminder list. It automatically transcribes my speech into text. If it's long, I'll make a short heading, and put details in the note field within that reminder, or make a separate note in a note taking app. For quick reminders, I use an *In Box* category where I put new things without having to think about specific categories. I reassign them when I go through my In Box. Some people like to audio record their inspirations.

A *checklist* is something you use whenever you repeat an activity. For instance, if you give presentations, go food shopping, or go camping you may want to have a checklist of all the things you need to get, do, or bring with you when you do those things. With a checklist you don't forget anything. Once you've created these checklists for repeatable projects, you can use them again and again. It just keeps your life less cluttered. Checklists also work for checking off your healthcare activities. Some reminder systems can serve as both repeatable checklists and reminder lists – everything color coded and organized by category.

To Do Systems are more extensive than simple reminders. They often contain the many steps required to complete a certain project. The idea behind a to-do list is to get the backlog of all the things that you've been wanting to do out of your head and into a system – your goals, projects, and tasks to get you where you want to go. Businesses often use project managers to manage complex projects, but most of us don't need anything that sophisticated. A good choice is a hierarchical to-do list where you can assign categories to any item and order them easily.

In its most basic form, a to-do list or task list is simply a very flexible outliner. It's your life planning system where you make a list of your goals, projects, and tasks (to-do's), then drag them around to easily organize them. At the top level is your list of goals, then projects to fulfill your goals, then the tasks and subtasks to complete various projects. The list can be collapsed or expanded to see any portion of it. In a hierarchical to-do list, you have Goals>Projects>Tasks>Subtasks, even SubSubtask as deep as you want to go. All the tasks and subtasks are prerequisites before the goal is fulfilled or the project is completed. Any goal, project, or task can have many levels under it, as many as you need. There are usually no dates or times attached to tasks.

They just need to be done. Often, they need to be done in a particular order, that is, they may have dependencies.

Tasks shouldn't go in a calendar unless they are time sensitive, because usually they don't need to be done on a certain day or at a certain time. Likewise, they don't fit into a reminder system, because you would have too many reminders to track so many items. They would get disorganized. What you need is a big list of your to-do items, which becomes your planning system, categorized by your unique categories, goals, or projects with all the stuff you need to do. Schedule a reminder to review your To-Do list once a week. When you're ready to work on a project, move a few of your next-to-do actions, next tasks, into your active reminders (or calendars if they're time sensitive). In the meantime, your plans, your organized goals, projects, and to-do items, are neatly tucked away, always ready for you to review. Ideally, this to-do list should be reviewed weekly. I use the free open-source TaskCoach program for this purpose.

Try to find a to-do list manager that works well for the complexity of your life. Some people need a more complex system, others can get by with something simple. But don't think you don't need a system. There is a tendency to think, "Oh, I want to be spontaneous, I don't want any rigidity in my life." Having a list to work from does not have to detract from spontaneity. At any moment you can make any change you want, depending upon opportunities and circumstances, but at least you'll know what you're doing and have a helper guide when you want it.

Also, if you find that your list is becoming congested with things you never get around to, you can decide not to fulfill them and purge them from your list. You don't need the extra baggage of items that have become irrelevant. Just because you put them on the list doesn't mean they have to stay there. Trim your list down to the things you really want to commit to. There's no need to overcomplicate your life, but trying to oversimplify also doesn't work.

Note Taking is about capturing inspiration and information related to your goals, projects, and tasks. Some people carry 3 x 5 cards, a small notebook, or simply use an app on a portable device. Note taking is also for capturing your great ideas and inspirations just like you can do with reminders. You always want to grab such inspired ideas when they're fresh. Note taking apps can be more feature rich, giving you the ability to sketch or draw ideas. Many new devices allow you to speak your notes as either an audio recording or transcribed speech-to-text. For sketching, sometimes just a napkin or piece of paper does the job. Capture it NOW, any way you can. Put it into your system later. You have so much power available to you today, if you will just use it. Be sure to add a reminder to review your notes weekly, otherwise your notes could get buried. Note taking applications are useful when you're doing research at a library or attending meetings. Later, you'll need to edit, condense, and move that information to where it will finally be used within your system. Review your calendars, reminders, to-do lists, and notes weekly.

I also use *timers* and *alarms* on a regular basis. I use timers to time meditation, cooking, equipment charging, etc. Timers often have both stopwatch and countdown functions. Alarms can be set to repeat on certain days of the week. Calendars, Reminders, Timers, and Alarms are all very handy "hard working" personal assistants.

The first thing to put on your to-do list is to set up your systems. Do that now. Search the Internet and find the systems you want to work with, or schedule a visit to an office supply store for a paper system. Many applications are system dependent. Since I use Apple products, my app list looks like this on both my computers and portable devices: Contacts, Calendars, Reminders (also for Checklists), TaskCoach (PC, Mac, Linux, iOS), Notes, and Clock (for alarms, stopwatch, and timers). All of these applications are free except for TaskCoach on iOS portable devices (99¢). So there's virtually no expense. It's just a matter of learning how to use your computer and your portable devices. All these applications sync automatically (or with an easy sync interface). I always have access to my organizing system. It's totally flexible and I can change anything at any time, and often do.

On Windows, many people use Outlook. All modern calendar applications allow multiple calendars. Practically every modern computer calendar will sync with portable devices. All devices come with reminder and alarm apps. Task managers or to-do lists can be created with any outlining program. Find the apps you need on your system of choice. Many cloud-based apps are free. Check http://www.appappeal.com or similar cloud app review sites. The important thing is that you have a consistent, reliable, automatic reminder system, plus a multiple alarm system that you can set to predefined intervals. Find something that works for you.

These tools are like having a personal assistant, servant, employee, coach, guide, helper, and friend to keep you on track. Make this life organizing project an adventure. Have fun with it.

,uggestions: On your healing calendar, mark the days of the week and the ,imes of day you're going to devote to improving your health. For instance, you might set aside some time to collect some healthy recipes. You could mark out time to do a physical cleanse. You might schedule an exercise regimen, or create reminders to take supplements or herbs at certain intervals. You might set aside time for meditation or yoga. Whatever you decide that you need for your healing, based on the information you are learning, along with your intuition, and perhaps an Internet search, set events or block out time for them in your calendar, set alarms or reminders, or put them on your to-do list.

If you haven't already done so, create a To-Do list, not only for healing but for life planning in general. Investigate systems like GTD, *Getting Things Done* by David Allen. It's a great stress reducer to get everything out of your head and into a system. GTD, and others like it, are quite useful. There are also many free open source systems. As I mentioned, I use TaskCoach. In your system, clearly define your priorities. What are your goals? What projects will get you there? What is critical? What is essential? What is important? What is desirable? What is mere fantasy? What should go on the back burner?

You may wonder if it's really necessary to go through so much bother to create an organizing system. It is! The reason is the tendency in all of us to sabotage ourselves. We forget. New habits are difficult to form. If you don't have a reminder system, if you are not organized, you will invariably fall flat. So set one up now on your computer and on your portable devices. If you don't use computers or portable devices, then set up the best paper system you can manage. You can use a digital kitchen timer as an interval timer. Dollar stores often have them for $1-2. Even simple mobile phones often have timers and other useful apps.

As you work through the book, start entering items into your Calendars, To-Do lists, and Reminders lists. Every time you come across something you don't understand or something interesting that you want to know more about, put it on a list to learn more about it. For instance, you may learn that certain food additives are dangerous. Put it on your list to learn more about which ones to avoid.

Setting Goals

One of the first things you may want to do with your new Calendar, Reminder, and To-Do systems is to set some goals. It's good to have some targets. You can set goals for all aspects of your life. Goal setting is important because it gives you a positive direction for your life, but don't get too serious. Enjoying the journey is also important. Put some initial goals into your system now to address the major items listed below. As you learn more, you can add projects and action items to accomplish your goals. A few examples for goal setting:

Healing Goals on Five Levels (Suggestions)

- *Physical*: An attractive, well-proportioned, healthy body, at your ideal weight, free from pain and illness, flexible, strong, tremendous vitality. (Upgrading your physical structure is a great goal. An example action item would be to learn some yoga asanas. Perhaps one vinyasa.) *Sensory Acuity*: Sparkling clarity of the senses – richness of color and sound, complete control of the senses. The sense of sight, hearing, taste, touch, and smell beyond ordinary limits. (An example action would be to schedule a short fast that will un-fog your senses, or to practice really listening to every sound.)
- *Bio-Energetic*: Bio-energetic vitality and magnetism with much higher life force. Virtually unlimited energy to do what you want. (An example action item would be to clear an embedded stress in your energy body.)
- *Emotional*: Lightness and joy, unshakable peace, unbounded love and compassion for all life, enthusiasm for life, friendliness, and a supportive/devoted attitude. Perfect emotional balance and stability, no depression or emotional chaos, no cravings, no addictions, total self control. (An example action item would be to choose one positive emotion to culture this week.)
- *Mental*: High intelligence, great concentration, perfect memory, great creativity, powerful decision-making ability, increased IQ, great ability to focus. Openness to new ideas. Perfect mental health and mental stability, great clarity of thought, elimination of mental patterns that have held you back. Powerful discriminative ability. (An example action item would be to learn a memory system like the Link Method.)
- *Conscious Awareness*: A profound connection to your inner conscious self that gives you access to the highest experiences of life. A return to your natural status as being one with the creative energy behind all phenomena. Perfect connection with the intelligence, energy, and consciousness that is this universe. (Action item - learn meditation.)

Home Goals

- *Home Environment*: Highly organized, beautiful, and functional living space, well-designed spaces appropriate for each purpose. (Action: Organize your home: Gather, sort, purge, group, and store.)
- *Home Upgrades and Repairs*: Gardens, landscaping, hardscaping, home and property repairs. (Action: List, prioritize, & schedule)

Work Goals
- *Work Environment*: Noise, ergonomics, lighting? Prioritize & schedule.
- *Work Goals*: Make a list, prioritize, choose first goal to pursue.

Service and Volunteer Goals
We should all do something to give back to society, something for which we have no expectations of gain or return.

- *Service Goals*: Make a list of organizations, places, or people you care about. What goals you would like to pursue with them?

Doing some kind of selfless service can actually provide deep healing, more than many people realize. When you live unselfishly, doing something to enrich others, you are also enriched, even without asking for it.

Relationship Goals
Harmonious, fulfilling, and balanced relationships. (An action item would be to choose some way to enrich each person in your life.)

Financial Goals
Sufficient wealth to meet your needs, sufficient wealth to fulfill your purpose. (An action item could be to review finances and plan for how you can contribute something of value to others; improve your work.)

Now that you know how to get answers through intuition, and you have a practical system to keep yourself on track, you're ready to begin your journey into extraordinary healthcare and transforming your life.

Action Plan - Introduction and Chapter I
1. Decide to take control of your health and your life. Decide to learn how to heal every aspect of yourself and others.
2. Develop your intuition. Get answers to your questions. Practice.
3. Organize yourself with a system that works for you – Contacts, Calendar, Reminders, Checklists, To-Do List, Notes, Timer, and Alarms. You may already know how to use many apps – just add a healthcare focus to your existing system. If you are not yet electronically organized, learn to use your computer, tablet, or smartphone to be your digital servant. Or choose a paper system.
4. Set goals, decide on projects, start putting action items into your system. As you go through the book, you'll have valuable resources to add.

Chapter 2
How Healthcare Was Compromised

How We Got Where We Are Today

We need to understand how we got into trouble. If you grew up in America, eating the typical diet, I must tell you the honest truth, your body has been severely compromised. There's just no good way to put it. Anyone living on the typical Western diet of fast food, soft drinks, saturated fat, junk food, restaurant food, processed food, "refined" food, and devitalized packaged foods has been cheated, lied to, and led down the path to an early and painful death.

Cancer has skyrocketed from the #8 killer to #2 in just 10 years. A hundred years ago, it was virtually unknown. C. Everett Koop, M.D., former Surgeon General of the United States, said, "Out of 2.1 million deaths a year in the United States, 1.6 million are related to poor nutrition." That's 76% of all deaths!

Most food manufacturers, restaurants, and grocery stores don't seem to care about your health. They sell what makes money, what people will buy. They sell what tastes sweet, has the flavor you want (artificial or not), and gives the most "comfort." They sell marketing hype. Nutrition and health are last on the list, really not even a consideration for the average business.

Using sophisticated television marketing – promoting convenience, taste, color, sex, and anything else they can come up with – these marketers and manufacturers, in effect, lie to you and your family. Truly, it's a crime foisted on all of us through their greed and our ignorance. If you want to heal, you must now purify, cleanse, and detoxify your system. The first thing you must do is stop putting junk in.

The detailed knowledge of proper nutrition and diet is the subject of another chapter. I'll just say here briefly that your best bet is to minimize all packaged foods and fast foods, ideally, none at all. At least that way you'll minimize the disaster that most people are creating. Prepare healthy meals from scratch, especially using lots of fresh raw fruits and vegetables. Focus on fresh foods which are delicious in their natural state.

There's a lot of unlearning and clearing to do. It will take some time to completely regenerate your body – about one month for every year of age! If you're 35 years old, it will take about 3 years once you begin in earnest to apply all the information. Don't worry, it won't take very long to feel much better or to feel incredible benefits. Many long standing problems will disappear within a few weeks, certainly within a month or two. Most regeneration will happen the first year, but it keeps getting better the longer you apply regenerative principles. The result of just a few years of regeneration is a youthful physiology, with astounding health.

Universal Mis-education

You never got the knowledge you needed. Almost everything you were taught since childhood about health and well-being is not accurate – if you were taught anything at all. The poor health that we see in the United States and around the world is not an accident. It is intentional, not necessarily in the sense of a conspiracy, it is just plain old corruption, greed, politics, and complicity. You have never been taught the essentials of how to maintain either your mental or physical health.

This is why over 30% of adult women today are taking tranquilizers, antidepressants, and other psychoactive drugs such as Xanax, Paxil, Prozac, and many more. Every year, anti-anxiety drugs alone account for 250 million prescriptions, over 60 doses for each man, woman, and child in the U.S. – drugs for health is an addiction business. According to the Kaiser Health Foundation, the average adult takes over 11 prescription drugs. Drug costs now exceed $1 trillion per year. Prescription drug abuse is epidemic. The fundamental cause is the lack of knowledge of how to naturally create and maintain physical and mental health. This is why over 65% of adults are overweight and over 35% are obese. Health misinformation, disinformation, and absence of natural health knowledge is the cause.

I won't go into specific details here because there are many well-documented books and movies on the subject. Here's a short summary:

You were never taught the natural diet of the human. Most of what you've learned came from industry propaganda provided to public schools for free (Four food groups, etc.) and from advertisements on television. You were never taught how to protect your mental state: How to handle stress, how to keep yourself motivated, how to prevent destructive mental patterns, or how to heal your mind and body. Our educational system failed us by failing to teach us how to care for ourselves and how to protect ourselves from corporate and political interests.

The Depleted Food Industry

The food industry, in general, is not designed to promote or protect your health, it's designed to make money. The food industry discovered that by packaging convenience foods they could charge 10-20 times as much for the same food. In addition, all kinds of cheap fillers could be included simply because you can't see them. Also included are taste enhancements designed to promote addiction, referred to in the food industry as "cravability." Sometimes they even use addictive drugs. When Coca-Cola could no longer use cocaine, they switched to caffeine. The idea behind all mass marketed foods is to sell more food. The food industry as a whole cannot be trusted. Buyer beware. Read the labels. If you don't know an ingredient, don't buy. I have a thorough section on food and diet in a later chapter.

The Toxic Medical Industry

Likewise, the medical industry is not designed to promote health and well-being. Actually, medical intervention itself is the third leading cause of death, after cancer and heart attacks. These deaths arise from medical negligence and mistakes, wrong prescriptions, botched surgeries, hospital and doctor induced infections (35-40% of all disease), wrong diagnosis, and toxic therapies. Mostly, it's designed to make money. It's not the fault of doctors. They have been miseducated as well. For instance, in medical school, rarely were doctors given any information on nutrition. That may come as a shock, but they often know less than you do. As mentioned before, doctors are taught that health comes through drugs and surgery. They have virtually nothing else to prescribe. The medical myth of drugs for health expanded greatly through television advertising – now at 80 ads per hour!

Watch the evening news and make a note of all the drug ads. Most ads are pharmaceutical or medical insurance ads. Unfortunately, doctors and nurses were never taught other forms of healing from the world's great healing traditions. They've been kept in the dark just as you have, yet the industry is always promoting some new "magic bullet," some new drug that you can try now (for some outrageous price), or will be available sometime in the future. I have met people who have actually spent over a million dollars trying to solve basic health problems that could easily have been solved for free.

One promising development in the medical world is a newly found focus on regenerative medicine. For instance, in dental medicine they are developing techniques to grow new teeth naturally. It may also be possible to regrow failing organs. As we develop higher consciousness, we may be able to do all of these things ourselves with no outside intervention. The possibilities for healing in higher states of consciousness are unlimited.

The Toxic Agricultural and Chemical Industries

The agricultural industry is trying to promote genetically modified foods (GMO's) so foods can be grown with internal poisons and so massive amounts of poison can be sprayed without killing them. There is no way to avoid these poisons once they become part of the plant. The agricultural poison industry even targets home gardeners. These poisons are not beneficial to your health; they're designed to kill. Poisons will never create better cells. Recent studies in France show that GMO corn causes cancer. Many countries are now banning GMO products, (not yet in the United States). So far, there are no long term studies that show that GM foods are better for you in any possible way. They just create a more polluted, poisoned environment.

There are huge chemical industries designed to take whole natural foods and taint them with colors, flavor enhancers, stabilizers, preservatives, and other artificial ingredients. Chemical industries, whether for food additives, home cleaning products, personal care products, garden products, or agricultural pesticides, are all designed to make profits, not nurture your health and well-being.

The Toxic Dental Industry

The dental industry has been using toxic mercury compounds for decades. Mercury is a known neurotoxin used in the amalgam for dental fillings. The claim that it does not enter the body after compounding is not true. Scientific tests prove it does. Fluoride is the main ingredient in rat poison. The aluminum smelting industry couldn't figure out what to do with fluoride wastes, so they decided to put it in our drinking water and toothpastes. Many countries are banning these practices. If you need dental work, be sure toxic heavy metals are not used. Avoid toxic chemicals in your toothpastes and water as much as possible. You will need to do research. Not all ingredients are listed. Markets are changing rapidly. Look for Ayurvedic and natural alternatives. I include a simple toothpaste recipe in the Resources Chapter.

Miseducation Summary

The result of our miseducation is that we are confused and misguided. We simply don't know what to do or what the truth is. In most cases, the educational system, the food industry, the medical and pharmaceutical industries, and the chemical industries are working against us. The only solution is to educate yourself, which is the purpose of this book. Rarely is accurate information presented to the public through any of our institutions. Media programming and commercial advertising compound these problems. Drug advertisements, food advertisements, and restaurant advertisements are all designed for one purpose, to make money. You have to protect yourself from this onslaught. Children especially need to be taught to protect themselves. Otherwise, in their innocence, they believe advertisements are telling the truth.

There are no advertisements on how to create healthy cells, how to prevent disease, how to build a strong immune system, how NOT to need the services of doctors and hospitals, how to become self-sufficient for mental and physical health. In ancient times, this essential education was part of the culture, but today we no longer have a culture, we only have commerce.

The Effects of Media on Health

Television is perhaps both the worst invention and the best invention of the modern era. It's the best invention because of its ability to reach millions of people. It's the worst invention because of its programming. Most television programs are designed to accentuate fear, violence, lust, and greed. The potential of television has been almost completely lost. By promoting instinctual drives, particularly adrenaline and infatuation, we are driven into addictions.

Mental and emotional addictions are not trivial. On an unconscious level, you are made to believe the world presented on TV is real. The more you buy into it, the more real it becomes. Our whole society has been programmed. The typical method is to promote fear and greed, and then promote a solution, usually drugs or violence. You are kept in a state of drama and fear, based on unreal, abnormal fantasies.

Studies prove you're not immune. When you show violence to children, they become violent. Children mimic what they see, whether at home or on television. The more violence that is presented, the more angry and violent our society becomes. Likewise, the more that greed, sex, and infatuation are presented, the more greedy and infatuated our society becomes. These destructive emotions dramatically damage your health.

The best way to protect yourself and your family, at this point, is to simply turn the television off and disconnect from the companies that have a vested interest in promoting mental and emotional addictions.

Television has a huge potential to benefit society. It can be an excellent instructional tool for showing how to do things. Television could also show us how to become more compassionate and loving beings, but that is not yet available. In the meantime, your best educational tools are the Internet, books, especially inexpensive ebooks, carefully selected Internet video, and enlightened mentors. These resources are the basis of a new system of education. They will be the basis of your future learning for health, or any other subject you may be interested in.

The Future of Education For Health

Healthcare is intimately tied to education in surprising ways. To create a healthy society, we need to completely rethink our educational system and the cultural values that it instills. We need to create a cultural transformation for many other reasons as well. Education is the way to do that. Extraordinary healthcare requires extraordinary re-education. This book is a comprehensive start, but you will want and need more education. Ebooks, recipe books, audios, and videos are needed, not only for healthcare, but to redesign your life towards greater fulfillment.

There have been great advances in learning since the advent of computers, the Internet, and now, with new portable tablet devices. Computer-based instruction has the power to completely redefine your own education and your children's education. It can provide superior instruction and completely eliminate the need for classroom instruction, which is highly inefficient and for many, quite intimidating. It provides self-paced learning so students never get lost or fall behind. Laptops and tablets provide access to all kinds of media: texts (ebooks), databases, graphics, photos, and videos.

These powerful learning tools are becoming inexpensive, especially considering that classroom education in the United States costs roughly $8000 per child every year. A computer or tablet that costs a few hundred dollars is an extraordinary bargain. Studies by Sugata Mitra, Professor of Educational Technology, showed that self-education is far more potent, relevant, and faster than classroom education. Many studies prove that computer-mediated education is often at least twice as fast and effective as classroom education. Watch his "TED Talks" on the Internet.

As radical as it sounds, Dr. Mitra proved that children, once they can read, can teach themselves almost anything when given: 1) Access to the Internet, 2) permission to interact with each other (their peers), and 3) the absence of teachers! He and others proved, time and again, that education is best when self-motivated and self-guided. You can only learn something when you have an interest and a reason to learn. All great minds do this. Steve Jobs and Bill Gates never finished college, yet they were highly educated. Lest you think they are anomalies, twenty percent of America's millionaires never attended even one day of college. That doesn't mean you don't need education. No, it means there are other ways to get it. Self directed ways.

Access to free education is already available. Harvard and MIT and other prestigious universities are making their classes available for free. New websites featuring the best instructors are already online. To get a glimpse of the future, take look at these websites. https://www.edx.org – https://www.coursera.org – http://www.udacity.com – http://www.khanacademy.org

Public education costs could be reduced more than 75% using these principles. A 50% shortening of learning time alone gives a 50% cost reduction. A massive reduction in classroom space leads to more cost reductions. Any state or regional government could fund the development of textbooks (e-books) and online video courses that could drastically reduce the cost of education. Many school facilities could be repurposed. Existing classrooms could become walk-in mentoring centers that combine mentoring – peer to peer, adult to child, and child to adult – plus include research services offered today by public libraries. Public libraries are a valuable asset. You might want to learn to use your library's research services and interlibrary loan services for books, ebooks, and other media that are not locally available.

Our Outdated Educational System

In the United States, there are massive numbers of students "graduating" from high school who cannot even read proficiently. Students are passed from grade to grade without mastering basic skills. It's all about money. Schools are paid for each child enrolled, so dropouts don't bring in money. How bad is it? Journalists who researched the issue claim that in New York City, 80% of "graduates" can't read well enough to enroll in a community college without remedial education. The same is true in other cities. But it isn't really the fault of teachers. It's the system.

If you study history, you'll find that our current educational system was derived from the Prussian military and then adopted by the British. Essentially, it was designed for war. It was designed to teach how to take orders, not how to think for yourself. It was designed to suppress your natural curiosity and creativity, suppress enthusiasm for your own interests, suppress your uniqueness, and to make each of us a standardized product.

This absolutely kills the vitality and self image of children. The system was originally designed to crush self worth, independence, and uniqueness in order to make good soldiers.

Essentially, educational systems worldwide are designed to be an assembly line that manufactures a standard robotic product, dull machine-like humans to do the work of commerce, industry, and military. It does not nourish our uniqueness or happiness. It is inhuman. In many ways, it is worse than death. In fact, among teenagers, suicide is the third leading cause of death. Tens of thousands per year. Worldwide, many teenagers commit suicide when they don't make the grade on standardized tests. Entire countries decide their fate by their standardized test scores. The laws of the country dictate what opportunities they have, what educational opportunities are available, what possibilities they have. Students feel that their whole life has been ruined, their life is over, if they don't score high on certain standardized tests. How does this destruction happen?

Here is how it is done. As soon as you create a system of grading students and then force them on to newer concepts without mastering previous concepts, you destroy them. Once a child makes a C, D, or F, it is an irrevocable scar, permanently stored in the system. It is on their record and can never be undone. They now consider themselves a C, D, or F person. This absolutely crushes the child, crushes their self image and self worth. This should never be done. Schools should immediately abandon competitive grading. The purpose of testing is to discover what you don't yet know, or have not yet mastered, so that you can return to your studies to master the techniques and knowledge where you are not yet proficient. How else can you achieve mastery? Only test to reveal what you need to learn.

Every student gets to retest as much as they want until they "make an A" in every subject they want to explore. Let them take as long as they need to master a subject or even skip over a subject, according to their interests, enthusiasm, and ability. There is no rush. When they are interested, they can master any subject in 1/2, or even 1/3 of the time spent today.

Grading destroys self image and self worth. It causes many of the healthcare problems we have today – physical, mental, and emotional. Once people are demoralized, discouraged, and disempowered they no longer take care of themselves properly. Their mental and emotional qualities degrade. They often take to alcohol and drugs. They lose curiosity and enthusiasm to explore life in all its fascination. They are easily manipulated by commercial interests. Gradually, their physical health deteriorates.

Unfortunately, the school system is not likely to change in the near future. There is too much vested interest. Having personally taught in the public schools and observed the effects of the current system of education on children, I can only recommend that if you have children, take them out of school and begin homeschooling. Find out what your children want and empower them to learn it themselves. If you are unable to empower your children towards self-motivated, self guided education on your own, gather with other parents and form a cooperative homeschool and work together.

The main value of parents working either alone or together is to inspire and nurture children. Self image and encouragement are far more important than detailed instruction which, once they can read, children can get on their own. Children are naturally curious, creative, and enthusiastic. You only need a few other parents to help out with encouragement, occasional mentoring, learning resources, and opportunities. Given resources, encouragement, and collaboration with their peers, children will excel beyond your limited dreams for them. They have their own dreams and a deep knowledge of their purpose.

To educate yourself and your children, only three skills are needed:

1) Effective reading comprehension – the most critical skill of all, 2) Information search and retrieval skills – understanding how search engines work, including keywords and Boolean logic, 3) The ability to discriminate between what is valuable and what is rubbish. Discrimination prevents us from being conned or programmed, and helps us to avoid being driven by instinctual drives and addictions. Everyone should learn how to get their information from the highest sources possible. This comes with experience and constant intuitive discrimination. Teachers have other opportunities.

Great Opportunities for Teachers

If you are currently a teacher, you have great opportunities as a facilitator, mentor, and coach – the parental role. Take over for parents who are unable. You could be part of a walk-in mentoring group for both parents and children at existing facilities, or create your own mentoring facility. You also have great opportunities for creating the media that will be used by millions.

Skills for Extraordinary Healthcare

Self-education skills apply to your own healthcare. 1) Learn how to search and retrieve information (Tip: Ask librarians how to search, or Google the words: "effective web search"), 2) Learn how to recognize value when it's being presented. Use your intuition, logical assessment, and common sense

– does the source have a hidden agenda? and 3) Learn how to keep yourself out of trouble physically, mentally, and emotionally. This is an essential skill in the world today. The techniques given on intuition will be invaluable. When in doubt, check your intuition.

Healing ourselves is not like fixing a broken machine. It's important to understand that you are not a machine. You are a living being with the ability for self repair. You can heal directly. I don't know of any limits to your healing possibilities. I do know that we are currently using only a fraction of our potential. Use your time wisely to learn how to expand possibilities for yourself and your family. You are NOT going to expand your potential by indulging in the currently available television and radio media. You need to look at new sources of information, new concepts, and be willing to explore more of your potential.

Summary of Education and Media on Healthcare

Today, both our educational system and the commercial media industry are almost entirely stress inducing. High stress makes us recoil into a state of fear and powerlessness. The vast majority of media creates these stress-inducing reactions for drama and sensationalism – television, print, video games, and music. Media industries foster destructive thinking habits and destructive emotions. They promote wrong assumptions about life and, indirectly, are the cause of many diseases and psychological disorders.

For instance, TV advertising promotes the idea that we are the innocent victims of germs that only pharmaceuticals can tackle. It promotes the idea that only specialists can take care of us. It promotes the purchase of products and services which are life damaging. Commercial media as a whole is dangerous to life. It would be wise to avoid all its forms. Instead, seek out the new life-supporting, life-enhancing publications and media that are popping up to fill the growing interest in positive expressions of life. There are new magazines, books, and Internet sites that are doing good work. Use your sleuthing skills to find the ones you need.

The best use of your time is to learn the skills cited above. Stay away from mass education and mass media with their destructive, commercial interests. Learn to self-educate yourself and your family. There is nothing to stop you from becoming more educated, intuitive, intelligent, and self-sufficient in every way. In the future, medical services may not even be needed, except for injuries. Every family will have one or more people who understand extraordinary healthcare, who can heal virtually every condition. Emergency services and specialist in the medical field will still be necessary, but on a very limited basis.

Action Plan - Chapter 2, How Healthcare Was Compromised

1. Learn to defend yourself against the onslaught of commercial interests.
2. Purchase only healthy, unpackaged foods, and natural, personal care and home care products made from simple ingredients.
3. Turn off your television and cancel cable services. Locate new sources of inspiration. Read inspirational books. Have more gatherings with friends and family instead of programmed media.
4. Join the future of education. Develop a self-education program for yourself and your children. Forget about public education. It is a failure. Just look at the results – generations of obese, stressed, depressed, prescription-drug addicted adults! It's time for a change.
5. Develop self learning skills: 1) Effective reading comprehension, 2) Internet search and retrieval skills – keywords & Boolean logic, 3) Intuitive discrimination of what is valuable and worthy and what is not.
6. Avoid commercial media – TV, print, video games, and music. Learn to use libraries, including interlibrary loan for printed books, ebooks, and media. Discover the positive, but often hidden, new media that fosters self empowerment – new magazines, books, and Internet sites that are doing good work.

Chapter 3
Symptoms of Degeneration

Self Diagnosis:
Strengths, Weaknesses, and Causes

A New Kind of Diagnosis

Your system is always telling you when something is wrong and alerts you that corrective action is needed. It has its own language that you can easily learn. Each symptom indicates a weakness that needs to be corrected. In this system of healthcare, we don't try to diagnose diseases directly. Instead, we diagnose the precursors of disease, which are non-medical.

Evaluating Your State of Health

How healthy are you? There are many ways to know. Maybe you've been to a doctor and been diagnosed with some problem or even have a serious disease. If so, you already know you're in trouble. If not, there are other ways to know your state of health. Your body "talks" to you all the time! The language it uses is the language of pain, visual indicators, sensations, and intuition.

When degenerative forces begin to dominate, you get signals. For instance, you're always tired and weak. You have aches, pains, pressures, bloating, and other sensations. Even without obvious symptoms you often "just know" that something is wrong. Your intuition is telling you to take action.

The symptoms listed below are indicators that you're in trouble. They're signs of degeneration. They're an immediate red flag to take action. The usual reaction in Western countries (abetted by industry advertising) is to ignore these signals. Ads tell us to take painkillers. An arthritis ad says, "You can even go dancing all night!" That's like ignoring or unplugging the oil light in your car! The consequences are disastrous. Avoiding the signals your body gives you leads to greater breakdown, increasing weakness, worsening of disease, greater pain, more suffering, and premature death. Here are some self-diagnostic exercises you can use right now. Don't worry if you find problems. You'll be able to reverse them.

Diagnosing Weakness

There are at least 4 ways to diagnose your health: 1) Observing Symptoms 2) Iridology - Iris Analysis 3) Fasting Reactions, and 4) Pain and Pressure Sensitivity.

Observing Symptoms

First, look at your daily experience. Any pain, pressures, or other sensations show you're in trouble. Here's a checklist of symptoms. Quickly skim this list and rate your own state of health. The more symptoms you have, and the more severe they are, the more you need to take action. A healthy body has NONE of these symptoms.

General Symptoms:

- Pain Anywhere in the Body
- Pressure Anywhere in the Body
- Swelling or Bloating
- Headaches
- Low Energy
- Insomnia
- Anemia
- Shortness of Breath
- Faintness Between Meals
- Weakness
- Poor Stamina
- Heart Pain
- Fast Heartbeat
- High Cholesterol (above 200)
- Hyper Sensitivity
- Frequent Illness
- Frequent Fevers or Infections
- Poor Skin Quality (fungal infections, skin eruptions, etc.)
- Inability to Gain or Lose Weight
- Excessive Hair Loss
- Premature Gray Hair
- Uncomfortable, No Matter What
- Blurry or Unclear Vision
- Deteriorating Eyesight (requiring corrective lenses)

Digestion/Elimination

- Food Allergies
- Constipation (<1-2 BM/day)
- Persistent Flatulence or Gas
- Bloating
- Stomach Pains
- Diarrhea
- Loss of Appetite
- Intestinal Pain
- Intestinal Irritation
- Difficulty Breathing After Eating
- Adverse Reactions After Eating
- Burning Sensation in the Stomach
- Overeating and Still Hungry
- Cravings For Sweets or Alcohol
- Lack of Appetite
- Distress From Eating Fatty Foods
- Bleeding Gums
- Discoloration of Gums
- White Coated Tongue (especially upon arising)
- Cold Sores
- Bad Breath
- Undigested Food
- Indigestion, Stomach Upset
- Hemorrhoids
- Acid Reflux

Joints, Muscles, Extremities, & Skin

- Pain in Back, Thighs, Shoulders
- Slow Reflexes
- Leg Cramps
- Numb Hands or Feet
- Pale Skin
- Age Spots
- Stiff Joints
- Varicose Veins
- Easily Bruised
- Yellowish Face
- Wrinkling and Aging of Skin
- Ridges on Fingernails/Toenails
- Fungus on Fingernails/Toenails
- Cracking Around Lips
- Clammy Skin
- Dry Skin
- Muscle Pain
- Muscle Cramps
- Cold Hands or Cold Feet
- Pain in the Joints
- Injuries Slow to Heal

None of these symptoms are normal. Later, you'll learn how to reverse them. Here are some deeper explanations:

Pain Anywhere in the Body

Pain is the language of your body. It has no other way to talk to you. It should be an immediate red flag that something is wrong and needs to be corrected. Society teaches us to either ignore it or cover it up with painkillers. Neither approach is successful.

Tiredness

Tiredness is an indicator of weakness. It means you're out of balance. It is often due to congestion. Not getting healthy nutrition is another cause.

Headaches

Headaches are just another form of pain to tell you something's wrong and that you should take action. Even occasional headaches are not normal.

Allergies and Hypersensitivity

Allergies and hypersensitivity mean that your body is congested and not able to eliminate toxins and overload, due to a systemic imbalance. Allergies also have emotional causes. There may be environmental toxins.

Breathing Difficulties

Breathing difficulties arise from congestion and emotional trauma. Asthma is one example. Labored breathing indicates the need for internal cleansing. There may be toxins in the air.

Digestive Distress

Digestive distress is one of the leading symptoms of degeneration. Some alternative practitioners believe that all disease begins in the colon. Related symptoms include nausea, constipation, undigested food, constant hunger, bloating, swelling, stomach aches, heartburn, acid reflux, and others. Generally, it's the result of wrong diet and overeating.

Body Odor

A foul odor indicates foul conditions inside your body. These include body odor, bad breath, odorous gas, odorous body wastes, odorous ear wax. A healthy body does not have foul odors.

Congestion

Congestion manifests in many forms: Overweight, bloating, swelling, coated tongue, skin rashes, difficulty breathing, weakness, numbness, stiffness, skin discoloration and eruptions, allergies, sinus congestion, phlegm, discharge from your eyes, coughing, sneezing, poor vision, cravings, poor digestion, and others.

Mental Symptoms

Memory loss, confused thinking, poor concentration, learning limitations, lack of creativity, difficulty staying focused, difficulty comprehending, difficulty recognizing and interpreting things – these are all symptoms of mental degeneration.

These mental symptoms are the result of never learning how to manage your mental life. We're never taught the right use of imagination, how to avoid destructive thinking, or how to use the power of our mind to advance ourselves. Success in life requires clear mental organization. For most people, their inner mental condition is one of chaos, confusion, and destructive mental habits. There are also physical causes for mental problems – nutrient deficiency, hormonal imbalances, and injuries.

Emotional Symptoms

Common emotional symptoms include depression, anxiety, anger, fear, frustration, and instability. These emotional symptoms arise from mismanagement of our mental life. They lead to addictions to drugs, alcohol, food, sex, or work. They are responsible for untold relationship problems. Virtually all the problems of society are caused by mental and emotional mismanagement and the lack of practical guidance and tools for managing our inner mental and emotional life. Mental and emotional mismanagement leads to hormonal imbalances, which cause powerful "instinctual" drives towards excessive passion, greed, anger, and violence. Essentially, all the problems of the world are due to lousy instruction.

The result of this widespread miseducation is that we have a society in chaos. It's simply not enough for our educational systems to teach reading, writing, and mathematics. Our educational systems should teach us about life and how to use our mental and emotional resources to create an extraordinary life of health and the flowering of our mental and emotional capabilities.

Emotional problems can also be caused by physical imbalances. Body, mind, and emotions are not separate. They are related to each other. Imbalances in one can cause imbalances in others.

Self Diagnostic Methods

In addition to symptoms, there are other ways to assess your well-being.

pH and Health

You may remember from school that pH is the measure of acidity or alkalinity. It varies from 0, extreme acid, to 14, extreme alkaline. Neutral pH, like water, is a pH of 7. Vinegar is acid, baking soda is alkaline. Your body also has a pH. Physically, the single most important factor influencing your health is the pH of your body. Babies are born with a pH of 7.36, slightly alkaline. All degenerative diseases take hold when the body becomes acidic, therefore, the single most important test is to test your saliva or urine pH. If it is below 7.0, you are in trouble. If it is below 6.0 you are in big trouble.

How to Measure Your pH

It's easy to measure your pH. Get pH paper that measures in .1 or .2 increments from values 5.5 to 8.0. Graduated colors indicate the pH, often using shades from yellow (most acid), to green (neutral), to blue (most alkaline). In North America a good source is Micro Essentials Laboratory, item #1606. You may find it locally at special pharmacies that serve hospitals and doctors. The company web site is https://www.microessentiallab.com (or call them at 718-338-3618). Amazon also has it. Health food stores sometimes carry pH paper. Ordinary pharmacies rarely have it. There may be other brands that are just as good. You can make the pH paper last longer if you cut the paper tape into short test strips (hold with tweezers). Give some paper to friends to test their pH. You could save their life.

Saliva test: Not having eaten for two hours or more, swallow the saliva in your mouth three times. Then take a drop of fresh saliva and touch it to the pH paper. DON'T put the pH paper in your mouth. Wait 30 seconds and check the color.

Urine test: Capture a bit of urine in a cup and touch a drop of it to the paper. Wait 30 seconds and read the color. For the most accurate reading, collect urine for 24 hours and test the mix. If you have a urinary infection, the reading will not be an accurate indicator of your body's pH.

These tests can vary quite a lot from morning to night. Morning is most acid. Your pH should measure not less than 6.5 and not above 7.8 for any length of time. Do the test over several days to get a sense of how your body is managing pH. If your pH measures well below 6.5 (4.5 to 6.2), you're in big trouble and need to alkalize your body rapidly.

Examine the Iris of the Eye – Iridology

Iridology is a window into your body, a kind of free do-it-yourself CAT scan. The colors and textures in your iris indicate your body's strengths and weaknesses. To look at your iris in detail, shine a flashlight from the side of your eye. In a mirror, you'll see all the detail including areas that are dark or light. If the iris is smooth textured, like fine silk without spots or discoloration, then your constitution is strong. If there are dark spots, discoloration, and a coarse texture like burlap, then your constitution is weak. All very dark areas indicate major troubles. Most people are somewhere in between these two extremes, in which case health is moderately compromised. Search the Internet for "iridology" then click on IMAGES to see lots of color photos that show how weak organs manifest as visible shapes, patterns, textures, and colors in the eye.

A practical system of diagnosis was developed by Dr. Bernard Jensen. Through observation and autopsies, indicators in the eye were correlated with known diseases. It's a whole science you can study if you want to. Using this system, you can identify a weakness before it becomes a disease.

Some health practitioners photograph your eyes and give a detailed analysis. However, in my experience, it's enough just to get a sense of where you are with your health. Then watch the changes take place in your iris as you heal. It's exciting to watch your body heal! If you want to diagnose specific weaknesses, there are charts that you can purchase online. Dr. Bernard Jensen, the developer of iridology, has several books available for in-depth research. Charts correlate each location in the iris with certain organs of the body. There are apps for smart phones and tablets with charts. Search your app store for "iridology."

Reflexology

There are over 72,000 nerves that end in your feet and hands. The location of these nerve endings correspond to organs throughout your body. The degree of congestion and sensitivity of these nerve endings indicate problems with the corresponding organs. Reflexology is both diagnostic and therapeutic. By clearing the congestion of these nerve endings, the corresponding organ is stimulated, balanced, and healing influences are directed to that organ. Such diagnostic and therapeutic methods have been used for centuries, sometimes with dramatic results.

For instance, massaging the tip of the little finger on the left-hand has been used to reverse heart attacks. Massaging the base of the ring and little fingers has been known to reverse deafness in some cases.

It's a good practice to keep the hands and feet clear of congestion through reflexology massage on a regular basis. Once or twice a week is sufficient. You can massage with your fingers or use any blunt object. As you massage, you'll notice your body becoming calmer and more balanced.

Locate a reflexology chart. Search the Internet for "reflexology chart" or visit a natural food or health food store. I have a fairly detailed reflexology chart that you can download from my web site. There are inexpensive, sometimes free, smartphone apps with colorful reflexology diagrams. Make a note of any locations on your hands or feet that are especially sensitive. Those correspond to areas where your body is weak.

Acupressure as a Diagnostic Tool

Just as there are maps on your feet, hands, and eyes, your whole body contains a map of all organs and systems. Life force energy and information flows from one part of your body to another by way of definite channels, different from the nervous system. These flows of energy are called meridians and are widely studied in Eastern medicine. Along these meridians are many points that correspond to different organs and functions of the body. By keeping these points clear of congestion, organs are strengthened and the health of your body is maintained.

Acupuncturists use needles to stimulate and clear congestion at these points, but pressure also works quite well. By simply massaging these points, you can discover places of weakness. Every sensitive location is a place of imbalance. Normal pressure should not produce any discomfort or pain. You can use your fingers, thumb, knuckles, or any smooth, blunt object to explore the meridian system. Take time to map out your sensitivities. Press on every square inch of your body. Then draw a body map, a gingerbread or cartoon figure is sufficient, and mark your sore spots. Use this map as a guide to maintaining your health. It's fun to watch your body change as you clear these points and meridians.

You don't have to study acupressure or acupuncture to use this system because you can directly feel any areas of discomfort or sensitivity. Of course, if you wanted to work therapeutically on others, you would need to know the points and their corresponding effects. Just discovering sensitivities is enough to help yourself. Working out these energetic kinks provides more therapeutic value than is generally realized. It can have dramatic effects in improving physical, mental, and emotional health.

Not only is the entire meridian system a therapeutic map for your body, but several locations contain complete whole-body maps. I've already mentioned the maps on your hands, feet, and eyes. There are additional maps on your ears, face, lips, tongue, and the top of your head. All these places can be used therapeutically. In the chapter on bio-energy healing, I'll go deeper into acupressure. I also provide a link to a detailed chart if you want one. But for now, just experiment with pressing on different parts of your body and notice how some places are sensitive and some are not. The left and right side of your body often differ. If you're curious about what organs or body systems are influenced by certain points, there are acupressure smartphone apps detailing the points and their effects.

What Happens When You Fast?

Another way to get a quick sense of your health is to simply stop eating for a day or two. Fast. You can drink all the water or juices you want, but no solid foods. If you can't skip a whole day of eating, or even a single meal, without feeling weak, tired, sleepy, congested, or have a major reaction, then your system is weak and your health is substantially compromised. You don't actually have to fast to know your state of health. If missing a single meal makes you uncomfortable and begins to bring on these symptoms, you know you need to start a natural healthcare program.

Fasting is recommended in all spiritual literature (mentioned about as often as prayer in the Bible), so it must have importance for spiritual and physical well-being. Your ability to sustain a short fast, without symptoms, indicates how healthy you are. Before beginning a long fast, you must learn how. You can get into trouble if you don't have the proper knowledge. How to fast is discussed later. Some conditions such as diabetes are not favorable for fasting. If you have a condition you suspect may preclude fasting, see a healthcare practitioner.

How Life Works - Diagnosing Your Life

Life works in patterns and cycles. Life is always trying to help you become the best that you can be. The problem is, you've probably never been taught how to listen. You are always being guided, but most of us often miss the cues. There are generally seven opportunities for change.

Quiet Intuition – There's always a part of you that knows everything. The discussion earlier on intuition applies here. If you stay aware and listen to your inner guidance, then you don't have to learn everything the hard way. Your first opportunity to improve your life comes through quiet knowingness. Listen.

Dreams – Most dreams are not revelations, but just an expression of your underlying stress, hidden emotions, and embedded patterns. Occasionally, you can get guidance through your dreams. It's rare. Generally, the content of your dreams shows you what you need to work on, the hidden aspects of yourself that need upgrading. In that sense, they can guide you regarding what you should avoid, and what positive influences you may want to introduce into your life. As your system becomes clear of stress, emotional turmoil, and mental patterns, you will return to dreamless sleep.

Environmental Cues – You may be sitting at a cafe and listening to a conversation nearby. You know it's not polite to eavesdrop, and yet you find yourself listening intently. In such situations, what you are hearing is exactly what you need to hear. It applies to you. The universe brings information to you in mysterious ways. While browsing a bookstore or library, a book may jump out at you. Friends or even strangers mention a topic, a book, or a person you need to investigate to learn more about. If you pick up on these cues from the environment, you can be led to your next step, but we often discount these serendipitous events. If you encounter something more than twice in a short timespan, definitely check it out.

Emotional Pain – Because we often don't listen, life becomes a little more painful. It's nature's way of telling you that you're off track, you need to make a correction. What usually happens is that we get caught up in the pain, not understanding the lesson. If you still don't pay attention, the universe begins to talk to you a little louder.

Physical Pain – Emotional pain or mental anguish eventually develops into physical problems. You have physical symptoms: pain, pressure, tightness, inflammation, queasiness – some kind of physical reaction. These are just deeper and louder wake-up calls for you to pay attention. It's time to change the direction that you're going. If you still don't pay attention, symptoms become more obvious and develop into something more problematic.

Disease – Eventually the wake-up call becomes a disease, something you can no longer ignore. Now you *have* to pay attention. But our society teaches us to cover up symptoms and the expressions of disease with drugs. Most drugs rarely heal anything and often drive the disease deeper into your system. Disease is an opportunity to explore yourself in a deeper way, to come to terms with how you are violating some laws of nature. It often means letting go of old conditioning and patterns, old ways of seeing the world. It's time to seek deeper truths about how you should live your life.

Near-Death – If you still don't pay attention, then life continues to degenerate until there is not enough life force available to keep you alive. You always have every opportunity to turn everything around. You've probably heard about people who were on their deathbed, but suddenly healed. This kind of spontaneous remission is always due to a deeper transformation. An inner change took place and a lesson was learned.

These seven opportunities happen to all of us and offer us the potential to change. Whenever an uncomfortable situation arises, it's time to be more aware. Sometimes you can figure things out rationally, systematically. Sometimes your memory reminds you that you are in a loop, a pattern, and it's time to jump off the merry-go-round. When there is no precedent, the only source of help is your intuition or the guidance of someone who can see more deeply into your predicament through their intuition.

Overcoming Obstacles

There are many obstacles on the path to better health, but they can be easily overcome if we understand them. These obstacles are also the causes of poor health. They include:

- Lack of knowledge
- Lack of effective tools for inner or outer change
- Excessive ego
- Unwillingness to change
- Unwillingness to take responsibility
- Unwillingness to let go (appropriate surrender)
- Misuse of power
- Unwillingness to learn
- Unwillingness to properly use your power
- Resignation, disinterest, laziness, preoccupation
- Lame excuses: No time, too busy, too many distractions

The main thing is to be aware. Awareness itself is healing. Fighting with or indulging in problems rarely brings a solution. Problems are rarely solved at the level they were created. Usually, you have to make some kind of jump.

You have to confront your familiar comfort zones. You often need to adopt new habits, new knowledge, new ways of seeing the world, new ways of understanding yourself, and make different choices. All these things are difficult only if you are egoistic.

The 7 Fundamental Causes of All Disease

Here is a quick overview of the fundamental causes of virtually all diseases. Your inner environment is the underlying cause. These are some of the different ways that the environment is disturbed.

Chemical and pH Imbalances

Many people have abnormal body chemistry due to poor diet and other bad habits. The typical diet is far too acid forming (pH well below a neutral 7). Chemical and pH imbalances are a major cause of pain and degenerative diseases such as cancer, diabetes, kidney disease, and more.

Congestion

No system can function when it's clogged. Congestion is caused by wrong diet and a sedentary lifestyle. It's the precursor to a vast number of diseases. It affects all systems of the body. Even people who don't think they're congested often have congestion at the cellular level.

Toxicity

In these times, we're exposed to unnatural chemistry and poisons in food, air, and water. These toxins must be removed from the body, otherwise normal metabolic processes can't work. Most people are highly toxic.

Parasites

Thousands of parasites can invade the body: Viruses, Bacteria, Flukes, Worms, Fungi, Mold, and Yeasts. Your body can't function normally with these parasites stealing nutrients and doing damage.

Poor Nutrition

Your body needs certain nutrients to fight off disease and build healthy tissues. Without them, your body loses strength, becomes chaotic, and cannot defend itself.

Energetic Disturbances

There are invisible energy systems in the body. Eastern medicine works with the meridians and acupuncture points. There are energy fields surrounding the body (aura) and special energy vortexes that feed subtle energies into the body (chakras), which must also be strong and stable. These 3 systems, 1) meridians with their energy points, 2) the aura, and 3) the chakras, form the energy systems of the body. These must work together in harmony. Even with a perfect physical body you cannot be healthy if these systems are out of whack. These systems constitute the life-force systems of your body. Without life force, you are dead.

Mental and Emotional Stress

Emotions such as anxiety, depression, confusion, and other chaotic or depressed states severely affect your health. If your mental and emotional health suffers, your physical health will suffer, too. You need to heal on all levels to be really healthy.

The Ultimate Cause

Ultimately, your underlying physical symptoms and problems are due to unconscious choices that you made because of the concepts and beliefs you have about yourself, your self identity. That identity itself is based on the unique collection of experiences that you have become identified with. This mis-identification is the fundamental cause of all suffering. In later chapters, I'll go deeper into this false matrix, this false identity. As soon as that fabricated identity is dropped, your body can self correct miraculously. It's a cognitive shift that can free you from a multitude of problems and suffering.

Summary

The focus of this chapter was to look at symptoms of degeneration so that you can take stock of where you are. I covered symptoms and general self diagnostics for physical health, mental health, and emotional health. Go through each section of this chapter and make a list of your symptoms and understand their various causes. Carefully work through the action plan below so that you are not ignoring anything. As you heal, you will be able to refer back to this chapter to see how far you've come. In later chapters, I'll introduce methods for overcoming these problems.

Action Plan - Chapter 3, Symptoms of Degeneration

1. Diagnose weakness in yourself, friends, and family by using the list of symptoms provided in this chapter.
2. Purchase pH test strips and test the pH of yourself, friends, and family.
3. Examine your iris and show friends and family how they can explore their own health. See how everyone's eyes are different. Note any weaknesses.
4. Locate a reflexology chart and experiment with reflexology on yourself. Make a note of sensitive areas. Those correspond to places in your body that are weak.
5. Experiment with acupressure to locate sensitive places on your body.
6. Try a one-day fast and see how you feel.

7. Examine your life history in relation to the seven opportunities for change. Notice how you missed certain cues. Look at what's happening now and discern how you may be missing current cues. The seven stages are: 1) Quiet Intuition, 2) Dreams, 3) Environmental Cues, 4) Emotional Pain, 5) Physical Pain, 6) Disease, 7) Near Death.

8. Review the obstacles list. What is holding you back? Lack of knowledge, lack of tools, ego, unwillingness to change, unwillingness to take responsibility, unwillingness to let go, misuse of power, unwillingness to learn, unwillingness to properly use your power, resignation, disinterest, laziness, preoccupation, lame excuses: no time, too busy, too many distractions. Make a note of your weaknesses. Next to each weakness, list one or more ways to overcome it. Don't focus on problems, focus on solutions. Use your intuition.

9. Understand the seven fundamental causes of all diseases. 1) Chemical and pH Imbalances, 2) Congestion, 3) Toxicity, 4) Parasites, 5) Poor Nutrition, 6) Energetic Disturbances, 7) Mental and Emotional Stress, 8) The Ultimate Cause

Chapter 4
Environmental Healthcare

Your Environment at Home and Work

Environmental Concerns

Anyone who has traveled to a large city and experienced smog knows that we live in a toxic soup. What most people don't know is that the indoor environment is commonly 5 times worse and often 25-100 times worse. Chemists have produced tens of thousands of chemicals without regard to safety, chemicals with many different toxic effects and side effects. Most people are significantly contaminated with at least 700 chemicals. Our homes and offices may not be safe places to live, but with care you CAN create a safe environment in your home and your workplace.

There are types of mold that are so highly toxic they can render a house or office totally unlivable. Some homes still have lead paint and asbestos. Another major problem is that there are literally thousands of chemicals in cleaning and personal care products that add an additional toxic load to your body. You breathe in fumes from these products when you use them. Your skin absorbs them directly. Some people have become so chemically sensitive they cannot live in an ordinary house or work in an ordinary office. These people are our "canaries in the coal mine." They are a warning signal to all of us that we need to change our ways.

Pure Air

It's possible to make indoor air more pure than outdoor air by avoiding toxic products and by using devices to purify the air. The new-house and new-car smell that you have experienced is really an outgassing of often toxic fumes. The best solutions for cleaning the air include: Electrostatic Filtration, UV Light, Negative Ion Generators, and Photocatalytic Oxidation (PCO), the technology used by NASA. Electrostatic Filtration is useful to capture particulates. UV light can destroy viruses, bacteria, allergens, and mold spores circulating in the air. PCO can neutralize many chemical toxins. It's a more recent breakthrough technology. Negative Ion Generators can neutralize some chemicals and clears particulates out of the air. Every home and office should have an air purifier, even if only an inexpensive negative ion generator. Search online for "negative ion generators" and "PCO air purifiers" There are ion units for under $20. You don't need to spend a lot of money, but you may need more than one since ion generators usually have a limited square footage they can cover. Check for the coverage area on any unit you plan to purchase. Truck stops often have units for your car that plug into your lighter socket. If you drive a lot, they are worthwhile. Avoid units that combine synthetic deodorizers.

For your home or office, the more comprehensive solution is to get a unit that combines all four technologies. Most newer units do. They cost between $150-$300, but are well worth it if you have any respiratory problems. There are also houseplants that help purify the air. NASA did studies on how to filter the air on space stations and recommends the following 18 plants:

1) English ivy (Hedera helix)
2) Spider plant (Chlorophytum comosum)
3) Golden pothos or Devil's ivy (Scindapsus aures or Epipremnum aureum)
4) Peace lily (Spathiphyllum 'Mauna Loa')
5) Chinese evergreen (Aglaonema modestum)
6) Bamboo palm or reed palm (Chamaedorea sefritzii)
7) Snake plant or mother-in-law's tongue (Sansevieria trifasciata 'Laurentii')
8) Heartleaf philodendron (Philodendron oxycardium, syn.Philodendron cordatum)
9) Selloum philodendron (Philodendron bipinnatifidum, syn.Philodendron selloum)
10) Elephant ear philodendron (Philodendron domesticum)
11) Red-edged dracaena (Dracaena marginata)
12) Cornstalk dracaena (Dracaena fragans 'Massangeana')
13) Janet Craig dracaena (Dracaena deremensis 'Janet Craig')
14) Warneck dracaena (Dracaena deremensis 'Warneckii')
15) Weeping fig (Ficus benjamina)
16) Gerbera daisy or Barberton daisy (Gerbera jamesonii)
17) Pot mum or florist's chrysanthemum (Chrysantheium morifolium)
18) Rubber plant (Ficus elastica)

Take this list to any garden center and choose a selection of plants for your home. If you are not a gardener, ask for easy care plants from this list. You will need 15-20 plants, one 6-8" potted plant for each 100 sf. Obviously, larger plants are better.

Mold in Your Home or Office

If you discover mold, you need to take action. Mold can be a trigger for asthma and many other bronchial conditions. It can even be fatal. Mold shows up in damp conditions, such as found in bathrooms and basements. It appears as a black splotchy stain. It is often caused by a water leak. If you

have mold in your home or office, you need to do repairs. If you can't
professional mold remediation, here's what to do.

1. Before working on it, purchase an N-95 respirator, which costs from
$12-$25. Make sure it seals well. You don't want to breathe mold spores.
Wear rubber gloves for your hands and unventilated goggles for your eyes.
Spray the affected area with oxygen bleach (sodium percarbonate), it's a
powder that you dissolve in water. It's just hydrogen peroxide, which you can
also use. Avoid chlorine bleach, which is toxic in itself.

2. Purchase a negative ion generator or one of the better air purifiers and
put it in the room near the affected area. This will chemically neutralize
toxins in the air and cause particulates to rapidly settle out. It would be a
good idea to install a purifier as soon as you discover mold, but that won't
stop the problem. You have to get rid of the source.

3. Tear out every bit of sheet rock that has mold on it and put it in a large,
heavy-duty, contractors trash bag for disposal.

4. Fix any leak that was keeping the area damp or wet. Anything that you
cannot remove, spray thoroughly with oxygen bleach. Then paint those areas
that can't be removed with hydrated lime whitewash. To make whitewash,
use hydrated lime and fine salt (5:1); mix into water to make a thick paint.

The traditional formulas used slaked lime which gets very hot when
mixed with water. Always add quick lime to water, never pour water onto
slaked lime. Hydrated lime is safer to use and is available at any building
supply. Wheat paste can be an additional binder, but not necessary.

Wear gloves and eye protection. Protect sensitive surfaces from the caustic
mix. The caustic nature of hydrated lime will prevent mold from coming
back. Whitewash has been used for centuries and is a safe alternative to
chemicals.

5. When all is dry, complete the repair with new building materials.

It is absolutely essential that you do not have mold in your living space.
Do not put off making repairs.

Pure Water

Cities go through extraordinary measures to provide water that is safe for
drinking. Sediments are filtered out and the pH is balanced. The problem in
the United States is that in order to prevent the growth of microorganisms,
water companies use chlorine, a highly toxic chemical. Many countries have
banned chlorine. One reason is because when it reacts with organic matter,

disinfection byproducts (DBP's) are formed, such as trihalomethanes. DBP's can be 10,000 times more toxic to humans than chlorine itself. Instead of chlorine, many countries now use ozonation, which is completely safe. Another highly toxic chemical added to our drinking water is fluoride. There is no excuse for continuing to use fluoride. It has no benefits for human health. It can cause teeth to become mottled, discolored, and is a needless expense. It is a poison. Needless to say, avoid toothpastes that contain fluoride.

Your drinking, bathing, and shower water needs to be filtered due to this contamination. The best filters contain at least three elements: a coarse sediment filter, an activated carbon/silver filter to destroy microorganisms, and KDF, a compound that can remove chlorine and other contaminants. KDF does not work with monochloramine, a type of chlorine product which is now used by some municipalities. Check. All chlorine disinfectants in water supplies should be banned worldwide and replaced with ozonation.

Countertop devices often use standard-sized filter canisters. Definitely purchase a unit that uses a standard filter canister. Some newer canisters have 10 filter stages and do an excellent job of purification. Countertop devices are available at any big box home improvement store, but you may have to shop around for a better filter canister. A good countertop unit should sell for around $100. They can often be installed under the sink to avoid losing counter space. Natural food stores often carry the better units, and especially, the better canisters. There are also devices that attach to your shower head to filter shower water. You absorb one-third of your daily intake of water when you shower. Shower units are often available at natural food stores and possibly department and home improvement stores. They won't work if your water company uses monochloramine as a disinfectant. You would need to use a whole house filter with a large activated carbon component.

If your water comes from a well, it is a good idea to have it tested. Wells can also be polluted. In fact, many cities have had to close down wells due to excessive pollution. Bottled water is not a very good solution. Bottled water is often just filtered tap water, which you can do for yourself much cheaper with your own filter. If you live in a city, your best choice for drinking water is your own countertop or under-the-counter filter. Fill your own bottles for travel and work, and attach a filter to your shower.

Lighting

Light pollution can become a medical problem. Your body heals in darkness and produces a different chemistry. If you don't sleep in darkness, your metabolism will become imbalanced. The rhythms of nature are important for your well-being. It's also important to be exposed to full-spectrum sunlight during the day. Fifteen minutes of sunlight per week can provide all of the vitamin D you need. 10 minutes of bright sun on your skin will produce 10,000 IU's of vitamin D, far better than any supplement.

Home and office lighting can be another source of pollution. The widely used and highly promoted fluorescent lights and CFL bulbs contain mercury, which is a highly toxic neurotoxin. If you break one, you should immediately vacate your home or office for 3 to 6 hours. The space should be aired out and special care should be taken when cleaning up:

• Get everyone, including pets out of the house. Close off the affected area and turn off air handlers to prevent spreading the toxin. Open windows in the affected area to let in fresh air. Don't step on broken glass or the mercury powder.

• Wear an N-95 respirator. Use disposable rubber gloves, duct tape, stiff paper or thin cardboard, and damp paper towels to collect the residue. Place all waste in a sealable container with a lid, (or at least a zippered plastic bag). Carefully examine the area to get everything. Finally, vacuum the area (don't use a beater). If the CFL broke on carpet, you should replace the carpet. Mercury left behind even after cleaning can be released as vapor when children play or sit on it.

• Take the wastes and any exposed items, such as bedding, fabrics, clothing, cleaning materials, and vacuum bag, to a special toxic waste center. Call your local government for locations. Fluorescent lights should never be discarded in normal trash. They should always be taken to a special toxic wastes disposal center. Obviously, it would be best not to use them at all. Avoid switching to CFL bulbs which can cost even more to dispose of than to purchase. There are better options on the horizon.

• After cleaning the area, everyone in your family should do a mercury cleanse using cilantro and parsley (covered in the next chapter).

New Lighting Options

New, safer, affordable lighting technologies are available or coming soon. LED is available now and is becoming more affordable if you shop carefully. Research is continuing at a rapid pace for incandescent bulb replacements.

Incandescent bulbs will still be available, but are required to be more efficient. You can save money by choosing a lower wattage.

Sound Pollution

Sound pollution is another problem. We all need rest and silence. Later, I'll talk about the need for meditation. It's good to have someplace to go where you can relax, free from the bombardment of noise. If you don't have a place at home, find a quiet place like a library or meditation center where you can stop in and recuperate in silence. Foam earplugs can be useful in excessively noisy environments, not only to protect your hearing, but to provide much needed relief. They are available at any big box home improvement store. They're sold for hearing protection for power tools.

Your Inner Environment

The environment inside your body is more important than the outer environment. You also have more control over it. There is so much talk today about ecology, climate, and other problems with the environment. That is nothing compared to the problems we are having inside. Being at the top of the food chain, we accumulate all the poisons.

Toxic Foods, Personal Care and Household Products

There are toxic heavy metals and thousands of poisons in our food, air, and water. Foods often contain pesticides, herbicides, insecticides, fungicides, antibiotics, and a host of processing chemicals. Many personal care and cleaning products have unnatural chemistry that should be avoided. Cleaning products for home and office are often highly toxic. There are three categories to deal with: 1) Foods, 2) Personal Care Products, 3) Home and Office Products. Here's how to protect yourself.

Toxic Foods

Many people believe that governments protect us through agencies like the Food and Drug Administration and the Environmental Protection Agency in the USA. Everyone knows about food labeling laws, and we assume that these laws are there to protect us, but the reality is that virtually all governments throughout the world are run by corporations. Practically all the policies of governments are designed to help corporations. Many, many products are produced which are extremely unhealthy, but since most are at least minimally labeled, we can generally protect ourselves.

A good rule of thumb – *If you don't understand every ingredient on the label, don't use the product.* When you're shopping, read every label. If it sounds like a foreign language, don't buy it. One way to learn about ingredients is to take a picture of the label with a digital camera or smart phone. When you get home, look up every ingredient on the Internet, then decide if you want that chemical in your body. It's sad that we have to go to such lengths to protect ourselves and our families, but we need to do it. Avoid products with undesirable ingredients. You don't know how such ingredients interact and neither does anyone else. It isn't being researched. It's too complex. Yet, we are having epidemics of degenerative diseases that didn't previously exist. Connect the dots. Simple, natural foods are best.

Actually, the only foods that are really healthy are fresh foods and foods that have been dried at temperatures below 115°F (46°C). Especially when you're trying to heal, avoid all processed foods and previously cooked foods, even foods you cooked earlier in the day. Any food that was dried at high temperatures or canned is not very healthy. Only fresh raw foods are full of vitamins, enzymes, bio-available minerals, and life force energy. Old foods sitting in the fridge, canned foods, processed foods, and virtually all restaurant foods cannot build healthy tissues because they lack essential nutrients. Foods which are tainted with chemicals are not fit to eat. Basically, if it comes in a package with a long list of ingredients, it's not fit to eat. In a later chapter, I'll cover the best foods for health.

Wise Shopping

Most developed countries are pervaded by processed foods, that is, foods with high calories and very little nutritional value. These are the foods responsible for obesity and disease. I think they should be considered poisonous. They should at least have warning labels. Essentially, you and your family should live on foods that do not come in packages, that are not processed. To find the healthy foods that truly nourish your family, you will need to find new places to shop.

The absolute best place to shop for fresh fruits and vegetables is your local farmers market. These markets have produce that is often *weeks* fresher than what you find in most conventional food stores. You can talk with the growers to find out how their food is grown and get to know them. When you shop local, you also support your local economy.

For bulk foods, do an Internet search for "natural food stores" in your area. (Delete all the vitamin & pill shops.) Put this list of healthy food stores in your contacts list under an appropriate category and set a reminder to check them out. Natural or health food stores often have bulk bins to provide low-cost whole grains, legumes, nuts, seeds, and more. If you are not used to shopping this way, the store personnel will show you how to shop from these bins.

Unfortunately, many natural food stores have also gotten into the business of highly marked up, processed and packaged foods. They are high profit items. Avoid those foods and those stores. If you have a natural food co-op in your area, shop there. They're a better choice because profit is not their central motive. Some of the larger natural food chains have been bought out by conglomerates. They may not be a good choice because their values are now based on the corporate bottom line. They are in business to make the most money and often no longer promote simple foods in their natural state. Such stores are bloated with packaged and prepared foods.

Many natural food stores carry organic produce, which is great. Another source of produce, much of which is organic, is Asian and Indian markets. Do an Internet search for (use the quotes) "ethnic food stores," "Asian food stores," and "Indian food stores," plus "*your city*." These stores are sometimes the only source of great, high-nutrition Chinese vegetables such as bok choy, tatsoi, and many others. Asian and East Indian people living in the West often know better how to find good values in basic foods than most Westerners. These markets cater to this crowd.

Indian markets are the best source for spices. These spices are often Ayurvedic blends. Although they come in packages, they are just spice blends without additives, and do offer some convenience. Avoid the ones that are too hot or contain onions and garlic (which have steroidal properties and often cause agitation). Read the labels, learn the ingredients, make sure they are not tainted. Once you understand how these blends are made, you can make your own blends.

Some regular food stores are starting to carry organic produce, which can be helpful. Be aware that ordinary commercial food stores are designed to entice you with unhealthy, high-profit products usually placed in the path to the produce section – cakes, brownies, donuts, fudge, pies, chips – every kind of high sugar hydrogenated product. Shoppers beware! They don't have your health interests in mind. Commercial food stores are designed for highest profit. Fresh, locally produced food from local growers is much better. The absolute freshest and best food is from your own organic garden.

Toxic Personal Care Products

There are many personal care products on the market that I believe are not safe. Thousands of chemicals are added to products. Some massively used chemicals are known to be irritating, toxic, even cancer causing. Some are used in practically every shampoo. Thousands have never been tested sufficiently. Not all chemicals are labeled on personal care products, so it's impossible to know what's there. To find out how toxic your personal care products are, search the Environmental Working Group, http://www.ewg.org/skindeep/. Look at the ingredient list on every product and look up each ingredient. You will be amazed.

Another good source of information is the Organic Consumers Association. Check out their list of the 10 worst chemicals, visit http://www.organicconsumers.org/bodycare/toxic_cosmetics.cfm. Chemicals on your skin could be even more dangerous than when eaten! Your digestive juices have enzymes that break down many chemicals, but chemicals put on your skin are directly absorbed. The word "natural" doesn't mean anything in personal care products. The Organic Consumers Association found at least one cancer-linked chemical in over 40 percent of products that claimed to be "natural." Multiple chemicals together cause a chemical cocktail, the effects of which are not known and have not been studied. The safest bet is to keep your exposures to a few simple, truly natural ingredients.

The best source of information is the Environmental Working Group, http://www.ewg.org – you can search this website for practically any chemical, and you can look for brands that you can trust. They have special web pages for personal care products, cleaning products, and more. This is your best source for up-to-date information on toxicity in the marketplace. EWG estimates that about 20% of cosmetics may be contaminated with a cancer-causing agent.

In many cases, you can make your own healthy personal care products easily. Shampoos, deodorants, face creams, body lotions, and most cosmetics can all be made from healthy ingredients at a fraction of the price of store-bought goods. Most are very easy to make. There are formulas in the Resources Chapter.

Healthy Personal Care Products

In the same places you shop for healthy foods, shop for healthier personal care products. To learn what to buy, go to the website of the Environmental Working Group and locate products that will be of value to you. Remember, in our society, and in societies trying to mimic Western trends, only products with high profit potential are promoted, not necessarily products that are good for you. In many cases, you'll have to create your own, but it's often very easy.

For example, suppose you want to improve your skin quality. There are thousands of products on the market, expensive products that often have tons of junk in them. You probably don't need any of them. You can make a wonderful skin care product with one tsp of powdered vitamin C, 3 Tbsp of water, and 2 tsp of vegetable-source glycerin (a 5-10% solution of vitamin C). Put it in a dark bottle to protect it from light. Apply it to your skin after your shower. It helps to create healthy glowing skin.

You might also want to add a little essential oil to a carrier oil, like olive, coconut oil, or shea butter to protect your skin from drying out. This may be all you ever need for skincare. Your skin knows how to regenerate itself when it has the right nutrition.

You can combine both ideas into an emollient. Blend the liquid vitamin C/glycerin formula with olive oil, coconut oil and/or shea butter. Add vitamin E from a capsule for more protection.

Likewise, look for simple natural products for dental care, hair care, and other needs. I include simple recipes in the Resources Chapter. The Internet is your friend when you know how to effectively search. Do searches for how to create the products you need from simple ingredients. You may already have what you need around the house. Keep your life elegant, simple, and safe.

Home Care and Office Products

Just as personal care products are often toxic and carcinogenic, products for home and office are even worse. There are over 78,000 chemicals used in such products. Many have never been tested for safety. Many are known to be highly carcinogenic. As mentioned, indoor air pollution is often 25-100 times worse than outdoors because of this. For instance, air fresheners sometimes contain chemicals that deaden your sense of smell. You can avoid practically all of these toxins and pollutants by educating yourself and using simple DIY products. Baking soda, borax, white vinegar, lemon juice, hydrogen peroxide, plain vegetable-based soap, eco-enzymes, and washing soda can satisfy all your cleaning needs. Eco enzymes are DIY enzymes, also referred to as "garbage enzymes" that are made from kitchen scraps and brown sugar. The ingredients ferment and eventually turn into an amazing vinegar-like cleaner. It also has uses in the garden. I make our household cleaner out of citrus peels and a little rice flour or other starter. Use about 10 parts water, 3 parts food scraps, 1 part brown sugar, and 1/4 part rice flour or any probiotic starter. Do not keep air tight as gases must escape. Search the net for recipes: "eco enzymes" and "garbage enzymes."

All household and personal care products can be naturally scented with essentials oils from the health food store.

These are just a few of many recommendations for avoiding toxic exposure. There are whole books dedicated to toxins in our environment and how to avoid exposure. Do the best you can. When your body is stronger, it can deal more easily with our contaminated environment. In the Resources Chapter, there are formulas for green, environmental, and nontoxic living.

Even new cars and homes can be highly toxic. Some people have had to park their new car in the garage for months, with windows down, to air out toxins. Many people cannot move into a new home without ill effects due to the toxins used in construction. Clothing is often tainted with many kinds of chemicals. You may want to consider using only natural fabrics such as cotton, ramie, silk, linen, wool, bamboo, hemp, rayon, and lyocell (Tencel). Even so, it's better to wash clothing before wearing the first time. Many chemicals are applied to clothing to improve salability, but will wash out with the first washing. When dry cleaning, ask if they use oxygen-based cleaners and eco-friendly methods.

Be aware that all fabrics are flammable, but synthetics melt to your skin and are difficult to remove if ignited, often causing terrible scars. Some synthetics produce toxic fumes. Natural fibers char rather than melt. Very lightweight fabrics burn more rapidly.

Radiation Exposures

We are all exposed to many different frequencies and intensities of electromagnetic (EMF) radiation and nuclear radiation. Lets look as radiation exposures.

Nuclear Radiation Exposure

Any building with a basement is subject to nuclear radiation pollution from radon gas. If you have a basement at home or work, you should test for radon gas. Search the Internet for testing kits.

Avoid all foods from the ocean, particularly the Pacific Ocean, due to the meltdown of the Fukushima reactors. Current observation shows a massive die off of marine life in the Pacific Ocean. It is not being reported in the major news outlets as of this writing, and we don't yet have scientific studies to report, just observations. We do know that background radiation on land has doubled or tripled on the West Coast of America. It's better to be safe than sorry.

Many navel personnel who helped with the Fukushima relief efforts, who showered aboard ship with desalted ocean water, are dying from radiation sickness and cancer three years later. Nuclear radiation has a half-life measured in decades, even centuries. It may be decades before anything from the ocean is safe. For many nuclear isotopes, there is no safe level of exposure. The official public government position is that the massive radiation being dumped into the ocean by the Fukushima reactors is diluted enough to be safe. The problem is accumulation in the food chain. Fish accumulate heavy metals and are unfit for human consumption on those grounds alone. Radioactive pollution from nuclear testing, illegal dumping of toxic wastes and nuclear wastes in the ocean, and nuclear generating plant meltdowns make seafood unsafe. Tuna and other fish now have higher measurable radiation. Later, I'll give other reasons for avoiding seafood.

EMF Radiation Exposure

Electromagnetic radiation is all around us in the form of radio broadcasts, computer emissions, power line emissions, and wireless telephone emissions. If you live within 100 yards of a high power transmission line, you should consider moving. At least test your property for excessive exposure. Cell phones, because of their close proximity to your brain, produce excessive EMF exposures, especially for people who use them a lot. Consider using a separate earpiece so that the antenna is not near your head or avoid using cell phones altogether. For the same reason, stay away from cell phone towers, which have much more powerful transmitters. Wireless computer connections and cordless home phones also use high frequencies, which many authorities consider damaging. Try to minimize your exposures. It's also not a good idea to use electric blankets due to EMF radiation. Comforters are much better and are very affordable. They also work when you lose electric power. Flannel sheets are a joy to crawl into on cold winter nights.

Our bodies are very sensitive to unnatural EMF exposures. Quite a lot of research has been done to show that these exposures have damaging health effects. All of the controlling activities within your body are electrical or energetic in nature. Your heart rhythm and EEG brain activity are common examples. You should protect yourself from disturbing this delicate system as much as possible. One of the best ways is to ground yourself.

Earthing or Grounding

Clinton Ober recently rediscovered the protective and rejuvenating health effects of being connected to the Earth. He and his associates researched the phenomenon for several years and promoted the results through the book, *Earthing: The Most Important Health Discovery Ever?* I wouldn't say it's the most important health discovery ever, but it does have some merit. Their research is available at http://earthinginstitute.net. I suggest that you review their research and watch some YouTube videos to learn about the impact this can have on your well-being. It will motivate you to use this information. The flower comparisons are amazing.

They found, as have others before them, that you can protect yourself from many kinds of EMF exposures plus boost your health by connecting your body to the earth, either by walking barefoot on the earth, or connecting to the earth through a copper wire. This is called "grounding" or "earthing." The wire transports energies that have beneficial health effects. Many people are familiar with antistatic mats used for working with sensitive electronics or at your computer. This is similar, but in fact, antistatic mats are not good for this purpose. Their resistance is too high. The valuable contribution of Ober and his associates is the scientific research they have done on the numerous health benefits. Here is a short list.

- Reduces or eliminates inflammation. (Inflammation is the precursor to most disease. When you reduce inflammation, you create a tremendous boost in health.)
- Reduces or eliminates chronic pain.
- Improves the quality of sleep. Makes it easier to fall sleep.
- Increases energy.
- Lowers stress, increases calmness, rapidly soothes the nervous system.
- Reduces stress hormones.
- EEG instantly normalizes when your body is grounded.
- Normalizes biological rhythms.
- Improves blood pressure and flow, naturally thins the blood.
- Eliminates clumping of red blood cells.
- Relieves muscle tension and headaches.
- Reduces hormonal and menstrual symptoms.
- Accelerates healing.
- Reduces/prevents bedsores in bedridden patients.
- Reduces/eliminates jet lag.
- Protects against potentially damaging EMFs.
- Accelerates recovery from intense athletic activity.

There are few things that are as simple and as easy to do that produce such a profound impact on health. You can get these health benefits by just sleeping while grounded! The reason that grounding works is because the Earth provides energies that your body needs. For example, the Earth provides electrons that function in the body like antioxidants to reduce the damage of free radicals. The Earth and the ionosphere are two polar opposites of tremendous electrical charge. The Earth holds electrons in vast quantities. It provides other life supporting energies that are, as yet, not understood. There is also the natural Earth oscillation known as the Schumann Resonance that has human impact.

The human body evolved in contact with the Earth. It still requires those energetic resources. Here are two ways to do it.

1. The easiest way to connect with the Earth, is to walk on the moist bare earth with your bare feet. No doubt, in the ancient past we all lived this way. Some cultures still go barefoot. Thin moccasins are almost as good, especially when they're a little moist and become more conductive. Try walking barefoot on the earth at home, at a park, at the beach, or while hiking or camping. You will feel a lightness, a joy, an energetic boost. You may recall how good you felt when you were at the beach on vacation.

Unfortunately, modern shoes are all insulated with synthetic materials. They don't work to transfer the energies. You need to be barefoot or wear special conductive footwear. When you walk barefoot on the earth, you receive electrons from the charged Earth as well as other vital Earth energies. In India, they categorize at least five different kinds of pranic energies, life-force energies, within the human body. The earth provides its contribution of these energies.

For most people, modern lifestyles don't allow us to go barefoot very much or to sleep directly on the earth. It's just not practical, especially during harsh winter weather.

2. A more practical solution is to run a wire from the earth to your body while indoors. It's really simple. You just need a grounding kit. A kit includes only four simple items: 1) a ground connection, 2) a resistor, 3) a wire, and 4) a pad, mat, or other material to contact your body. The earthing researchers created a business to sell such products. They sell silver-threaded conductive sheets to sleep on, conductive rubber mats for feet or hands, grounding hardware, wires with a resistor, and more. Their kits vary in price; some are expensive. If you have the money, you could get their products and support them. If you don't have extra cash, you can make a kit for little or nothing (see below).

Once you have a kit, plug the wire directly into the earth (or a grounded outlet), and connect the other end of the wire with its pad touching your skin. The conductive mat or pad completes the connection to your body. Nothing could be easier. The best location to connect to your body is K1, the acupuncture point near the ball of your foot, so a foot connection is ideal. K1 is centered just under the ball of the foot. K1 balances and feeds all the meridians of your body. Search the Internet for "acupuncture point K1," if interested. Don't worry about the precise location, you'll use a fairly large pad to connect.

There are various ways to sleep and work while grounded that are described in the next section on making your own kit. Get the PDF from my web site with more details for scrounging a no-cost, low-cost kit. The cost of a kit is low and the potential health payoff is high. The whole world is suffering with inflammation, both physically and psychologically. This simple approach could improve health around the world at practically no cost. It can reduce stress, anxiety, and inflamed mental states, which could even lead to greater world peace. Consider making kits for family and friends.

Making a Ground Connection Kit

If you're a little bit industrious you can make a grounding kit for free by scrounging materials or for less than $5 if you purchase materials. A kit includes:

1. A ground connection to the earth.
2. A resistor to prevent high currents. A resistor is a small electrical part with two leads. It limits electrical flow. In this case, it protects against electrocution if you were to touch a faulty device, like a shorted lamp. It costs a few pennies wholesale or in bulk.
3. A thin, flexible, insulated wire from the resistor to your body.
4. A conductive pad to place against your body.

Let's look at the simplest approach. Download a more detailed version from my website.

Connecting to the Earth

You can connect directly to the earth by inserting a 1-2 foot metal probe into the ground outside your window. The probe could be galvanized tubing or heavy copper wire. A direct ground connection is ideal, but for most people, not very practical. There's an easier way. All modern homes and offices have grounded outlets connected to a copper rod buried deep outside your home or office. In North America, the round holes on your outlet are grounded. It's perfectly safe to use them. In other countries you need to determine which prong is grounded. If you don't have grounded outlets, you need to use the direct earth connection, or connect to a metal water pipe that goes into the ground.

To use an outlet, insert a 3/16" round metal prong into the hole, (scrounge any 3/16" metal object). The simplest choice is to buy a "standard banana plug" at your local electronics or audio store (ask for it by name, or search the Internet). It's almost a perfect fit, (you can widen the prong if necessary). You can also connect using the faceplate screw on any grounded outlet or use any screw on the chassis of any grounded equipment, like a computer or stereo (anything with a three pronged plug). Loosen the screw to make your connection. This only works when using 3 prong outlets. Old two prong outlets or equipment with two prongs won't work.

Connect a Resistor to Your Ground

To protect against high current, as a safety against a rare electrical failure, like a shorted lamp, use a small 1/4 or 1/2 watt resistor. You may not know anything about electricity, but that's okay. If you have 120V wiring (standard in the USA and many parts of the world), just ask for a 27K (27,000) ohm resistor at any electronics store, like Radio Shack, or go online. Use 47K in countries with the 240V standard. A resistor is not needed if you connect directly to a ground probe, AND you're away from any electrical appliances that could fail. Connect one lead of the resistor to your ground by wrapping it around the screw on the banana plug, faceplate or chassis. Tighten.

Connect a Wire to Your Resistor

You need an insulated wire to run from the free lead of your resistor to your body. Thin speaker wire works best. You only need a single wire for each kit. Split the two-lead speaker wire to make more kits, or attach them in line for a longer run. Speaker wire is available at most department stores. The thinnest wire is okay. Twist the free resistor lead to one end of the wire. If you want to get fancy, or if you're making lots of kits for family and friends, there are all kinds of electrical wire connectors – ring, star-ring, spade, in-line, and fork terminals. They are available at home improvement, hardware, electronics, and auto parts stores. Search for IMAGES of "electrical terminals", "electrical connectors", and "wire disconnects" on the Internet to see how they work. Crimp-on types don't require soldering. Connectors are similar to the way speakers, trailer lights, and auto wires are connected.

Connect the Wire to Your Body

To connect the wire to your body you need a pad. You can make a pad or buy one. Thin sheet metal or screening 2x2 or 2x3 inches works well. Avoid metals that are toxic such as nickel, lead, or aluminum. Plastic window screen obviously won't work. It's non conductive. Building supply stores have sheet metals and metal screening. Jewelers and metal sculptors know about metals and where to find them. Use galvanized sheet metal, copper, brass, stainless steel, or iron. Even a large "fender washer" will work. Of course, anything gold or silver works. Some people have reactions to metals. Choose one you are compatible with.

Cut sheet metal or screen with "tin snips" (heavy-duty shears). Round the sharp corners. Avoid sharp edges by filing or taping them. Drill or punch a hole in the corner to connect the wire. Tape it in place.

You can also buy bio-compatible pads made from conductive carbon rubber, fabric, or silicone. Conductive pads are marketed as TENS or muscle stimulator pads. 2x2 inch pads can be found for roughly one dollar each. http://www.tenssystem.com is a U.S. supplier with decent prices. Search Amazon or the Internet for "TENS pads." These pads have a sticky surface, much like a Post-It note. For this purpose, the pads will still work even after the sticky surface is no longer functional. You could wash them to remove body oils or dirt, and continue to use them by tucking them under clothing or using an elastic band. They come with either snap or pin connections. Pin connections are less bulky. Be sure to put a connector on your wire that will match your pad. You may have to search for it. Ask the pad supplier for the details of the connector it uses.

You have several places to connect to your body: K1, ankle, calf, wrist, forearm, or waist. To hold the pad in place, if it doesn't have a sticky surface, insert it into a sock, shirt sleeve, or at your waistband. It will even stay in a sock at K1 while you sleep. If your health is in any way compromised, it's worth the little bit of hassle.

Now you can make a kit that meets your comfort, aesthetic, cost, and hassle-factor requirements. Start with any low-cost, no-cost materials you have. Upgrade later as you like.

Is your outlet wired properly? Almost 100% of the time it is. Occasionally, ground and neutral can be reversed. You can test with an outlet tester, but outlet testers won't find other problems. You can test better with a multimeter. Digital multimeters cost less than $10 at discount stores like Harbor Freight. Many people keep a meter handy to test voltage, resistance, fuses, light bulbs, batteries, and circuit continuity in your home and car. It's a better choice than a dedicated outlet tester, much more versatile. It can be fun to learn to use a meter. To test with a multimeter, download the earthing kit PDF from my web site or visit http://ecmweb.com/content/diagnosing-power-problems-receptacle for more instructions.

Action Plan - Chapter 4, Environmental Healthcare

1. Take stock of your home and office. How toxic are they? If necessary, have your home tested for toxins such as mold, asbestos, or lead paint.
2. Consider the purchase of air purification devices such as electrostatic, PCO, UV light, and negative ion generators.
3. Purchase a countertop water filter if you are on city water. Find a high quality insert for the filter. Install a shower filter. If you're on a well, have your water tested.
4. Minimize toxins in personal care and household products. Read the labels on all your existing products. Look up every ingredient you don't understand. Mark the products that are dangerous and safely dispose of them. Visit the Environmental Working Group and the Organic Consumers Association for better options.
5. Be cautious when purchasing new homes and cars. In general, be more aware of toxic conditions in every environment. Purchase natural clothing, as much as possible.
6. Minimize sources of radiation. If you have a basement, test for radon gas. Look for sources of electromagnetic pollution in your home. Get a separate earpiece for your cellular phone if you use one. Don't use electric blankets; get a comforter. Be careful with florescent lights. Avoid them if you can. If one breaks, follow the instructions in this chapter and then do a Mercury cleanse for the entire family (covered in a later chapter). Avoid sound and light pollution as much as you can. Avoid products from the Pacific Ocean until extensive scientific research shows otherwise. Be safe.
7. Create an earthing or grounding kit for everyone in your household.

Chapter 5
Physical Healthcare

Purification Removes Congestion and Toxicity

Benefits of Purification

This section on purification is not really fun, but I have to lay the facts bare, because you need to be able to make intelligent decisions. I wish I could make it more fun, but the reality is that the subject itself is just not feel-good, cozy stuff. I have to talk about how to get probably decades of garbage out of your body. That's the downside. The upside is, when you get the garbage out, you'll feel incredible. Your agility and stamina will reach new highs. You'll awaken the life force in you and you'll have incredible energy and aliveness. Your senses will become brighter and stronger (you'll sense the beauty of a rose as never before). You'll never want to trash your body again.

When your body is pure, free from congestion and toxicity, you'll feel wonderful, beyond language to express. When you purify your system, you'll lose excess weight. You'll avoid the primary cause of premature death. You'll have more energy, less stress. Innumerable pains will vanish. Your body will become nimble, supple, and light. Your mind will become clear and your heart will sing. Your senses will explode with new sensations, new colors and tastes. You will be renewed, revitalized, and made whole again. Is that enough inspiration?

In a sense, it's like getting a brand new body, made to order. Your body can be molded, almost like clay, into a perfect or near perfect form through a series of steps that begin with purification. What a delight it is to have a body that works for you rather than weighing you down! Keep these images in mind. Let your spirit soar with possibilities, because that is what will sustain you when, at times, purification taxes your will to change. You need to strengthen your resolve for the journey ahead, and the best way is to remember the goal. In this crucial step, the goal is a body with beauty, grace, peace, energy, strength, vitality, and longevity.

Right now, while you are thinking about it, create the ideal image of how you want to look, feel, and be. Take a few minutes. See yourself the way you would like to be. Make mental movies. Envision yourself and your family in a state of peace and radiant health. You deserve it. Solidify this image in

ʌind's eye. You'll need it to guide you into the future. Take a moment
ɔ write it down as a goal. Keep it near you. Frequently visualize this
ɪ... ;e during the day. You want to *fasten* yourself to this new self image!

Steps to Strengthen Your Physiology

I've organized the cleanup process into step-by-step methods starting
with the most important actions first. Use your common sense with each of
these steps. Remember, you are the one who is responsible for your health.
You are the one making the decisions. Be wise. Here are the steps:

Get more Rest

When you rest, your body has more reserves to heal. If you continue to
push yourself, you will have few resources to heal what ails you. Every effort
you make requires nutritional resources, enzyme resources, life-force
resources, and more. Reduce mental stress, also. Take complete mental
breaks from your usual regimen. Play more. Lighten up. Worry less. The first
rule in natural healthcare is DON'T GET TIRED. Don't worry and fret
yourself into a weak state. Go to bed earlier, sleep later, take more breaks, be
at peace. Later, I'll explain meditation techniques that will help immensely.
The reserves you build by letting go of crazy schedules, overcommitment,
and unrealistic expectations will pay huge dividends. Rest, stay peaceful. Be
closer to the slower rhythms of nature. Whenever you feel taxed, STOP.
Breathe deeply and relax, even for a minute or two. Do not push yourself
into an early, painful death. Relax into healing and rejuvenation instead.
Later, after healing yourself, you'll be able to take on more responsibilities
with less effort.

Drink more Water

Drink therapeutic amounts of water with a pinch of unrefined sea salt in
each 8-ounce glass. Every day, drink 1/2 ounce of water for every pound of
body weight (metric: 6.5 centiliters per kilo). The water must be pure, room
temperature or slightly warm (body temperature). NOT chilled. Drink small
amounts throughout the day. When you first wake up, start with two glasses
to rehydrate from a night without liquids. Avoid drinking very much right
before meals or within 2 hours after a meal. Sip 4-6 ounces of water with
meals. Nothing else counts. Only water. For every other beverage you drink,
you will need to add that much MORE water. If you drink a soft drink or
coffee, you will need vast quantities of water to undo the damage (about 20
glasses for each glass of soda). Remember, these are therapeutic amounts.
When your body is pure, you won't need so much. For 125 pounds of body
weight, you need 64 oz of water, one half gallon, eight-8 ounce glasses.

(Metric: 58 kilos: 2 liters) Only use water that has NOT been heated to boiling, or even above 180° F (high heat destabilizes normal molecular clustering which reduces its healthy, cleansing action).

Water is the universal solvent. Without sufficient water your body becomes dehydrated and cannot function normally or remove wastes. Nutrition can't get to where it's needed. A 5% level of dehydration is severe. You simply must get used to room temperature water as your primary drink. You can add a bit of lemon if you like. No sugar.

A little salt is necessary. Claims that a low salt diet would help reduce blood pressure and be a health benefit proved not to work out in practice. Probably, that recommendation only applied to purified table salt, pure sodium chloride, which is known to cause health problems. Sea salt contains both sodium and potassium chloride. Chloride ions are needed to produce hydrochloric acid for digestion and the alkaline metals are necessary for producing alkalizing chemistry (bicarbonate) for later in the digestive process to neutralize stomach acids. Natural sea salt also contains dozens of trace minerals, which are absent from our soils and foods. These trace minerals are essential for health. Refined, iodized salt, however, is not a healthy choice. Use whole unrefined sea salt in modest quantities. Kelp or other seaweeds also have valuable trace minerals, including iodine, but they must be from an uncontaminated source, free from nuclear radiation exposure.

Whole books have been written on diseases which have been healed by just drinking therapeutic amounts of water. Dr. Fereydoon Batmanghelidj, M.D., describes in his book, *Your Body's Many Cries for Water,* how even severe cases of heart disease were healed simply by drinking this amount of water with a pinch of sea salt, combined with a modest daily walk. Take this very seriously. After rest, drinking sufficient water is the single most important thing you can do to restore health.

You are dehydrated if: 1) Your nostrils are dry, 2) your eyes are dry, 3) your tongue is dry, 4) your mouth is dry, 5) your skin is dry and wrinkled. By the time you get really thirsty it is too late – you're already past the point of excessive dehydration. If you don't have much of a "thirst desire" anymore, you may be dangerously dehydrated. One sign of dangerous dehydration is loss of the sense of thirst.

You can't re-hydrate by drinking lots of water all at once. It has to come in measured amounts during the day. Sip water all day long in small amounts. This will also prevent having to run to the restroom frequently. It will take

30-90 days to re-hydrate your body to normal levels. It will only be possible to re-hydrate properly if you are not deficient in minerals. Since the vast majority of people *are* mineral deficient, you will want to re-mineralize your body as you drink more water. A pinch of sea salt helps. Restoring minerals is discussed in the section on diet and nutrition.

Wild Shaking and Gentle Bouncing, 5 minutes, 4-5 times per day

When you first arise in the morning you can wake up to a new level of life by activating the nadis (energy points) in your body. There are tens of thousands of these points. All you have to do is shake your body wildly, vibrating as many parts as possible for a minute or so. It's easy, fun, and it really works. It starts an amazing energizing and cleansing process. Just shake and move wildly. It activates the meridians, the nadis, and begins a cleansing process for every cell.

Another amazing health practice is to gently bounce up and down while breathing deeply. You can jump or jog in place on the floor (preferably on a carpet or mat), or use a rebounder (a mini trampoline – department stores often sell them for about $50), you could also jump rope. The idea is to jostle your body so that it experiences zero gravity then double gravity over and over. Schedule this gentle exercise several times throughout the day. As your body becomes hydrated again, your lymph system begins to function fully.

During each bouncing session, after about a minute or two, you will notice a strange sense of delight. That's your body talking to you. It's telling you that it likes the opportunity to cleanse the putrid, toxic phlegm and mucus out of your body. Any method to bounce and jostle your body is OK. Just make sure to jostle your whole body as much as possible. Create alternating pressure on all the tissues of your body to move the most lymph fluid you can. Here's why:

Your lymph system is the drainage system for your body, but it doesn't have a pump like the circulatory system. Most people are aware of the circulatory system with its huge system of veins, arteries, and pumping heart. The lymph system is even bigger – about FIVE TIMES bigger! That's how important the drainage or clean-up system of your body is. But without a pump, it depends upon differential (alternating) pressure to push lymph fluid through tiny one-way valves. This is how it circulates lymph fluid.

From the cellular level, the lymph fluid moves into progressively larger channels. It's stored temporarily in the lymph nodes and then moves into the central lymph channel behind the lungs where it empties into the liver. The liver purifies the fluid, discards wastes, and injects the purified fluid (plasma) back into the blood for another trip to carry nutrients to the cells and then returns again carrying wastes. This system of cleansing the body at the cellular level is essential for health. The more efficient the process, the "happier" your cells will be. Lymphatic congestion is always due to the lack of this essential, alternating, pressure-pumping action. It's especially a problem if you're dehydrated.

Lymph circulation keeps you alive. Without it, you would die in only a few days as toxic levels of congestion build up. That's why bed-ridden people have so many problems and die so easily. This is also why sedentary occupations are so dangerous. Vibrating beds, chairs, or swings could provide the oscillating movement necessary to pump the lymph for those who cannot get up and move on their own. You simply must move to heal. The lymph system will clean up your body and move wastes to the liver and colon to be detoxified or removed.

Bouncing is the best way to create alternating pressure which can even reach into the brain. Any physical movement will help: pressing, squeezing, stroking, rubbing, and muscle tension/release. Tension/release should be done by everyone who is bedridden. All these methods work, but bouncing is best. Don't get tired doing this. You're not interested in creating more waste products of metabolism. Do gentle, easy, non-tiring bouncing. As you bounce, breathe very deeply. It's easiest to exhale at the bottom of a bounce and inhale at the top.

Breathe Deeply

Schedule deep breathing sessions at periodic intervals throughout the day. Set aside 4-5 breaks during the day in which you focus on deep breathing for 3-5 minutes. Begin by taking eleven very deep breaths. Be conscious of your breathing during the day and whenever you feel tired, anxious, or out of balance, breathe deeply for a few minutes. Deep breathing cleanses the respiratory system, exhausts waste gases, and floods your body with oxygen and life force energy. An excellent idea is to breathe deeply and rapidly while bouncing. This floods your body with oxygen. It enables cells to throw off more toxins. At other times, breathe deeply and rhythmically.

Breathe from deep down in your belly. Due to stress, most people have become upper-chest breathers. But the good blood flow is at the bottom of your lungs, not the top. To re-learn belly breathing, lie on your back, put a book on your belly, and see if it moves up and down. You need to draw air deep into your belly to open up the lower lungs. Watch a baby breathe; copy that. The upper lung is the last to expand. You need to practice consciously in order to return to normal breathing. Upper-chest breathing is insufficient for a healthy body.

If you smoke, realize that it's possible to simply stop and never need another cigarette. If you've had difficulty stopping, see the section on eliminating addictions. Remember to bring to mind, inspiring images of perfect health. See yourself free and healed of ugly habits, create beautiful habits instead. Forgive yourself for having taken that route, but don't go back. The easiest way to change is to upgrade your self image. I'll talk more about self image in the chapter on mental healing.

Mechanically Cleanse the Digestive Tract

When the colon is congested, it's difficult to absorb nutrients and difficult to eliminate the cesspool-like conditions which make your body toxic. Much has been said about a high fiber diet, and it's true that a high fiber diet can help immensely, but fiber should come from natural foods, not artificial supplements. Digestive troubles are primarily due to poor diet and stress. As with lymph system circulation, diet plays a major role in natural healthcare. Poor diets cause colon toxemia and congestion. The same dietary advice applies. Minimize processed, packaged, junk, and fast foods.

There are two methods for cleansing the colon. The first method is to add additional fiber. In addition to a high fiber diet of fresh fruits and vegetables, there are commercial fiber products. Most of them are good, but only in the short term. Taking supplemental fiber should not be a lifestyle. They reduce nutrient absorption. The inexpensive route is to purchase whole *psyllium seed husks* at a natural food store. Put 1 Tbsp in a glass of water, swish, and drink quickly (before it expands to several times its size!) Follow with more water. Take this fiber twice a day, not with meals, for 2 weeks maximum.

Psyllium husks acts as an intestinal broom to sweep filth and impacted fecal matter out. This mechanical approach to cleansing the digestive tract can be very effective. Do this for only a couple of weeks at a time, then repeat the process a month or two later. The scrubbing action is hard on the cilia of the digestive tract. This is NOT a lifestyle. When you're clean, you won't need it. You may need to repeat this a few times, but don't rely on laxatives or excessive fiber to be regular, because you will lose nutrition and create a bad habit. Your body knows how to function without it.

Juice Fasting and Cleansing Options

Fasting is recommended in every spiritual tradition. It has tremendous health benefits. It's a good idea to do a short fast of 2-3 days with every change of the seasons and to do a periodic long fast when needed. Fresh vegetable juice and fruit juice fasts are the best to start with. Colonic irrigation combined with a fast can remove toxic conditions very quickly. Colonic irrigation is exactly what the name implies – irrigating the colon with water. This procedure can save your life in the case of extremely toxic conditions. It's well worth learning and doing.

Note: Some conditions preclude fasting. Check with a health practitioner if you have a known medical problem.

If you are food poisoned or have great bowel distress (with no access to medical) you can drink salt water (2 tsp/quart) and move everything through your body and out very quickly. Take salt water in and use colonic irrigation, an enema, to take everything out. Colonic irrigation is highly useful in cases of bowel distress, bloating, diarrhea, etc. In cases of chemical poisoning, call a poison help center. If you have access to medical help, use it in such emergencies.

If you feel weak during a fast, remember it is virtually NEVER due to lack of nutrition, certainly not in less than 30 days on a liquid vegetable or fruit juice fast. Weakness and other unpleasant symptoms are almost ALWAYS due to toxic congestion. Your body tries to dump all the garbage it can as quickly as it can. As toxins enter your blood steam and lymph system for elimination, it can make you feel extremely weak, dizzy, nauseous, headachy, or just down right horrible. You can QUICKLY relieve this horrible feeling through bowel irrigation. If you have the money, see a professional colon hydro-therapist ($35-75/hour). If you don't have the money, here's a way to do it cheaply and safely:

Your body needs to be clean on the inside more than it needs to be clean on the outside. Most people never consider an internal wash. But the real cleaning needs to be internal where toxic conditions undermine both health and psychology.

Colonic irrigation can be a spiritual, uplifting experience if you choose to make it so. It's not intrinsically fun, but it's extraordinarily valuable. If you want inspiration, read the small book "The Essene Gospel of Peace" (book 1), translated by Edmond Bordeaux Szekeley. This method of healing was practiced in the first century and brought about many miraculous healings. Here's how to do a colon cleanse:

To begin, you need a clean potable source of water. Tap water is fine in developed countries, although pure filtered water without chlorine, fluoride and other unnatural chemistry would be better. But the water isn't going to be in you for very long, so it isn't critical. Use what you have available, as long as it's not tainted with microorganisms.

You need a simple device you can make yourself. I'll describe a device that works well, but has no equivalent on the market. Get 15-20 feet of 1/2" (outside diameter) clear vinyl tubing – available at any home improvement or hardware store in the USA (get the equivalent in metric overseas). At one end of the tubing attach 12 inches of bicycle tire inner tube with rubber bands, plastic electrical ties, or string. You can get used inner tubes from any bicycle shop for free. Use only plain tubes, not puncture-sealing types with goo inside. Make sure it has no holes in the part you use and seals well to the vinyl tubing. This inner tube is going to stretch over your faucet, so find an inner tube about the right size (10-speed bike tube generally works well). Make the device ahead of time, before you start a fast.

The inner tube protects you from excessive pressure by expanding when pressure might build up. I don't know of any device on the market that gives you pressure-safe access to unlimited water supplies such as this simple device. Some devices on the market use a 5 gallon bucket and are quite expensive. Ordinary enema bags have too little volume. This device can be made very cheaply and is quite portable. (If I locate such a device pre-made, I'll note it on the web site.) Now the procedure:

Attach the tubing to a convenient faucet in your bath and seal it with rubber bands and/or string so that when you turn on the water it doesn't leak or blow off. Test that it works well when you partially stop the flow. Adjust the water so that it shoots up only about 2-3 inches (5-7 cm) when held vertically. No fire hoses here! Adjust the water to make it warm to the touch, but not hot. If the drain in your tub has a screen with small holes, remove it by taking out the screw in the center.

Light a candle and/or use essential oils to sweeten the air in your bathroom. You can think of this as a spiritual purification experience and make it as pleasant as it can be. Adjust the water as described and squat or lie in the tub, (obviously without clothes on). Place the vinyl tube at the rectum and allow the water pressure to create the path for insertion. You don't even need any special tip or lubricant. Flowing water under mild pressure works extremely well.

Insert only about an inch or so. Take in a small amount of water, then evacuate on the toilet to get rid of solids. Repeat once again to be sure all solids are out, then flush.

Now, if your tub also has a shower, you may want to start a "warm rain shower." It's not necessary, but it helps to wash any spill down the drain, and makes the experience more comfortable. Lie down and insert the tubing and take in water to your comfort level. You want NO PAIN or excessive pressure. You can always allow water out by relaxing the sphincter muscle at the anus. Only hold the water for a few seconds, then let the water flow out and down the drain. Then repeat. In fact, you want to repeat the process 15-20 times taking in as much water as is comfortable, then release. Don't hold the water in. Take in, release, and repeat over and over. Continue until the water leaving your body is pure and clear, then continue a few more times. Many toxins are not visible.

After 15-20 times you will come to a point when you begin to feel wonderful. That's your body telling you that you've done a good job. I remember once (over 40 years ago), starting a fast which lasted 23 days. Early in the process, on the third day, I felt absolutely horrible, nearly suicidal. In one session of cleansing I went from such a horrible feeling to near ecstatic bliss, as my body released the toxins. Interestingly, I had to repeat the whole procedure 3 hours later. In fact, I had to do the cleansing 5 times that day! I was very toxic. I went through the same cycle of feeling horrible, cleansing, then feeling wonderful. The next day I had to do 3 cleanses. The day after that, one cleanse. Then no more. My body was sufficiently pure to continue the fast for 23 days.

This procedure for internal cleansing of the colon is necessary ONLY IF you feel horrible due to toxic release from the purification that occurs from fasting. It can be an amazing experience which will allow you to rid yourself quickly of horrible conditions in your body. Use it to your health. Sometimes people really get into colonics and overdo them. Don't do that. Use it as part of a fasting system, and cleanse only if necessary. If you need it, it can do wonders.

A substitute for colonics is to use psyllium seed husks for intestinal scrubbing. It is not as powerful, but works well enough in many cases. Colonic irrigation can create amazing cleansing and healing benefits.

Abdominal Exercise for the Colon

There is another exercise for purifying and toning the colon. It's a simple exercise that comes from the yoga tradition. It takes a little practice, but it's very healthful for the colon. It improves digestion and elimination. It's called uddiyana bandha (search for videos online if you need them). In a standing position, knees slightly bent, lean forward and put your hands on your

83

knees. Exhale, then, holding your breath, suck your belly back towards your spine and lift up your belly towards your chest cavity. You are drawing your belly back, up, and in. Now alternate the pressure on your knees from one side to the other. You will become familiar with how the muscles in your belly tense and release. With a little practice, you can create a rippling motion moving from right to left to facilitate elimination (nauli kriya).

Fasting to Heal Many Problems

Fasting along with cleansing the colon is a powerful way to heal, even for problems not related to the colon. Fasting can be a wonderful experience when done correctly. If done without knowledge, it can be big trouble. Start with a one-day fast, then a 3-day fast, then 7 days, then 14 days, then 21 or 30 days (if you want a long fast). Generally, more frequent (seasonal) 3 to 7 day fasts are better than infrequent long fasts. Here's how to fast:

You can start quickly, but you must end very gradually. Simply stop eating solid food, but drink liquids. Water fasts are generally too taxing for most people. Dry fasts are dangerous. For your first fast, use only freshly prepared vegetable juices. You can have all you want. Later, you can try fresh fruit juices. A stronger fast is a citrus juice fast, diluted by half with water. Citrus, with a small amount of blackstrap molasses and a pinch of cayenne pepper is an effective fast. A little "fire" can be helpful.

Always come off a long fast gradually. Start with extra water, then citrus juices, fruit juices, veggie juices, then finally, begin solid foods. Take a week or more come off a very long fast.

Cleansing the Sinuses

Many people have sinus trouble and congestion. There are two easy ways to cleanse the nostrils. The first is to simply catch some water in your hands while taking a shower. Several times, snort a little, then expel. This will rinse the nostrils near the opening, but won't get far back into the sinuses.

Natural food stores and yoga centers often sell little pots called neti pots that look like a very small tea pot with a spout that fits the nostrils. These are used with salt water to thoroughly cleanse the sinuses. This method also comes from the yogic tradition. Put one teaspoon of sea salt in two cups (one pint, 500ml) of warm water (body temperature). Fill the pot with water and stir until the salt dissolves, then tilt your head sideways over a sink, and introduce water into the upper nostril. It will drain out of the lower nostril. Tilt your head slightly backward to irrigate deeper into the sinuses. Repeat until your sinuses are clear.

Although a neti pot is usually sufficient, this next method is more thorough if you need a deeper cleanse. Purchase at least 6 feet of flexible surgical rubber tubing at a hospital/surgical supply or at a home improvement center. It's sometimes available in the same location as the vinyl tubing. It's a natural rubber color— very flexible and pliant. The rubber hose gives easier control and you can use it in the shower instead of the sink and not worry about spills around the sink.

Get an empty one or two liter pop bottle to which you add two level teaspoons of sea salt per quart (or liter) of warm water (adjust salt and temperature to your comfort). Shake to dissolve the salt. Attach a string to the bottle so you can hang it near the sink, or in the shower, 2-3 feet above you (perhaps on a mirror or door in the bath). Insert the hose and siphon a little water out to get it flowing. Pinch the hose to stop the flow. Tilt your head to the side and slightly back. Insert the hose into the upper nostril and seal the nostril around the hose, un-pinch the hose and allow water to circulate and exit the lower nostril. It's a little exasperating the first few times you try, but soon you'll be able to do it easily.

Of course, you can't breathe through your nose while cleansing the nostrils, you have to breath through your mouth. This method of irrigating the sinuses gives incredible relief to those who have sinus trouble. Colloidal silver can be added to the water to reduce infections. A few drops of lavender and tea tree oil on a handkerchief can be inhaled to eliminate sinus infections also. (More on essential oils later.)

Cleansing the body at the cellular level is essential. You can't be healthy without cleaning up your body. As you fast and cleanse your body internally, you are removing congestion and toxins from all of your organs. This can easily add 10 to 20 healthy years to your life. Fasting also resets all your digestive and metabolic processes. Learn to fast safely. Remember, you can begin by simply stopping eating and living on juices, but when you return to eating, return to solid foods after several days of progressively denser juices.

Take Digestive Enzymes With Meals and Between Meals

Another way to remove toxic conditions in the digestive tract is with digestive enzymes. You can take digestive enzymes for 6 months to a year. Purchase good quality digestive enzymes. Buy only brands which rate their product in Activity Units. For example Protease 75,000 HUT, Cellulase 200 CU, Bromelain 100 GDU, etc. Products which list milligrams or mg could be worthless since their activity could be zero. Take these enzymes with all meals, and also between meals to digest and break up the crud in the digestive tract. If you've had digestive distress, take enzymes for a minimum of a few months. If your digestion is weak, also take Betaine HCL with meals (but not between meals) to increase the hydrochloric acid in the stomach. Take it until your digestion is normal and you have no undigested food in your bowel movements. Follow the label.

Most degenerative diseases begin in the colon with loss of nutrients and congestive waste buildup. Acidic conditions increase. The induced weakness hurts every other bodily system. Restoring health begins by eliminating congestion throughout your body, especially in the digestive tract.

Avoid Toxic Exposures, Eliminate Heavy Metal Toxicity

By far the worst metal toxin in the body is mercury. Mercury poisoning was and sometimes is still inflicted on children and babies through vaccinations. The most common preservative in vaccinations and flu shots was Thimerosal, a mercury-based formula which has been implicated in ADD, ADHD, and Autism. There is no safe level for metallic mercury in the body. I believe the industry has been lying about the destructive effects of mercury in order to avoid lawsuits. Mercury is a nervous system toxin – plain and simple. Efforts are being made to find substitutes, but in millions of cases, much damage has been done. You CAN repair the damage, but don't wait too long. Watch the movie *Autism: Made in the USA*. It's a very inspiring movie. Follow the recommendations in my diet section, which are similar to the movie.

Another source of mercury poisoning is amalgam ("silver") dental fillings. The mercury in these compounds will leach into the body, continually poisoning the unsuspecting victim. As soon as practical, it would be wise to have all of your mercury fillings replaced with quartz composites. Aware dentists, trained in safe methods of removal, specialize in amalgam replacement. Ask at natural food stores for recommendations in your area. In the meantime, existing mercury toxicity can be removed from the body with the following procedure.

How To Do a Mercury Cleanse

Take a handful of parsley and a handful of cilantro. Blend in a blender with water and drink it. Repeat every third day for 1 month (10 times). If it's difficult to drink with only water, mix it with any fresh vegetable juice (carrot juice is especially nice) or fruit juice. It doesn't matter how you get it down. You can even process it into salsa. That's a lot of salsa though!

Parsley and cilantro have been clinically proven to bind with mercury in the body and remove mercury toxicity. If you're continually exposed to mercury (amalgam fillings), repeat this procedure once or twice a year. My wife and I met a dentist who was dying from mercury poisoning. He had only weeks to live. He had closed his dental practice where he had been exposed to high levels of mercury. After following this procedure, he was completely cured of mercury poisoning and reopened his practice using much better equipment to protect himself.

It's interesting to note that dentists often have high levels of suicide. Aside from the high stress levels of a medical practice, these suicides and other mental problems could indeed be caused by high mercury levels. Remember, hatters went insane due to the mercury used in the hatting process, which is where we get the phrase "mad hatters."

Aluminum is another problem. Many toothpastes use aluminum oxide as the abrasive ingredient (NOT listed on the label!). I believe it's wise to avoid all commercial toothpastes that don't claim to list *every* ingredient. "Inert" ingredients are rarely inert and may not be safe. Companies often lie to avoid losing money. Aluminum has been implicated in Alzheimer's and other nervous system disorders. Avoid using aluminum cookware. Destroy it, don't give it away. After destroying it, take it to an aluminum recycler to be made into useful products, like airplanes.

In general, green foods remove heavy metals. Increase your consumption of dark green leafy vegetables. There are also natural products on the market designed to remove lead and other heavy metal poisons. If you know you've had high exposure to heavy metal poisons such as lead, cadmium, etc., check for products at a natural foods store. Otherwise, periodic fasting and green foods will reduce ordinary exposures. Colloidal gold will also reduce heavy metal poisoning.

These are just a few of many recommendations for avoiding toxic exposure. There are whole books dedicated to toxins in our environment and how to avoid exposure. Do the best you can. When your body is stronger, it can deal more easily with our contaminated environment. As time allows, we may publish our own formulas for green, environmental, nontoxic living.

Eat More GREEN foods
Green foods are the most healing. They remove toxic materials from the body and supply wonderful minerals needed for health. The darkest salad greens are best. They are highest in chlorophyll. Richly colored vegetables in

have the highest mineral and vitamin content. There are also special ated foods such as wheat grass juice, barley juice, or blue green algae. These foods are special therapeutic foods and are unnecessary as a continual part of your diet, but for a few weeks or months, you might consider using them. They're expensive. They sell for about $40-50 for a small can or box, about a month's supply for one person. The best green foods are fresh, tender, dark greens from your garden. Any pleasant tasting or even slightly bitter foods, high in chlorophyll, will have high nutrition and detoxification properties.

Action Plan - Chapter 5, Physical Approaches to Healing

1. Create a new self image that embodies all the qualities that you want for yourself. Visualize yourself with these qualities frequently throughout the day. Let go of your old image of yourself.
2. Purify your system: 1) Get more rest, 2) Drink sufficient mineralized water, 3) Use wild shaking and gentle bouncing to energize your body and cleanse the lymph system, 4) Schedule deep breathing sessions several times a day, 5) Cleanse the colon and sinuses, fast for several days and use colonic irrigation if necessary, do sinus irrigation with a neti pot as necessary, 6) Take digestive enzymes with meals and between meals for improved digestion and additional cleansing, take betaine HCl with meals if needed until digestion is normal, 7) Avoid toxic heavy metals, do a mercury cleanse with cilantro and parsley, 8) Eat green foods.
3. It's not enough to know what to do, you actually have to do it. You now have many methods for purifying your body of congestion and toxicity. It cost little to nothing. Right now, create an action plan in your calendar and reminders. Here's what to do: 1) Review this chapter, 2) Write down any items you need to purchase and put them on your purchase list, 3) Schedule the various cleanses in your calendar.

Now read the next section on diet and nutrition. You've got to know what to eat and why. There's TONS of misinformation and confusion about diet and nutrition. When you learn how to nourish yourself with high vitality nutrients, you'll have the most important component for healing on your side. Remember to use the positive mental imagery. See yourself healthy and vital in your mind's eye.

Chapter 6
Diet and Nutritional Healthcare
The Secret to Health, Fitness, and Longevity

"Out of 2.1 million deaths a year in the United States,
1.6 million are related to poor nutrition."
— C. Everett Koop, M.D.
Former Surgeon General of the United States
(76% of all deaths)

What to Expect

According to the former Surgeon General, Dr. C. Everett Koop, M.D., over three-fourths of all deaths are related to poor nutrition. Obviously, a better diet is the easiest way to reverse serious disease, reduce illness, and minimize premature death. This approach is clearly more attractive than expensive drugs or surgery. An added bonus is that the foods that truly nourish and heal us, also happen to be the most agreeable and delicious foods on the planet!

With this approach, excess weight will melt off your body. Your skin will become more radiant, alive, smooth, supple, and elastic. Wrinkles will disappear and the light will come back into your eyes. The inflammation and anxiety stored in your body will subside. You will be more at peace and have the energy and enthusiasm to attain your heart's desire. Beneficial and desirable things will happen when you rebuild your body with the right foods. Remember to keep a powerful image of perfect health in your mind. See yourself willing to change, keep your self image high. Choose the healthiest foods described in this chapter for rapid healing.

All these wonderful things happen because your body knows how to heal when it gets the right nutrition. Did you know that every cell in your body is replaced every year? It was once thought that it took seven years to replace bones, but new discoveries show that we get a new body about every year. A year from now, will it be a better body or a worse one? That depends on what ingredients are used to build the new body! Lousy foods give you an ugly, unhealthy body. Wonderful foods, with excellent nutrition, build a beautiful, strong body.

Have You Done Your Clean Up?

To absorb the best nutrition, it's essential to have an exceptionally clean body on the inside. If your system is clogged and poisoned, even great nutrition can't get through to construct healthy tissues. If your pH is wrong you also can't absorb nutrition.

Remember Your Goals

Earlier you created a list of the qualities you want in your life, things like: health, grace, peace, energy, attractiveness, strength, vitality, willpower, love, compassion, and wholeness. Come back to your beautiful self image of how you want to look, feel, and be. Remember to "play" your best inner movies several times a day. Techniques of visualization are very powerful.

Diet Religions

Before we start, you probably know that EVERYBODY has an opinion on diet and health. If you were to read a few hundred books and a few thousand articles, you would begin to make sense of all the confusion and claims. If you were to try out all the diets and nutritional claims, you would learn even more. I would like to save you the trouble. What follows is the best knowledge on diet and nutrition I've been able to discover through research over the past 43 years. I'll give it to you straight... but there's a problem.

People are attached to their food. Whatever they're currently eating, they think it's just the best. People don't want to change. It may be killing them, but they're NOT about to change. I've worked with people who would rather die than change, and because they refused to change, they died. Sometimes people still choose to die rather than choose life-regenerating nutrition. People still smoke cigarettes. I find this amazing! Why do otherwise intelligent people choose death over life? Suffice it to say that it seems easier to change a person's religion than change their diet.

But for those who are open minded, I'll present information on diet in such a way that it makes perfect common sense. It will be compelling. I hope you will be inspired AND be willing to change. This section on diet is a bit long, because most people need extensive information before they're willing to change.

Your First Visit to Planet Earth

Let's begin with a few stories. Let's try to understand diet and nutrition from a completely new perspective.

Just imagine that you are the very first person to be dropped on planet Earth. It's a beautiful pristine planet – here you come... Zzzzzzzzzzzzzz bzinggggg. You're here! You're in a tropical or semitropical environment. You look around. It's beautiful. But... you're kinda hungry. You look around again. What are you going to eat? Think about it.

If you're like most people, your first thought is to pick some fruit. Maybe a banana, a mango or some grapes. You might collect some berries. Great. You've just hit upon the first and most natural food for humankind. Fruit is the best, most compatible, easiest-to-digest food source for human nutrition. It's loaded with nutrition. Fruit even has more protein than mother's milk! Worldwide, there are over 300 different kinds of fruit – enough to keep you busy for a long time.

After eating fruit for a while, you get a hankering for something different. What else would you eat if you were the first person to arrive? Remember, you only have your hands.

Most people say they would pick green leafy foods that were pleasant and not too bitter. Greens! You've hit upon the second most natural food: Vegetables, especially green veggies. It's interesting to note that animals with almost identical digestion to ourselves, primates, live mostly on fruits and green leafy vegetables. So veggies in all their glory would be second on the list.

You might also discover nuts or maybe sunflower seeds which could be shelled, though a bit tedious. Melons would be an obvious choice, coconuts, too. There would possibly be other kinds of seeds such as grass seeds (grains) and maybe beans (legumes). If dry, they would be as hard as rocks. They would store well, but they'd be hard to eat. However, you could soak them. When soaked, they get plump and soft, even sprout. Then you could eat them easily, no problem.

Now, as an example, let's say you saw a little rabbit not too far away. First of all, do you think you could catch him? No, of course not, they're really fast. But let's say you did. Would you relish the idea of ripping open the flesh of that rabbit with your teeth, tearing the muscle off the bone of this living, squirming animal, and lapping up the blood? Did you just feel your stomach turn? Does this seem natural to you? It IS natural for a true carnivore. A wolf relishes the idea of getting that rabbit, killing it between its jaws, gnawing the muscle off the bone, eating the internal organs, and lapping up the blood.

What does this tell us about ourselves? Every fiber of our being tells us we are NOT carnivores. We do not relish what carnivores relish. Can you see yourself sneaking up on an animal, pouncing on it, killing it with your hands and teeth? Can you see yourself raiding a henhouse, like a wolf, and biting chickens through the neck to kill them? No one in their right mind would live like a carnivore. This instinctive reaction means that meat is a totally unnatural food for humans. Scientific research also proves that meat is the most acid forming, toxic, and disease producing food we can eat. Our teeth, digestive acids, colon, and stomach are nothing like those of a carnivore. They are those of a fruitarian and vegetarian.

More Stories

Let's take a different approach. Suppose you live in a beautiful house with a big field next to it. How would you like to have an orchard next to your house with peaches and blueberries? Good idea? YES. Most folks would love to have an orchard next door. What about a vineyard with grapes or blackberries. YES. We would all love to have a beautiful vineyard next door. Well, now, how about a slaughterhouse? Would you like to have screaming animals being pummeled to death, horrible stench, and rivers of blood next door? Do you see how strange we have become? At present, we humans are mostly a global society of meat eaters. Yet, every person I have ever talked with, without exception, finds the thought of having a slaughterhouse next door to be abhorrent.

We hide from ourselves the most obvious facts. We don't want to think of the pain, suffering, and carnage we inflict on the creatures of the Earth, tens of millions of animals daily. We don't want to think of how disgusting the facts are. Yet, we are responsible for it through our purchases. It's time to remember and decide. None of us, by nature, are carnivores. There's a long list of biological and physiological factors why we aren't. We don't need to know all those details. Just remember the thought of sinking your teeth into the fur of a live squirming animal and you KNOW you're not a carnivore. There is nothing appealing in it.

The diet that includes the bodies of animals also has disastrous psychological effects. When you eat animals, you not only consume their tissues, but you ingest their pain and suffering. You consume the hormones of fear and violence produced when they are killed. This leads to tremendous psychological heaviness and depression. No doubt, this is one of the major causes of violence and depression in our society.

We have been a world of hypocrites. Now is the time to put an end to it. You are a vegetarian by nature. You love to sink your teeth into an apple, peel an orange, or nibble some grapes. They're delightful and delicious. It's like returning to the Garden of Eden. Yummy. Now, let's learn about some very interesting scientific research that adds to your knowledge.

Amazing Experiments

Dr. Francis M. Pottinger, Jr. conducted some awesome experiments. He took two groups of animals, in this case ordinary house cats, 900 altogether. He divided them into two groups. One group of cats he fed their normal diet. The other group he fed the exact same thing, but cooked it first. So one group ate the raw food and one group ate it cooked. The first generation of cats eating the raw food lived to a ripe old age without any problems and with virtually no disease. But the second group, eating cooked food, began to have problems later in life. In fact, they began to get all the diseases humans get today… heart disease, kidney failure, cancer, lung diseases, etc. It was shocking to watch these animals die from degenerative disease. But then, the second generation…

The second generation of cats fed on raw food did extremely well, no problems. However, the group eating cooked foods began to have problems earlier in life than their parents. They fought all the time, had no peace. They were emotionally unstable. They contracted diseases early in life – cancer, digestive diseases, diabetes, every kind of degenerative disease. They did not live as long, but they managed to have kittens, and so another generation…

The third generation of cats on raw food did extremely well. No problems, no diseases, generation after generation. But the cooked food group had kittens that were born with deformities and disease, they contracted diseases early in life, they were emotional "basket cases" – fighting, scratching, and tearing each other up. They did not live long; they succumbed to diseases earlier than their parents. They lived horrible lives (like we see with many people today). Again, the only difference between the groups was cooked or raw food.

Now the fourth generation. For the cats on raw food, the fourth generation was as healthy as the first, no problems. Long healthy life. But the cats on cooked food? There was NO fourth generation! They could not even reproduce after three generations on cooked food! This experiment has been repeated with other animals and other researchers with the same results. This is the most amazing health research on the planet, but it is being ignored.

The Third Generation

Our human society is now in the third generation of a disastrous experiment. In the 1950's, the developed world adopted a diet of overcooked, processed, packaged, nutrition-less, junk-foods. Consumption of meat vastly increased. Most people today rarely eat fresh, raw, wholesome foods straight from the garden as our ancestors did. Earlier generations lived out of their gardens, orchards, and vineyards. Although they didn't eat 100% raw food, they also didn't eat 100% microwave meals, fast foods, and junk foods like many people today.

If you look at the emotional problems in the world today, especially in those countries which adopted this pesticide-laden, de-natured, cooked diet, it exactly parallels the disaster with the experimental animals. Perhaps worse, so-called developed nations have become addicted to drugs to combat emotional instability. In the United States, one-third of the children in many classrooms are on Ritalin or similar drugs. Adults take a wide assortment of antidepressants such as Prozac, Xanax, and other psychotropic drugs. Physical and mental problems, loss of reproductive capacity, and degenerative diseases are multiplying rapidly. The conclusion? It's diet. Plain and simple.

Our whole civilization is threatened if we continue this trend. A simple examination of recent trends: increased degenerative disease, increased obesity, increased depression, increased drug use, lower academic scores, increased suicides, reduced fertility, etc., all point to this continued social disaster. Obesity alone promotes innumerable complications: Increased premature mortality, adult-onset diabetes, hypertension, degenerative arthritis, coronary artery disease, increased cancer, lipid disorders, obstructive sleep apnea, gallstones, fatty infiltration of the liver, restrictive lung disease, and gastrointestinal diseases. When one condition has so many complications, think of the degenerative effects of multiple conditions pervading our population. We do not have time to waste. We must make drastic changes now!

What Caused This Disaster?

What was the problem with cooked foods? Why did they have such a disastrous effect? It turns out that there are vital nutrients that are totally destroyed by cooking. If we don't get these nutrients, we cannot be healthy or emotionally stable. Another doctor, Edward Howell, M.D., found through his research, that one group of destroyed nutrients were enzymes. Enzymes are catalysts. They're required for every chemical reaction in your body. You can't blink your eyes without enzymes. They are needed even to digest food. Enzymes begin to be destroyed at 104 degrees F. They're totally destroyed at 120 degrees. That's one of the reasons why YOU die if your body temperature gets to 106, 108, 110. No enzymes, no life.

Your diet requires these enzymes. You have to eat them. Your body can't manufacture all of them from cooked foods. There are THOUSANDS of enzymes. Bee pollen (taken from flowers) has over 10,000 different enzymes. Many foods have thousands of different enzymes. These nutrients can't be stabilized and put in a pill. There is simply NO alternative other than to eat fresh, raw foods. Older adults, on enzyme deficient diets, can have 30 TIMES fewer enzymes in their body than youths. No wonder metabolism slows and middle-aged adults become obese. Without normal metabolism, you can't burn off fat. Sufficient enzymes are critical for losing weight.

There are 3 major classes of enzymes: 1) Metabolic enzymes enable the body to function. They're produced by your body from the food you eat. 2) Digestive enzymes break down foods for assimilation. Foods contain many of the enzymes necessary for their own digestion. Digestive enzymes are also produced by the body. 3) Food enzymes come from living, fresh, plant life. Food enzymes are the primary basis for the others. We must eat foods in their natural raw state to get complete nutrition. There is no way around it. Otherwise, we become like Dr. Pottinger's cats. We get all the diseases and develop all the emotional problems we see rampant today. Now, what happens if we reverse the experiment?

The Experiment is Reversible

Dr. Pottinger continued his experiments. He wondered what would happen if he switched groups halfway through the experiment? Would the group with the failing health recover and the group in good health become diseased? Good question. That's exactly what happened. It turns out that the degenerative conditions brought about by a cooked-food diet are reversible. This gives hope to every person suffering from disease. Conditions are reversible with a massive infusion of enzymes and high quality nutrition. In the case of humans, additional measures can speed the healing process even more.

In fact, there are spas around the world that focus on enzyme nutrition. They serve practically 100% raw foods. They've had extraordinary success reversing every form of cancer and every degenerative disease. The problem is that they're expensive, often over $1000 per day. However, you can do it yourself at home. It's really very easy.

More Research – White Blood Cells

Other research shows another remarkable finding when comparing raw versus cooked food. The exact same food was fed twice to the subjects. In the raw form, there was no reaction, but with cooked foods, lots of white blood cells were produced. What do white blood cells do? They're the scavenger and defender cells. They react to invasions in order to protect you. The increase in white blood cells means the body thinks cooked food is something that must be defended against, an invader.

It takes enormous resources for the body to defend itself day after day. It depletes the body of huge reserves of nutrition and energy. It retards your ability to heal in many ways. As reserves are depleted, your body becomes weaker.

Modern Refined Foods

Dr. Weston Price, DDS, a dentist in the first part of the last century, wanted to know why we have so many cavities. He traveled the world studying cultures that did not have cavities or other dental problems. He noticed that when devitalized modern foods such a sugar and white bread were introduced into a culture, they rapidly began to have severe dental problems. Not only massive increases in dental caries, but even the skeletal structure, and the structure of the face and jaw changed within just a few generations. Eventually, there was no longer any room for wisdom teeth. Teeth became crowded, crooked, and many teeth were lost due to abscesses and cavities – just like we see today in "modern" societies. This was during the era when processed foods had just started. Now, food quality is much worse. Those cultures originally ate about 80% of their foods raw and unprocessed. Their vitality, bone structure, and dental health was extraordinary.

The loss of bone mass, loss of teeth, and the severe effects on jaw structure and dental health is directly related to the pH of the body. As the body becomes acidic from an unnatural diet, calcium retention is impossible. Your body robs calcium to try to balance the pH of the blood.

Ancient Societies

When people read ancient scriptures, they come across passages that claim people lived healthy lives to the age of 500 years, 700 years, 900 years and more. These are usually dismissed out of hand by most people. Yet, certain Dead Sea scrolls talk of the culture that Christ was born into. They claim that their spiritual advancement and longevity were due in part to a diet of completely raw foods. If you want, you can evaluate these scrolls for yourself and decide. There is no doubt the scrolls are authentic (they were discovered in the Vatican library). If you care to research on your own, the first scroll in the series is entitled *The Essene Gospel of Peace* translated by Edmond Bordeaux Szekely.

The information also tallies with current scientific research showing that raw foods can add decades to your life. It may not be that raw foods alone could increase longevity to hundreds of years, but it already demonstrates substantial life extension. It is also true that other nutrients are destroyed by cooking. Vitamin C is destroyed 100%. We still don't know all the nutritional factors in foods. We do know that animals that eat foods in their natural state don't have the health problems that we humans have.

The Solution

The only solution to these problems is to NOT eat cooked foods, at least not so much, especially when trying to heal or reverse diseases. All studies on natural healing eventually come to this conclusion. A diet high in raw foods substantially improves health. This is such a radical concept, that most people will not readily accept it. Yet, there is no way around the science and reality of it. The loss of enzymes, and many other nutrients, through a predominantly cooked-food diet, plus the constant wearing away of the body's defenses cannot be countered in any other way that I know of. This is one of the primary causes of premature aging and the high incidence of most diseases. We might live several decades longer. In fact, people living on 75-80% raw foods often live 40 years longer than average in near perfect health. It's unfortunate that we don't have societies today living on 100% raw plant foods for us to study.

Reactions

Most people when they first encounter this information are shocked into disbelief. In fact, it's often disheartening, because most folks don't feel they can accomplish such an ideal as a 100% raw food diet. Plus, they don't want to! As mentioned earlier, it's probably easier to change a person's religion than it is to change their diet. We've all grown up with our favorite foods. Now, to find out that our favorite foods, in fact, virtually everything we've been eating for years, contributes to rapid aging, wrinkles, headaches, dysfunctions, and diseases... it's just too much! What are we to do?

We are attached to our food choices with unbelievable intensity. "I like my French fries. I like my pizza. I like my steak and potatoes. I like my cream-filled chocolate donuts!" Plus, the pressures of living in a society where cooked foods are the norm can be difficult, especially without a plan. Where will you go out to eat when you want a break? What do you do when invited to a friend's house for dinner? Will you lose all your friends who think you're too weird? What will you eat at work? Even though poor diets are known to cause disease, people still eat them. The pressures of the palette, social decorum, habit, and convenience can be substantial obstacles. In a sense, it's worse than quitting cigarettes because everyone wants you to eat what they're eating. These are questions everyone has to deal with who wants to truly heal their body and mind. When you realize that the requirements for healing are completely outside the norms of society, it's a problem that must be overcome. Here's how.

Overcoming Obstacles to Dietary Change

First of all, what's the choice? Do you forget what you now know and continue to do what you used to do? Do you continue to eat what you want, come what may? Do you just accept that it's okay to die an early and painful death from diabetes or some other degenerative disease? What are you willing to do to rebuild a life of health and happiness? Are you willing to be strong and different from the norms of society? Is there any compromise?

Many people ask, "How far do I need to go to get better?" What's the minimum I can do to restore my health? Could I eat 50% raw foods, 60%, 75%, and then do whatever I want the rest of the time? How far do I have to go? How much of a difference does it really make? Here's the bottom line.

If your health is severely compromised, it makes an incredible difference. If you want to heal, you need to do absolutely everything in your power. To rebuild a weak, diseased body as quickly as possible, you need to transition into a 100% raw food diet within a few weeks. Drink **raw** vegetable juices almost exclusively. Make raw smoothies, soups, slaws and other high enzyme, high mineral foods. If your health is already very poor, then seemingly minor compromises will have major devastating effects on your health. After you are healed, you'll have more flexibility.

This approach is your way out of immediate pain, suffering, and disease. If you only have minor health problems, you can improve by simply becoming vegetarian and eating 50-75% of your diet raw. However, you will improve more slowly and you won't create the extraordinary health we have been talking about. Your life will be extended in a much healthier state for a decade or more.

My research and experience shows that there is a HUGE difference between a 90% raw food diet and 100%. Apparently, it takes vast resources to make up for enzyme deficiencies and to create massive white blood cell *where this is a resource?*

defenses that are required when consuming even occasional cooked
don't like the facts either, but they're true, whether we like them or r
realize that there is no way for you to accept this without experiencii
You simply won't believe all the extraordinary benefits a raw food diet can
provide, unless you try it. So why not experiment? Just tell your friends
you're on a strict experimental diet for health purposes. One very
entertaining movie that can provide inspiration is, *Fat, Sick, and Nearly
Dead*.

Experimentation

You don't have to commit forever. Try some experiments. If your health is
not too compromised, you can experiment gradually. Make Mondays raw
food day. A week later add Tuesdays, and so forth. You can always go back to
your old ways. Build up to 100% raw for a trial experiment. Once there, try
it for at least 30, preferably 90 days. Take a month or more to gradually work
into it. No matter what percentage of raw foods you adopt, it really helps to
make some days all-raw-food days. Even a single full day of raw juices can
do wonders.

A suggestion: Don't look at what you're giving up, look at what you want.
Suppose there was some food that was amazingly delicious, but it made you
ugly in two weeks? Would you still want it, no matter how delicious?
Wouldn't you rather look around for something that is also delicious, but
makes you attractive, happy, and healthy? What you really want is a fit body,
perfect health, a clear mind, and a joyous heart. If something you eat
contributes to the opposite, do you really want it?

Pleasure and Pain

We all make choices based upon pleasure and pain. We choose what gives
us the most pleasure and least pain, if we can. But what if the choices are
conflicting? What if the choice gives immediate satisfaction but future pain?
Over time, our experience teaches us to avoid it. This is something lots of
people have trouble with because they don't understand it. They don't know
how to give up immediate pleasure to avoid future pain, to have greater
long-term future happiness.

Junk food provides immediate pleasure because it's sweet, but the
consequences are undesirable. When you switch to a raw food diet, old
habits will nag at you, but you soon learn that the old choices don't actually
make you feel good in the long run. When you eat a meal, notice how it
makes you feel on three occasions: When you're eating it, 2 hours later, and

the next day. Keep a food diary. You will be able to see the connections between food and how you feel.

Overcoming Old Habits

To create a new habit requires consistently choosing the new habit in place of the old for reasons that are meaningful to you. Here's how it works. Focus on cause and effect and do the things that create the best effect. Actually, you have always been choosing what you want, but you have not been getting the effects you want. With this new knowledge, you can decide to let go of something that makes you feel worse by switching to something that makes you feel better in the long run!

Four Options

We really only have four options when choosing experiences:

1) Things that feel good now, but have disastrous consequences, like street drugs, junk foods, etc.

2) Things that sometimes feel bad, especially at the beginning, like fasting or exercise, but have wonderful consequences later. Better health, more joy.

3) Things that feel good now and also have good consequences, like delicious, fresh fruit.

4) Things that feel bad and ARE bad, like painful injuries.

We don't have trouble with number 4; we all avoid pain that has no benefit. We also don't have trouble with number 3. If it feels good and there's no negative, we quickly go for it. The problem is with 1 and 2. People become addicted to drugs and foods that kill them, because the immediate attraction is greater than the realization of consequences. People avoid number 2, because they don't realize how much better life would be if they accepted a little "deprivation" for a long term benefit. When you're deciding about things in your life, keep these four options in mind.

Sometimes people tell me that humans have been cooking food for centuries. How can it be so bad? Excellent question. Actually, we have not always cooked food to the extent we do today. Past civilizations, such as the Essenes and others had segments of their societies that did not eat cooked food at all. Civilizations that lived the longest cooked their food the least. The Hunzas today eat an 80% raw food diet. They commonly live to 130 years old even in harsh conditions. In fact, it doesn't really matter what went on in the past. You are living today. The science and experience of today reveals the same truth. Raw foods provide the highest level of health that is attainable from food. Try it.

Many, many diseases have been cured just from a raw diet alone. Type II diabetes is often cured in 30 days or less. Even type I diabetes has been cured, though it takes longer, six months to a year. Virtually every health condition is either healed or improved substantially for several reasons. 1) massive availability of enzymes and other nutrients that are ordinarily destroyed by cooking, 2) greater nutrient density and bio-availability of nutrients, 3) no need to create defenses, which use valuable resources that could otherwise be used for healing. If you are diabetic taking insulin, or have any condition for which you are taking drugs, work with an open minded medical practitioner to reduce your medications. Raw food nutrition operates so quickly that you want to keep on top of any need for taking medications. The need usually drops rapidly.

Human Possibilities

This is a true story. You can research it if you feel compelled. As an experiment, a man was checked into a hospital in New Delhi, India. He was put under observation in a locked room, with closed circuit cameras watching him 24 hours a day. He had no way out and no access to food or water. He happily survived with no food or water for weeks. Doctors were studying him. In fact, he had lived without food or water for 40 years! He was able to live on just air and sunlight. This man is not unique. There are others who have refined their physiology to such a degree that they no longer need food. Amazing as it sounds, these people have been found and studied. It's real. We don't really know the extent of our human possibilities, but we do know they are incredible. This also means that all of the food and nutrition recommendations promoted by government agencies and researchers are just averages that only apply to people with an unrefined physiology eating the typical, average diet. Individual requirements can and do vary greatly.

Even the concept of calories is practically meaningless. We all know of people who eat very little and yet easily gain weight. I also know of people eating 3000 to 4000 calories of raw food a day, up to 30 bananas and lots of dates, yet achieve substantial weight loss. It all depends upon the state of your mind and physiology, your natural metabolism, the kind of food – whether cooked or raw, and what your body does with the food. People today have huge individual variations due to differences in physiological refinement.

pH Revisited

I talked about pH in Chapter 3, *Symptoms of Degeneration* and recommended that you test your pH. In this chapter on Diet and Nutrition I'll explain the effects of pH on health.

Have you ever tried to grow a garden in poor soil where the pH was either too acid or too alkaline? You certainly met with catastrophic failure. Plants can only take up nutrients if the soil has the proper pH. As you remember from high school, pH is a measure of acidity or alkalinity. If too acid or too alkaline, you create either burning or caustic conditions where life cannot easily exist. Ordinary hand soap is free from bacteria because it is highly alkaline. Generally, the ideal range for pH is between 6.5 and 7.2 for plants, and not much different for humans. Blood has to be very close to 7.38, or you die. The normal, slightly alkaline pH of the body is an extraordinary finding that is virtually never utilized in medical treatment. This also explains why blood tests are a very poor measure of health. Your body will do almost anything to keep your blood practically perfect. By the time something shows up in a blood test, you have been in a disease-promoting situation for a long time.

In nearly every disease, the body is in a highly acidic condition. This is true of cancer, diabetes, MS, osteoporosis, and many, many other diseases. In an acid state, your body can't absorb or utilize nutrients, just like the garden. Oxygen transport decreases by orders of magnitude. As a result, the body withers and dies, just like the garden. When pH is normalized, the body heals rapidly. This takes us back to what Beauchamp said. The environment of the body is everything.

Essentially, an acid pH is a signal throughout nature that it's time to recycle that organism. When a tree falls down in the forest, it becomes acidic. Nature then sends all of her recyclers to attack the log lying on the forest floor: fungus, mold, yeast, bacteria, viruses, critters of all sorts. These recyclers tear the organism apart and return it to its primordial state as nutrients for the next cycle. If you don't want to be recycled, you have to keep your pH alkaline.

What causes this acidic condition? Primarily, it's the consumption of meat, sugar, white flour, and cooked foods. There are many tables and charts that show the acid or alkaline reaction in the body caused by different foods. Search the Internet for: "most acid forming foods".

You can correct your pH and help your body recover even faster through mineralization. It's faster than using raw foods alone. Mineralization also helps with enzyme nutrition, because many enzymes require trace minerals to function properly. Essentially, you use the same methods you would use in the garden – the addition of minerals.

Major Minerals

Four elements in the body are most active: Sodium (Na), Potassium (K), Calcium (Ca), and Magnesium (Mg). Of these, Calcium is the most biologically active. It generally coexists with magnesium, just as sodium and potassium complement each other. We almost always get enough sodium, but not in an organic form. We often don't get enough potassium. If we flood the body with bio-available alkalizing minerals containing – Ca (calcium), Mg (magnesium), Na (sodium), and K (potassium), we can change the pH rather quickly. Some of the higher alkalizing elements such as Cesium and Rubidium have profound alkalizing effects. Another simple alkalizing substance is sodium bicarbonate, ordinary baking soda. Dr. Tullio Simoncini, MD claims that cancer can be cured with it. He makes his protocols available for free (curenaturalicancro.com). Unfortunately, the cancer industry is unwilling to research simple inexpensive therapies, even with massive case histories of success.

Supplementation is useful, but only if the body can absorb them. Most products on the market are not absorbed well, because humans can't convert inorganic mineral salts to useable forms very well. They must be combined with a carbon atom. Ruminating animals CAN do it, because in their multiple stomach chambers, plant materials combine (chelate) with salts from a salt lick, a source of valuable mineral salts. Chelated minerals are more absorbable, but also more expensive to purchase. If your health is poor, you could take chelated alkalizing minerals daily until your pH is normal. A natural food store can provide product recommendations for chelated major minerals. This is not necessary, but it's useful if you need quick results. It can be done very successfully simply with new food choices, without any supplements. Be aware that just taking mineral supplements cannot compensate for a bad diet.

Minor Minerals

You must also ensure an adequate supply of minor minerals in organic form, supplying: Iron, Iodine, Silicon, Fluorine, Copper, Manganese, Zinc, Selenium, Cobalt, Molybdenum, Chromium, Tin, Boron, Nickel, and Vanadium. Minor minerals have extremely valuable functions in the body. You cannot live without them, but you don't need them in large quantities. They can even be poisonous at high levels.

Trace Minerals

Most people don't realize what's happened to our soils. In the United States, we've depleted our topsoil from a starting point of 2-3 feet of very fertile soil to a current average of about 6 inches of mineral depleted topsoil. Like every civilization throughout history that destroyed itself, we too have destroyed the soils we depend upon for life. The U.S. government, in Senate Document 264 from the 74th Congress (1936) stated:

- "The alarming fact is that foods – fruits, vegetables, and grains – now being raised on millions of acres of land no longer contain enough of certain needed minerals, are starving us – no matter how much of them we eat!"...

- "It is bad news to learn from our leading authorities that 99% of the American people are deficient in these minerals, and that a marked deficiency in any one of the more important minerals actually results in disease. Any upset of the balance, any considerable lack of one or another element, however microscopic the body requirement may be, and we sicken, suffer, shorten our lives."

Remember, this was back in 1936. It's much worse now. At the 1992 Earth Summit, North America led the world in soil destruction. Statistics showed 85% soil mineral depletion. The cause is modern agriculture. This should be a warning to the rest of the world NOT to follow our lead.

The agriculture industry realized they could grow big plants – indistinguishable from healthy, nutrient rich plants – by adding 3 elements, Nitrogen-N, Phosphorous-P, and Potassium-K (NPK fertilizer). But humans need many trace minerals, roughly 70 minerals altogether. Our farmers removed 70 minerals from the soil through repeated cropping without mineralization. For generations, they've put back less than a dozen minerals. It's been especially rampant since the 1940's.

This means that commercial produce is severely mineral deficient in minor minerals and trace minerals, a loss that must be corrected for us to be healthy. The depletion of minor minerals and trace minerals is considered by some experts to be a primary cause of disease, perhaps even more significant than the lack of enzymes. The body can manufacture many enzymes, but it's not so easy to create fundamental elements that are missing.

Modern societies don't recycle human wastes or animal wastes back to the land, we flush them into the ocean. Plus, thousands of years of rainfall have washed many minerals into the sea. The ocean is the repository of that vast mineral wealth. The easiest way to get trace minerals is to go where they are

now. The ocean has never been mined or cultivated. The best direct
of minerals from the ocean are sea salt and seaweeds such as kelp and
Kelp has the ability to take in only useful nutrients. Even in polluted wat
it won't take up heavy metals very easily. Still it's better to find sea salt and
sea vegetables harvested from pristine locations. The nuclear meltdowns in
Japan make us question whether the ocean is safe for harvesting either plant
or animal life. I suggest not using kelp harvested from areas exposed to
nuclear radiation. With regard to fish, it's not natural to eat them anyway.
Can you see yourself jumping into the ocean and stuffing a bunch of fish in
your mouth? Think of how you would naturally live.

We could fertilize our gardens with kelp and dulse or utilize it directly as a
food supplement. Add a tablespoon or more of powdered kelp or other
seaweeds daily to your salad dressings and smoothies. You hardly know it's
there. Trace and minor mineral nutrition are an extremely important need
in human health and nutrition. Trace minerals include most of the
remaining elements on the periodic chart. They often have biological effects
thousands of times more potent than their concentrations would suggest.

How To Get Your Minerals

Here are your options: 1) chelated minerals, 2) dehydrated whole food
supplements (green powders), 3) sea vegetables such as kelp, dulse, and
others, 4) organic foods from a grower who understands minor and trace
minerals, or 5) grow organic foods yourself (Be sure to mineralize your soils
with a variety of rock dusts, so you have a complete complement of
minerals). In order to be healthy, you absolutely MUST have the basic
elements that your body needs in a form it can use. There is no alternative.

The very best way to get minerals is from high mineral plant foods,
because the particle size of minerals in plants is extremely small. Plus, the
minerals are biologically active and powerfully vital in living plants. Green
foods have remarkable healing powers. If you have a large family, but
perhaps little money, you can grow greens in a small garden, even a
container garden. A modest garden can supply a large family with all the
greens and most vegetables a family needs. Just make sure that the garden
soil has all the minerals required for human health. It's not hard to do. For
calcium and magnesium, you can buy a 40 pound bag of dolomite at a
garden center for less than $4. Rock dust provides a full complement of
valuable minerals as microbes and humic acid break it down. Sea vegetable
powders, such as kelp or dulse also add trace minerals. I cover more

information on natural gardening later. Avoid synthetic commercial fertilizers which can destroy microbial life in the soil.

Soil amendments are available through organic gardening suppliers. Sea water contains all the minerals the human body needs in almost identical proportions. But we can't just drink sea water, it needs to be in an organic form. Diluted sea water (10:1) contains all the minerals for human health and has been used directly on gardens to provide valuable minerals. Dehydrated sea water (true sea salt) is available as a soil amendment. It's even used in hydroponic growing. Rock dusts are the best, low-cost trace mineral supplement for plants. All of the longest-lived people on the earth lived on mineral rich soils. There is no substitute for minerals. Search the Internet for "blue zones" and learn about long-lived people in relation to soils. For the most part, these people lived on a plant-based diet, but the interesting thing is that the volcanic soils where they live are extremely high in minerals.

Healthy Digestion Requires Good Bacteria
There are good bacteria that are supposed to live in the digestive tract to aid digestion. They're called probiotics. They minimize candida yeast (a destructive pathogen) and keep the gut healthy. Fermented products like fresh sauerkraut have many of these bacteria naturally. There are also supplements available. Buy and use them. Check with your natural health food store for recommendations. Products are improving all the time, but one the best products is homemade sauerkraut. A "how-to" is in the Resources Chapter.

How to Choose Healthy Foods
The easiest way to get healthy foods is to shop only in the produce section. Preferably buy organic or grow it naturally yourself. Buy locally, whenever possible. Produce from supermarkets is often over 12 days old before it is even displayed. Commercial produce is already mineral deficient. Shipping and storage times destroy many more nutrients.

A good rule is to avoid all foods that come in a package, can, or bottle. Virtually all packaged foods have been processed, sterilized with heat (or nuclear radiation!), hydrogenated, or denatured in some way in order to preserve color and shelf life. All bottled and canned goods have been sterilized and are therefore totally without enzymes, natural vitamin C, and are highly mineral deficient. Below is a detailed list of foods to avoid and the reasons to avoid them. Natural substitutes are mentioned. Many additional substitutes are covered in a later section on the natural diet of the human.

Foods to Avoid and Why

1. Meat – causes putrefaction, poisons the body, contains pesticides, antibiotics, and other toxins. It is unnatural for humans and is highly acid causing.

2. Eggs – same as meat, when cooked, proteins turn to a rubber-like substance that is difficult to assimilate.

3. Dairy products – No non-organic milk, butter, cheeses, or yogurt. Dairy today contains antibiotics, unnatural injected hormones, and pesticides. It is pasteurized and therefore dead. Dairy is implicated in many allergies. Most adults cannot digest dairy products. Most cheeses are made using scrapings from the inside of a cow's stomach (rennet). Most human races, especially blacks and orientals, lose the lactase enzyme for digesting milk at about age 4, as do all vegetarian mammals. Even adult cows won't drink milk. Only carnivores handle milk well. Organic fermented milk products can be useful if the source is not denatured or contaminated. There are natural cheeses, butter, and yogurt which are organic and not tainted, but you will have to search for them. Even so, many people do not handle them well. To re-establish intestinal flora use fresh unpasteurized sauerkraut or supplements. Milk does not protect from calcium loss. American women drink about thirty times as much cow's milk as the New Guineans, yet suffer forty-seven times as many broken hips.

4. Sugar – Avoid all white sugar and sugar products, corn syrup, or refined sweets of any kind. Occasional use of whole, dehydrated cane syrup, gur or jaggery (from India), or whole natural syrups may be acceptable in some cases, in small amounts weekly. If you have candida yeast or any other yeast infestations, or if your health is compromised, use NO sugars at all until you are well. Avoid pasteurized fruit juices (virtually all commercial fruit juices are pasteurized). If your health is compromised, avoiding sweet foods, especially sucrose and glucose, is a necessity. Avoid all foods that are high on the glycemic index. You can get current lists of high glycemic foods from the Internet. Basically, all white processed foods are unhealthy. Here's a partial list:

Glycemic Index

Classification	Glycemic Index	Examples
Low	35 or less	Most fruit & veggies (not potato), whole grains, whole rice, lentils

Classification	Glycemic Index	Examples
Medium	40 - 55	Brown rice, semi-sweet fruit, grapes, whole wheat pasta
High	55 or more	Sugar, corn syrup, dextrose, sweeteners, syrups, white flour products, corn flakes, baked potato, milled rice, very sweet fruits, melons

The glycemic index indicates how fast carbohydrates convert to glucose sugar. Fast conversion is harder on the body, which must increase insulin dramatically to counteract abnormal rises in sugar. Generally, eat low on the glycemic index, preferably below 50. Water has no carbohydrates (= 0), white bread (= 100) and bakery products convert to glucose rapidly and are trouble making, with values between 70-100, or more. The index doesn't take into account total calories or nutrition. It also doesn't take into account what is called the glycemic load, which is affected by food combinations and dilutions. If you have blood sugar problems, it would be wise to research this field in more depth.

Below are common foods and their typical glycemic values:

Grains and Beans / Index Value
White flour products/70-100+, Whole grain products/40-70, Beans/25-40

Fruit
Apple/40, Banana/50, Cherries/22, Grapes/43, Mango/50, Melons/50-80, Orange/48, Peach/40, Pear/40, Pineapple/60, Plum/24

Dried Fruit
Dates/103, Figs (dried fruit generally)/61, Raisins/64

Vegetables, Nuts, and Seeds
Potatoes/100, Most Vegetables/under 40, Nuts and Seeds/under 40

In general, if you avoid white starchy foods and all processed and packaged foods you will be safe from high glycemic-index foods. If you mix fruits, green leafy vegetables, soaked nuts and/or seeds in a green smoothie, you will create a blend that is very healing. Raw food recipe books have wonderful recipes. I also include basic formulas in the Resources Chapter. Now, continuing the list of foods to avoid...

5. White table salt – Use whole sea salt.

6. All white flour and white flour products, without exception, all "vitamin enriched" products. Useless synthetic vitamins are added that we cannot assimilate or utilize well – due to wrong enantiomers (left/right handed molecules) and missing co-factors, valuable natural nutrients are

removed during milling (to increase shelf life) and are fed to animals, which benefit greatly!

7. Alcohol – None of any kind, in any amount. The "benefits" attributed to wine is in the grapes, especially the pigmented skin, not alcohol. Alcoholic beverages have no human benefit.

8. Nicotine – NO smoking, no chewables. No human benefit. It's a good insecticide.

9. Caffeine – NO coffee, colas, commercial chocolate (raw chocolate powder is a healthy food, but not ordinary chocolate products), or black tea – depletes adrenals, causes caffeine withdrawal headaches.

10. NO soft drinks, without exception, even diet varieties – causes mineral imbalances, destroys enzymes. Extremely acidic pH. High sugar and caffeine creates an addictive reaction much like heroin. Destroys tooth enamel. They drastically depress and disrupt the immune system. Like cigarettes, soft drinks should require warning labels.

11. NO frozen foods – flash heat preserves color but destroys enzymes, they are devitalized, denatured, with at least 1/3 of enzymes lost. They are better than canned foods.

12. NO microwaved foods or water (devitalizes, denatures, and distorts subtle energies). Microwave ovens are banned in some countries. A nurse once used a microwave to warm blood for a blood transfusion instead of the slower method. It seems to have caused a blood clot that killed the patient (among other unknown potential causes). Microwaves are known to denature organic molecules more than other heating methods. From my research of the literature, I have concluded they are an unnecessary, unsafe technology.

13. NO hydrogenated oils in any foods (denatures the oils) – use primarily olive, coconut, avocado, sesame, walnut, and flax (for omega-3's) plus safflower, sunflower, in small amounts (Must be cold pressed). Remember, liquid vegetable oils don't occur in nature and we could never eat the quantity of oil we eat today. They generally require lots of processing. It's better to get oils naturally from avocados, coconuts, fresh tree nuts, and seeds. Oil has about 120 calories per tablespoon. One serving of a typical "American" dressing could contain 400 calories.

14. NO additives such as artificial flavors, artificial colors, artificial sweeteners, or preservatives – unnatural chemistry for the human body.

NO tap water. Drink spring or filtered water. Also, bathe in filtered
r if possible. Shower filters are available. You absorb 1/3 of your daily
water intake from baths and showers. Bathe in healthy water.

By Now, You're Probably Wondering What You CAN Eat!

The Natural Diet for Humankind

There are seven food groups to choose from, 6 basic tastes to consider,
many aromas and flavors, and many textures. These combine into millions
of possible food choices. In the Resources Chapter I include simple recipe-
formulas you can use for making delicious, healthy meals.

The 7 Food Groups

Depending upon how you group foods, you could even say there are only
three food groups natural to humans. 1) Fruits, 2) vegetables, and 3) seeds
(grains, beans, and nuts are all just seeds). We can divide the plant kingdom
into more groups to make the selection of foods easier. There are also
subgroups. Fruits, for instance, can be divided into citrus, sweet, stone, vine,
dried, etc. I use seven primary divisions because it's a simple, easy system to
work with:

1) Fruits – The product of a tree, bush, or vine. They have seed(s) inside.
Sweet tasting fruits go well together.

2) Melons – Sweet, watery, vine fruit with a hard rind, digests a little
differently. Melons are best eaten alone as a meal, but they can also work
with other fruits.

3) Vegetables – Leaf, root, or stalk. Many "vegetables" are actually fruits
but are used as vegetables including tomatoes, squash, cucumbers, etc.
Essentially all non-sweet fruits go well with vegetables. In a raw form, most
fruits and vegetable mix well and can be blended into smoothies, soups, etc.
Leafy vegetables contain chlorophyll and an abundance of minerals. They
are really super foods.

4) Nuts – From trees, have a hard shell. They're packed with essential
nutrition. Use soaked*. Raw nuts that you can add to your diet include
almonds, cashews, walnuts, black walnuts, pecans, filberts, hickory nuts,
macadamias, pignolis, pistachios.

5) Flower & Vegetable Seeds – From various flowering plants such as
sunflowers, sesame, poppy, flax, chia, hemp, and also pumpkins, squashes,
or other sources. I group these together and call them Flower Seeds, though
technically all seeds come from flowers (which make the fruit). These seeds
are packed with vital nutrients. Use soaked* or sprouted.

6) Grains – From grasses. Wheat, barley, rye, rice, corn, millet, quinoa, and amaranth are examples. Use soaked* or sprouted.

7) Legumes – Beans from a vine – either fresh, dried, soaked* or sprouted.

* Caution: I noted earlier the vital importance of enzymes. All seeds from the four categories described above 1) flowers, 2) nuts, 3) grains, and 4) legumes, have the characteristic that when they dry and become dormant, they produce enzyme inhibitors, phytates, tannins, and other anti-nutrients which stay active and interfere with digestion. They disable other enzymes – a bad thing. It's their way of protecting themselves from being digested internally or being broken down in nature before it's possible to grow. Many people have trouble digesting nuts and other seeds for this reason. Also, different kinds of seeds have different combinations of anti-nutrients. Some require more processing than others to bring out the highest digestibility and nutrition.

Become An Expert with Seeds

All seeds need to be properly prepared. You should not eat raw seeds without at least soaking them. Soaking begins the process of bringing seeds to life. Most enzyme inhibitors and other anti-nutrients dissipate within 24 hours and many other changes happen to greatly improve nutrition. Here's how to prepare all seeds:

1) Soak seeds in water until plump (2-6 hours depending on size and hardness). Discard the soak water. Some seeds like flax and chia become so gelatinous they cannot be easily drained of the soak water, but it's also not a problem with most flower seeds. They have fewer anti-nutrients such as tannins, and don't need rinsing.

2) Rinse at least 2-3 times during the day (~ 3-4 hr intervals). Seeds you are not going to sprout and also nuts, should be soaked and rinsed a few times.

3) Let seeds sit overnight in soak water if you're not going to sprout them. Don't keep seeds you want to sprout underwater. Excessive soaking prevents sprouting.

4) If you're not sprouting, do a final rinse, cover with water, and refrigerate. Storing underwater prevents oxidizing and mold. They'll be good for several days.

After soaking until plump, you can allow many seeds to sprout by continuing to rinse a few times a day while exposing them to the air to activate them. They become tiny sprouted plants in just a few days. Sprouts have amazing nutrition. For instance, broccoli sprouts have been shown to have 50 times the anti-cancer properties of full sized broccoli. Sprouts have less bulk, and are more digestible. Sprouts often provide 1000 times more total nutrition than their full grown counterparts! Examples of sprouts you've seen in the store, that you can eat directly, include: sunflower, mung bean, clover, radish, broccoli, and alfalfa. When sprouted large enough to your liking, put them in the fridge to slow continued growth and for longer keeping.

This all may seem to be an excessive bother, but as you will soon learn it can be really easy with modern kitchen equipment. It's also extremely valuable nutritionally. Consider setting up a small sprout garden in your kitchen.

Cooking or toasting seeds, rather than sprouting them, not only destroys enzyme inhibitors, which is useful, but it also destroys all the valuable enzymes and vitamin C as well. More problematic, it does not destroy all phytates, tannins, or other anti-nutrients. Soaking grains and legumes in warm, slightly acidic water will neutralize phytic acid and improve nutritional benefits. Nuts and seeds soaked in warm saltwater activates beneficial enzymes and de-activates enzyme inhibitors. Sprouting is the best option for seeds that sprout, otherwise all seeds should at least be soaked to remove anti-nutrients.

Deeper Insights into Seed Preparation

For a more complete elimination of anti-nutrients (for seeds you don't intend to sprout), you can soak them in an acidic medium such as buttermilk, cultured milk, yogurt, whey, or even vinegar or lemon juice to activate phytase which breaks down phytic acid. Sour milk products provide lactobacilli that helps break down starches, tannins and difficult-to-digest proteins. Three tablespoons of acidic activator with 4 cups of water prepares 2 cups of grains or legumes.

It takes at least 8-12 hours to break down phytic acid and enzyme inhibitors. 24 hours is better. It's easy to soak grains for tomorrow while preparing today's lunch. Most grains and legumes benefit from changing the water a few times during the soaking process. You can make the last soak the acidic soak. After soaking they should be drained and rinsed.

Flours are obviously not easy to rinse. After soaking the flour (making a batter), allow it to ferment 12-24 hours, then continue with cooking or baking. Cover the batter to prevent it from drying out or insects getting into it. Traditional Indian dosas are made this way. Ordinarily, you prepare the batter in the evening for the next day – more on this method, later on.

Nuts and seeds can be soaked in saltwater. Use a 2 or 3:1 ratio of water to nuts or seeds with one tablespoon of sea salt for 4 cups of water. All nuts should be soaked 12-24 hours (except cashews, which become slimly if soaked over 6 hours). When soaking is complete, rinse well and discard the water (it contains enzyme inhibitors). You can dehydrate soaked nuts and seeds, such an sunflower and pumpkin, in a dehydrator to make anti-nutrient-free snacks. Let them dry in a dehydrator at no higher than 120 degrees so as not to destroy the beneficial enzymes and nutrients. It can take 12 to 48 hours depending on the nut. Taste for desired crispiness. Prepared this way, nuts and seeds have more flavor and far better digestibility. Store in the fridge for longer keeping.

A little salt helps activate beneficial enzymes that deactivate the unwanted enzyme inhibitors. For grains and legumes, an acidic solution reduces phytic acid. Nuts have less phytic acid, but contain high levels of enzyme inhibitors. The native peoples of Central America would treat their nuts and seeds by soaking them in seawater and then dehydrating. The Aztecs prepared pumpkin and squash seeds this way.

Seeds Made Civilization Possible

You need to understand why human civilizations gravitated towards the use of seeds for nutrition. All primates primarily live on fruits and vegetation, but it requires a large volume of food to provide enough proteins and especially carbohydrates. In ancient times, humans learned that they could provide higher levels of nutrition much more easily, especially proteins and carbohydrates, by utilizing the four kinds of seeds.

All seeds are powerhouses of nutrition because they contain tremendous nutrition needed for a new plant. The use of seeds gave human civilizations more time to think, work, and develop a higher culture without having to forage for food continuously. Without them, we would be forced to spend too much time finding, preparing, and eating much larger volumes of food to meet our caloric and nutritional requirements.

Another source of nutrition for adequate carbohydrates are the starchy vegetables, including: sweet potatoes, white potatoes, butternut squash, acorn squash, other winter squash, parsnips, rutabagas, turnips, water chestnuts, yams, and pumpkins. The primary grains that have sustained civilizations include: barley, wheat, buckwheat (kasha), millet, corn, oats, quinoa, amaranth, rice, and wild rice.

Today, we need this carbohydrate nutrition to provide for our
vital demands. The brain requires a lot of power nutrition. Later,
after physiological refinement, our ability to live on less food and
foods will be easier. At present, our ability to live on the lightest diet
of fruits and a minimum of other simple foods is limited by the current low
standard of our physiology, due to toxicity, congestion, and lack of
physiological refinement.

Practically every ancient civilization around the world discovered ways to
eliminate or minimize the anti-nutrients, anti-enzymes, tannins, and
phytates in seeds. Even today, every civilization uses seeds as the primary
source of proteins and carbohydrates. Corn and beans, rice and beans, wheat
and beans, pasta, soy products, etc., but we have forgotten the valuable ways
of processing all four kinds of seeds to provide maximum digestibility,
assimilation, and enable their full nutrient capacities.

As mentioned, in every case, soaking is the first step to minimizing anti-
nutrients. Obviously, don't use chlorinated water. When seeds become
plump, they drop enzyme inhibitors so that they can come to life.
Traditionally, seeds were soaked in a slightly acidic media, sometimes they
were soaked in mild seawater, oftentimes, just plain water. A couple of
tablespoons of lightly salted sauerkraut juice would be a great addition to
plain water.

Soaking not only reduced anti-nutrients, but led to healthy fermentation.
The interesting thing is, practically every civilization learned to ferment
seeds. Sourdough bread is one example – fermented wheat. Fermented soy
products like miso, tempeh, natto, and tamari, are other examples (but not
tofu). Fermentation is a benefit, because it breaks down the food, essentially
pre-digesting it, which provides higher nutrition. Some foods like pasta were
not fermented, but the seed flour was mixed with water, extruded, and
allowed to dry for hours. Cooking in water helps dissipate the phytates and
is discarded.

How to Work with Seeds in Practice

It's really very simple. 1) Soak any and all seeds until they get plump, 2)
Drain and rinse a few times (if they're not gelatinous), 3) after 18-24 hours,
cover with water and put in the fridge. Total working time is less than five
minutes. That's all you really *need* to do for flower or vegetable seeds, like
sunflower seeds, pumpkin seeds, etc. and also for nuts like walnuts,
almonds, and hazelnuts, etc. Blended with herbs, spices, and salted to taste,
these can be used to make delicious savory salad dressings, sauces, spreads,

etc. It takes only a couple of minutes in a blender or food processor. They can also be blended with natural sweeteners, cinnamon, cardamom, and a pinch of salt to make sweet toppings. Flower seeds and nuts are extremely versatile.

With grains and legumes (beans, lentils, peas, etc.), more processing is desirable. You can make sourdough products from both. Start with freshly cracked grain and legumes (made in a few seconds with a blender or food processor). I often use 2/3 grains, like rice and 1/3 beans. Rice and urad dal (from an Indian grocery) are a classic combination, but any grains and legumes will work. 1) Soak the coarsely cracked mix until the mix is plump and then rinse, 2) add more water and blend with a blender or food processor into either a thick or thin batter, according to your use 3) put the batter in a bowl, cover with a cloth, and allow the mix to ferment overnight, preferably at around 90° F. No starter is necessary, but you could use a couple of tablespoons of fresh sauerkraut juice, or whey, if you have trouble with natural fermentation, or add a little rye or rice flour, which naturally contain starter. In cool weather, you can put the bowl on a heating pad (on the lowest setting, slightly elevated above the pad). Overnight, this naturally fermented batter will become bubbly and expand. It will smell like sourdough (Don't use if it smells really bad – which is *extremely* unlikely). Once made, it keeps in the fridge for several days. It's easy to make 2-3 times a week and takes less then 10 minutes total working time.

Use the fermented batter to make sourdough roll-up wraps, flat tostadas, or Indian dosas using a little olive oil or ghee, cooked on a flat cast iron griddle. Dosas are like very thin savory "pancakes" or crêpes that you can use to hold various fillings. It's like making super healthy burritos or tostadas. Pour the batter in the middle of a preheated, pre-oiled skillet, and spread it out into a large circular crêpe using the bottom of a spoon. Cook on one side and then flip over using one or two spatulas and cook on the other side. You can add fillings such as 1) chopped/shredded raw veggies, 2) fermented veggies like sauerkraut, or 3) stir-fry vegetables. Make them extra delicious by topping with your own blended raw-seed sauces or dressings. They can also be filled to make a nutritious sweet treat, using sesame or almond butter (made easily from blended soaked seeds), bananas, cinnamon, and salt. If you use a little imagination there's an infinite variety of gourmet tastes awaiting you. I have recipe-formulas in the Resources Chapter. Modern blenders and food processors make this otherwise tedious preparation both easy and quick.

Note: Regarding nutrition: Weston A. Price, DDS was a pioneer in exposing the severely destructive impacts of the modern, processed-food diet. He helped revive an interest in fermented foods. Although Price made significant contributions in opposing our depleted, processed-food diets, I do not subscribe to many ideas promoted in his books and his followers, such as Sally Fallon Morell (*Nourishing Traditions*) and others that have become popular. His promotion of whole foods and fermentation is admirable, but I believe his emphasis on meat and organ meat products is cruel, completely misguided, and unnecessary. He lived in an era when we did not understand human pH requirements and made mistakes based on his Western habits of food consumption. Humans have lived successfully as vegetarians for thousands of years. Ayurveda, the ancient system of healthcare, as well as the higher teachings of the enlightened, only allows for meat consumption as a medication for rare treatment of certain conditions, not as a diet.

Fermenting Foods with Protective, Friendly Bacteria

Lactic acid-producing bacteria exist all around us, all the time. It is a protective aspect of nature. Lactic acid fermentation has been used for tens of thousands of years to produce healthy foods and to preserve foods for when fresh foods are not available. No one has ever been poisoned from making lactic acid fermented foods. In fact, lactic acid destroys existing dangerous bacteria, prevents the growth of dangerous bacteria, and creates healthy conditions in the digestive tract, healing many conditions. Only after canning was introduced over a century ago, did deadly botulism show up. Inadequate boiling destroyed the good, protective, naturally occurring lactobacillus bacteria, but the bacteria causing botulism survived.

One of the easiest fermented foods to create is sauerkraut, which is made from shredded cabbage. Use organic cabbage. Conventional cabbage can contain pesticides that destroy the good bacteria. Shred the cabbage in a food processor, making some of it finer. Then smash it with a large wooden dowel or plunger to make some cabbage juice. Add a teaspoon of sea salt per cabbage and only enough non-chlorinated water to cover the mash when it's pressed down. Compress tightly into a large crock pot, using a plate, a smaller crockpot, or a casserole dish that fits snugly inside the large crockpot. Keep it pressed down with a weight. Let it sit at a temperature of 75-85°F for 3-7 days. Check every day or two for sour taste. When done, salt to taste and eat. (Caution, sauerkraut can overflow the container as the pressure weight settles! Don't put your sauerkraut on top of cupboards without a tray underneath. Overflow juice can remove paint and destroy adhesives.)

All kinds of foods can be preserved by fermentation. The lactobacillus species, (the beneficial bacteria you have heard so many good things about in yogurt), exists all around us, on all plants in nature. It automatically ferments vegetables when they are submerged in water. Mild saltwater helps retard other bacteria. Any food can be preserved through fermentation. The most well-known are cabbage (sauerkraut), zucchini, cucumbers (pickles), kimchi, cocoa, and sourdough bread. Before the advent of refrigeration, fermentation was one of the most successful method of preserving fresh foods for long-term storage. It also made food more enjoyable and healthier by breaking it down and enhancing the flavor. Fermentation is what gives chocolate its flavor.

Fermented vegetables last for months in a root cellar. It's easy to create fermented vegetables. Simply submerge them in lightly salted water, making sure the food is totally submerged. Don't seal the top while fermenting, since gases must escape. The description given for sauerkraut works with all vegetables. It also works for seeds. Grains, legumes, and other seeds have been fermented for centuries. Sourdough bread is a classic example. In the resources section is a recipe for making naturally fermented sourdough bread. Another primary method of preservation, used throughout history, is to dry foods in the sun. Low-temperature dehydration remains an excellent choice. It's also a great method for changing the texture of foods, for instance, when making dried snacks with a kitchen dehydrator.

Other Foods

There are other foods to consider as well, such as oils, herbs and spices. Most vegetable oils are highly processed and are unfit for human consumption. They are often rancid, but the producers filter out the rancid smell so you can't tell. Consider only fresh cold-pressed oils, especially those kept refrigerated. Olive and coconut oils are best and don't go rancid. It's even better to get your oils from fresh foods such as avocados, olives, bananas, and soaked seeds or nuts. The best source of Omega-3 oils is raw vegetables, chia seeds, flax seeds, hemp seeds, and nuts (not fish oil).

A Summary of a Natural Healthcare Diet

A super-nutritious healing diet emphasizes fruits and green vegetables over other foods. These may be consumed as juices, smoothies, blended soups (uncooked, with fiber), slaws, or salads. Food combining rules, which some people adhere to when mixing cooked foods are not so important with raw foods. Fresh vegetable juices, especially emphasizing tender greens, are the most healing foods you can consume because they are alkalizing and rejuvenating. The small particle size of juices, smoothies, and blender soups increases the surface area of foods and makes it easy for the body to use the nutrients without much work.

If you can afford the high expense, many companies are now growing high-nutrition green foods such as spirulina, wheat grass, barley grass, and other high potency greens and freeze drying the juice for market. Powdered greens can improve health because they are concentrated and convenient. Check with your local health food store for recommendations. Products such as these are useful, but quite expensive.

Properly prepared nuts, seeds, and to a lesser extent, grains, and legumes make excellent spreads when combined with vegetables. Vegetables can be finely chopped for use as a garnish or finely ground and blended for sauces and dressings. Make nut and seed milks by blending with water, then add sweetener, vanilla, and a touch of salt. Sprouts make excellent toppings for salads and fillings for wraps.

For healing purposes and longevity, especially if your system is severely compromised, 100% of your food should be eaten raw. Ideally, use organic foods grown on mineral-rich soils. Depending on the soil, commercial foods can have a nutritional content hundreds of times less, especially for micro nutrients. A diet of raw green juices, smoothies, raw soups, salads, and slaws can do wonders. This approach is ideal for highest health and most rapid healing, but start at a pace you can enjoy. Healing too fast can cause uncomfortable cleansing reactions. Once you're healthy, a diet of 70 to 80% raw is generally adequate.

Research has proven that a light diet of high-nutrient foods is best for longevity. It's better to eat too little than too much. Overeating and obesity is a prescription for disease.

Grow a Supernatural Garden

Fresh foods from your own mineral rich garden will be better than most purchased foods in every respect. For the cost of purchasing expensive supplements for a month or two, you could create a fantastic garden. I call it a supernatural garden because it's super easy, provides super nutrition, and is totally natural. For an organized approach to garden layout, read Mel Bartholomew's book *All New Square Foot Gardening*. He minimizes work by constructing raised gardens without tilling the soil, then fills the boxes with a blend of soil mixes. No tillers or garden equipment is needed. He then focuses on planting in square foot blocks for easy management. I prefer a 3 x 6 format to his 4 x 4 layout for an easier reach to the center of the gardens.

Unfortunately, he does not emphasize the need for minor and trace minerals, so you need to augment the method with rock dusts or seaweeds. He also does not present information on soil life for maximum plant nutrition. Let's look at the fundamentals of natural gardening and nutrition much deeper, and understand why you would want to spend some time creating a supernatural garden for yourself and your family.

In order to develop and maintain your health, obviously you need great nutrition. It's especially needed as you refine your physiology. Most of us were raised on conventional foods – primarily cooked foods, fast foods, and junk foods. That puts us at a disadvantage. We never received the super nutrition that was possible for humans. Now, you need to undo that damage and replace your old cells with high quality new cells made from the best nutritional products. Unfortunately, our agricultural system is ill-equipped to provide us with super nutrition.

You can provide at least some super nutrition from your own garden. Everyone can have a garden, even a container garden on a balcony can produce an abundance of greens, one of the best superfoods. A sprout garden is possible even if you don't have a balcony or any land – not ideal, obviously, but sprouts have enormous nutrition. Assuming you have access to some land either in your yard or in a community garden, you can create a supernatural garden. Let's look briefly at the different agricultural and gardening systems. I won't go into the details of natural gardening in this book. Instead, I'll quickly give you an overview and then refer you to websites where you can learn more.

There are four kinds of agriculture practiced today:
1) Conventional "modern" agriculture
2) Organic agriculture
3) Natural agriculture
4) Low-cost, no-cost, natural agriculture

Conventional agriculture is dependent upon petrochemical fertilizers and pesticides. High ammonia fertilizers, toxic pesticides, deep tilling, and the absence of mulching, destroys practically all life in the soil – thousands of pounds of subsurface living organisms per acre! Conventional soils have virtually no earthworms, and minimal fungi or microbes. This creates an addiction to high-cost external inputs, with ever-increasing amounts of fertilizers and pesticides. Since the natural soil life is destroyed, products of conventional agriculture are substantially lacking in trace minerals and other health factors. It's like building muscles using steroids. It looks powerful, but it is not healthy. The final products are coated or infused with toxins, and the land is poisoned.

Organic agriculture is promoted as the savior against the demon of ammonia/nitrate/pesticide-laden conventional agriculture. While organic agriculture is an improvement, it is not any more sustainable. Like conventional agriculture, organic agriculture requires tremendous inputs from outside, such as soil-amending composts, animal manures, heavy equipment, and petrochemical fuels. It is also expensive because like conventional agriculture, it requires costly soil amendments, labor intensive methods, and complex integrated pest management. Animal manures require special selection to avoid antibiotic and herbicide contamination. Composting requires special equipment, substantial labor and knowledge to produce a useable product. Hot composting takes substantial time and destroys many nutrients. Specialized knowledge is required to prevent crop loss and damage. Organic agriculture is not the savior it pretends to be.

SuperNatural Gardening is Better Than Organic

Natural gardening, natural agriculture is superior. It also recognizes that soil is the basis of all life, just as organic agriculture does, but it realizes that in order to build the soil, an entirely new approach is needed. Instead of trying to use external manures and composts at high costs and labor, it uses microbes to create them in situ, right in the soil itself. Let me explain.

Obviously, manures are created when animals consume food. What if you could create high quality manures from wastes that cost little to nothing? It would also be wise to use the most productive animals. If we look at the "animal" kingdom, the species that produces the best conversion of organic matter to manures are also the smallest! For deeper insight, read the simple, but profound free ebook, "Turning Garbage Into Gold" http://www.wastetohealth.com/turning-garbage-into-gold.pdf by Dr. Uday Bhawalkar, Ph.D. This book lists the conversion efficiency of different organisms per 1000 kilos of equal body weight (Manure produced / 1000 kg), as shown in the chart below.

Organism	Conversion per 1000 kg
Elephant	4 kg

Human	20 kg
Mice	200 kg
Earthworms	500 kg
Fungi	2,000 kg
Bacteria	10,000 to 20,000 kg

Obviously, bacteria are the overwhelming winners. The smaller the organism, the greater the conversion efficiency. The advantage of using bacteria is that they are already in the soil (or easily supplied), and can multiply rapidly. They can double within an hour! They require no care. Plus, they are usually available in massive amounts, 500 to 5000 kg/per acre, or 1100 to 11,000 kg/hectare. A kilo is roughly 2.2 lbs. All we have to do is inoculate, activate, and feed the bacteria some organic wastes that are properly prepared to meet their requirements! Systems of natural farming are designed to do precisely that.

No expensive fertilizers are needed. Bacteria can be fed at the surface of the soil using prior crop wastes and recycled food wastes. Ordinary earthworms, already present in the soil, distribute the massive amounts of fertilizers produced by the microbes. Pest management is minimal and based upon repelling rather than poisoning. Stronger plants often require no pest management. Organic wastes are inoculated with bacteria that prevents odor and rapidly recycles the wastes into new fertile soil. The probiotic bacteria also protects plants from attack by pathogens.

Forget About Vermiculture

Probiotic microbes eliminate the need for other intensive methods of composting such as vermiculture. Vermiculture systems use redworms and large containers which must be managed to produce worm castings. It would require a lot of work and a huge, expensive operation to produce tons of vermicompost per acre comparable to what existing soil bacteria can do easily. Proper care, management, and sifting of the vermicompost product is required. If you don't feed redworms the right quantities, the worms can die or create odor problems. They are like having house pets. You can't just leave them unattended. You can end up with a gunky, smelly mess if done indoors. Redworms can't survive in ordinary garden soil. They have many other problems which you can read about, such as being a vector for spreading viruses. Why bother? Bacteria are 20-40 times faster and require virtually no work, no management, no expensive special equipment. The compost product is created in situ, unlike vermicompost which must be sifted and evenly spread mechanically.

Another interesting aspect of natural agriculture, is that massive amounts of material to make compost are not actually needed. Plants are 75 to 95% water. Many solids within plants are based on carbon and nitrogen, much of which comes from the air. Although food crops are heavy feeders, they may only require 3-5% solids from the soil. The secret to plant nutrition is intense biological soil activity that more efficiently prepares nutrients for growing plants. This is very easily provided with simple, natural, probiotic methods.

Origins of Natural Farming and Gardening

Natural farming first developed in India thousands of years ago. It is now being revived in India, Japan, Thailand, Korea, Bhutan, and many other places. There's good reason why such methods are being adopted. In India, over 200,000 farmers committed suicide because they could not repay the loans required for conventional agriculture. They also realized they had destroyed their soils with expensive chemical fertilizers and pesticides. They were promised by Western agricultural companies that the new modern methods would make them prosperous! There is now a huge movement away from poisonous agriculture, including genetically modified crops that are designed to be self-poisonous or encourage vast quantities of applied poisons. Unfortunately, our small-scale backyard gardens throughout America, and most of the world, use the same destructive, poisonous approach. Just visit any garden center and smell the chemicals and poisons. It's even hard to breathe in a garden center. You don't need any of those chemicals, especially the herbicide "Roundup®" or "Miracle-Gro®" a chemical fertilizer like those used throughout the chemical agriculture industry.

Stop Composting for a Better Garden!

The first step to an amazing supernatural garden is to stop composting! At least stop how you were taught to do it. It's way too much work. You don't need heat from a hot compost pile to destroy pathogens. You can do it easier and faster with probiotics. Here is a new way to manage your yard and kitchen wastes:

1) In the fall, leaves should be shredded. A leaf blower set on vacuum does it fast. Cover the garden soil with shredded leaves during the winter to protect it and encourage soil life near the surface. Hot composting is a lot of work and takes months, often over a year, to completely compost food

wastes, leaves, grass clippings, and other organic wastes. You can do the same job more safely, with less work, in a few weeks with microbes.

2) Kitchen scraps should be processed separately from yard wastes. If you've ever made sourdough bread, dosas, or sauerkraut, you know how rapidly lactobacillus bacteria and yeasts can work. You can transform all your kitchen waste into fertile soil using bacteria, without any bad odors. There is only the slight odor of sourdough bread or dosa batter when you open the container to add more organic matter. No ugly kitchen smells whatsoever. You can do it indoors in the middle of the winter. You can create massive amounts of friendly probiotic bacteria and pre-composted nutrition for your soil. This inoculated pre-compost does not look like soil or compost in the bucket, but when it is put on or under the soil, and covered with soil or leaves, it becomes rich soil in only 7-14 days, because it is pre-composted with bacteria.

The system is called bokashi in Japan. Bokashi is just kitchen scraps kept in a 3-5 gallon sealed bucket. Each 1-2 inch layer of kitchen wastes is inoculated with probiotics, especially lactobacillus bacteria, as you add new scraps. It works best with a floating cover on top of the scraps to prevent airflow (anaerobic). It is sealed with a lid to further reduce air and prevent pests and odors. You don't need a special bucket with a drain or spigot. Any plastic bucket will do.

Lactobacillus bacteria are the most powerful and protective probiotic species of bacteria. I talked about them in the section on making sauerkraut and sourdough bread. This is the bacteria that prevents bad smells. It's also the bacteria that protects your plants from destructive pathogens in the soil.

3) When you're ready to boost soil fertility, your pre-composted bokashi kitchen wastes are simply spread on top of the soil and covered with leaves, mulch, or more soil. It breaks down very rapidly, and ordinary earthworms distribute the nutrition.

Understanding Probiotics For Soil and Plant Health

Natural farming or gardening is based upon culturing probiotic bacteria, which are used to 1) increase soil nutrition, 2) protect soil life, 3) directly fertilize plants through their leaves (foliar spray), and 4) protect plants from insects and pathogens. Various natural gardening systems in different countries approach the production and use of probiotics in different ways. The differences include:

1) The selection and sources of probiotic microorganisms.

2) The feedstocks used to grow them.
3) The methods to culture and store them.
4) Natural supplements to augmented them.
5) The methods used to nurture and protect both soil and plants.

For ordinary gardening you may need to do nothing more than a simple bokashi system. Natural gardening and low-cost, no-cost gardening differ by whether you purchase microorganisms or collect them locally for free. I recommend that you use indigenous microorganisms that you easily collect, similar to the way you make sauerkraut, dosas, or sourdough bread without commercial starters. This is the system favored by the Indian and Korean approaches.

Indigenous microorganisms (IMO's) are better adapted to your locale and will survive the best. The Indian approach is more comprehensive than other systems because it uses more feedstocks for microorganism preparation. Particularly, they found that animals that chew the cud, and which have a stomach with multiple chambers (such as the native Indian cows), produce vast quantities and varieties of probiotic bacteria in their manure. A small amount is used for feedstock in their soil preparations. A single cow makes enough manure probiotics to inoculate 30 acres for an entire year!

How to Make Probiotics

Probiotics are made as a concentrate, but diluted before use. Dilute either immediately or later when taken from storage. It's stored either as a refrigerated liquid, or low moisture powder, flake, or bran. Both low temperature and low moisture retard continued growth of the probiotics, which would deplete the feedstock that maintains them. Probiotics need feedstock to grow, usually brown sugar, unsulphured molasses, or starch, and also need feedstock to survive long storage.

The concentrate or a dilution can also be used for pre-composting, as with the bokashi system. Here is a simple system you can start with. It can be quite fun and requires the least effort of any gardening system. It also will take care of all your kitchen wastes and thus save you time and effort in your kitchen. Remember, the whole point of this is to make life easier and healthier by providing the highest nutrition to heal and maintain your family or community. This is so simple, once your learn it. If you are already a gardener, this will save you so much wasted effort.

For our bokashi system, I use a homemade liquid concentrate inoculant, rather than a commercial bran/molasses product.

1) Mix a blend grain and legume flour (or cracked grain/legume mix) at a ratio of 3:1 or 4:1 of grains and legumes. I often use rice and/or wheat with lentil/urad/garbanzo. Mix and match as you like. It all works.

2) Add a quarter teaspoon of sea salt or kelp, and a generous amount of water to make a thin "dosa batter." I usually make a gallon at a time.

In the winter, to keep it warm at night, I place the bowl of batter on a tray that sits on two chopsticks, slightly above a heating pad (set on low). It takes 12-24 hours to ferment. If it goes long enough, it separates into "curds" and whey, like yogurt does.

Whey from yogurt also contains lots of lactobacillus bacteria, and is another source of probiotics instead of the dosa ferment. The Korean system uses rice-wash water as a probiotic starter. They place it outside, collecting other probiotics from the air, though it takes longer.

When fermented, the concentrate can be stored in the fridge for later use. I use it directly or diluted to inoculate the bokashi.

Any of these concentrates can be boosted for garden application by diluting the whey with water, adding natural sugars to grow the probiotics rapidly for a few hours, then sprinkling the soil or spraying plants. Supplements like kelp and rock dusts can be mixed in for the soil.

The Korean system mixes the liquid with rice bran, or other high cellulose wastes, and brown sugar to reduce moisture for storage. It is sprinkled on each bokashi layer. I store my liquid probiotic batter in the fridge. Probiotics are diluted for final application. Water and molasses (or brown sugar) are added to whey, dosa batter, or any probiotic stock, and then diluted up to 1000:1, but generally in the range of 40-200:1. This multiplies the probiotic bacteria within a few hours, which are then ready to apply to garden plants or soil.

Store liquid inoculant concentrate in the fridge. Keep your dry inoculant in a cool place like a cellar. It can store for weeks. Drizzle liquid inoculant or spread a dry inoculant on each layer of your bokashi.

Many kinds of supplements can be used to augment your bokashi and gardening probiotics to build soil fertility or protect soil and plants. I use dosa batter with kelp and rock dusts. The Korean system uses plant juices for growth enhancement and protection. The Indian system includes many other sources of augmentation and probiotics, including cow manure, cow urine, milk, buttermilk, yogurt, ghee, charcoal, fruit, jaggery, molasses, etc. The idea is to 1) incorporate as many varieties of probiotics as possible 2) dd sources of minor and trace minerals, and 3) add natural sugars to feed the probiotics. See some example formulas in the Knowledge Base below.

Your Gardening Knowledge Base

Below are sources for you to learn natural gardening.

Indian System
http://palekarzerobudgetspiritualfarming.org
Bhutan System (Includes Indian systems)
Training Manual on Low Cost Organic Agriculture (pdf)
This manual includes conventional organic practices (that are of lesser value) but also Indian microbial methods…
http://www.snvworld.org/es/publications/training-manual-on-low-cost-organic-agriculture
Korean System
http://gilcarandang.com/recipes/
Search the Internet for: "indigenous microorganisms IMO" and "beneficial indigenous microorganisms"
Japanese System
http://en.wikipedia.org/wiki/Natural_farming
http://en.wikipedia.org/wiki/Masanobu_Fukuoka
Permaculture System
http://en.wikipedia.org/wiki/Permaculture

Of these systems, the Japanese and Permaculture systems are the least developed. They are also the youngest. They employ more surface animals, such as chickens, ducks, guinea fowl, etc. Rudolf Steiner's biodynamic system, that some gardeners are familiar with, draws only partially from the Indian system, and is not explained scientifically. All except the Indian system are generally non-vegetarian. The Indian system is the most comprehensive, has the deepest intuitive knowledge, and the most extensive use of microbiology. The Korean system has practical methodologies for using indigenous plants for crop protection. These resources should be more than enough to get you started. Enjoy your garden!

Natural Seeds

Remember, you will also need to use natural seeds for your garden. After reading about natural gardening systems, explore sources for natural, open pollinated, and heirloom seeds. See the Resources Chapter.

Community Agriculture

There is a revival in agricultural and gardening systems for larger communities that require much less work by layering different kinds of plants together. These systems are variously called *Agroforestry, Forest*

Gardens, Permaculture, and *Edible Landscaping.* They are based on perennial food crops with additional annual field crops and gardens as desired. If you are interested in food abundance for a community, village, city, or region, it would be worthwhile to research these systems. These could all be considered an outgrowth of the ancient systems of forest gardens practiced in ancient times throughout Asia. They are designed to create permanent, local, sustainable, food abundance to ensure food security for generations. These systems come as close as we may get to recreating *Gardens of Eden.*

What Makes Food Delicious?

Certainly, food should be healthy and contain all the elements for great nutrition, but it should also be delicious and enjoyable. What makes it delicious? Let's explore meal preparation from a new perspective. 1) Tastes – choosing herbs and spices, 2) Aromas – exploring the world's culinary traditions, 3) Texture – how to change the texture of any food, and 4) Setting up your kitchen for efficient preparation. Of course, there are thousands of recipes books on food preparation. Here I can only touch the surface and point out a few cautions from a health perspective.

Tastes: Making Food Delicious

The best foods are the ones that are already delicious without additions. Yet, there are herbs and spices that have healing properties and can improve tastes, add aromas, increase variety, and produce balancing effects. In the West, most of us have not explored the vast potential of herbs and spices to any great degree. Mostly, we use salt, pepper, garlic, and onion. For condiments we use mustard, mayonnaise, and ketchup – really, a pitiful use of the world's great treasure of flavor opportunities.

Herbs and spices have been used throughout the world for both taste and health. Generally, the more mellow the herbs and spices the better. Strong pungent herbs and spices tend to have irritating, sometimes addictive properties. If you use those, use sparingly.

Onions, garlic, and hot green chilies have steroidal properties. They are not really foods, they're medicines. You'll notice that all the cultures that eat these foods daily have an inflamed population. They are generally more *Research* emotionally unstable, overly sexual, and often have issues of family abuse and violence. Try going without these foods for 30-60 days and you'll see what I mean. Everything in nature has a positive use. Not everything is intended to be used all the time. This is especially true of strong herbs, spices, and some foods.

The Six Basic Tastes

There are 6 basic tastes: Sweet, sour, salty, bitter, pungent (hot), and astringent. The last three are more medicinal in nature and should be used sparingly. Excessively sweet, sour, and salty foods can be addictive, especially in cooked form. Ayurveda recommends having some amount of all six tastes at every meal. This creates more satisfaction and less tendency to overeat. A mild, less spicy, less addictive diet is best for emotional balance and a clear mind.

Aromas: The Subtle Sensory Quality of Foods

The tastes you enjoy come not only from the six basic tastes, sensed with your taste buds, but also from aromas sensed with your nose. There is a huge variety of aromas that have not been classified in the English language. We have a few: flowery, sweet, stinky, acrid, spicy, fruity, earthy, fragrant, aromatic, and a few others, but these can't describe spices and herbs or even foods in any meaningful way. It would be hard to describe the aroma of basil or fennel. You can only learn to use herbs and spices by taste, smell, and experience.

Generally, the simpler your diet, the better. Gravitate towards foods that are naturally delicious. Foods that need lots of doctoring are usually a problem. A good way to get started with herbs is to explore herbal blends based upon traditional cultural usage: Italian blends, Indian curries and masalas, Chinese, Mexican, Greek, Thai, and other traditional spice blends. Visit a natural food store or talk with a friend who is a good cook. You can mix your own custom herbal blends. Curries don't have to be hot. You can mix herbs and spices to meet your own requirements. Also, be aware that in recent times ethnic foods and spices have gravitated towards more addictive qualities. As mentioned, strong pungent foods and spices like onions, garlic, and hot chillies, create a fiery temperament and addictive behaviors. The Resources Chapter includes extensive recommendations on food selection and spices.

Food Textures

Food textures vary greatly – from liquid to completely dry. They can be liquid, soupy, creamy, spreadable, a paste, firm, dry, or crunchy. You can process any food in your kitchen to have any texture by adding liquids, adding dry ingredients, or using a low-temperature dehydrator. Multiple textures can be created with kitchen tools like graters, blenders, and food processors. It's beyond the scope of this book to cover all aspects of food preparation. There are many raw food recipes books on the market, plus extensive online resources. Starter recipe-formulas are in the Resources Chapter.

A Fantastic World of Flavor, Aroma, and Texture

Many people enjoy the process of creating delicious meals from raw foods. There are literally millions of combinations of foods, herbs, spices, and textures to create an infinite variety of delicious healthy meals. Some folks like to keep it simple. Simplicity is easier, variety is more interesting. Balance complexity to match your interests. It doesn't have to be difficult.

My wife and I lived mainly on ambrosia fruit salads and vegetable salads loaded with soaked nuts and seeds for several years, sometimes adding sprouted grains and legumes to the veggie salads. We make fresh salad dressings drawing from over 50 herbs and spices in our kitchen. Our total meal prep time is usually around 20-30 minutes. We like gourmet tastes, but we do it quickly. We're not particularly domestic, so we minimize the effort. Green smoothies can be made in a few minutes and are delicious.

How to Set up Your Kitchen

There are a vast number of fancy kitchen gadgets on the market. Many of them are quite expensive. Some of them can be a good investment, but you really don't need much to get started. Here is a list of the basics:

Knives & Accessories – Good kitchen knives, an 8 inch knife and a small paring knife. Look for knives that give enough clearance for your knuckles. You will also want a cutting board, and possibly flexible cutting sheets that allow you to transfer freshly cut items to other places in the kitchen. Silicone spatulas are great and can often be found inexpensively at dollar stores. Bamboo spoons and spatulas work very well and last a very long time.

Blender – Our favorite blender is an Osterizer with a fusion blade. Most people don't realize it, but Oster blenders will accept most jars as a blending container – half pint and pint jars, even larger quart jars. Small jars can be used for grinding seeds and spices. You don't need a separate grinder. Blenders are used for making green smoothies, fruit smoothies, soups, salad dressings, nut and seed milks, and for chopping, and pulverizing almost any food, including ice. It's the most universally useful kitchen appliance. High speed power blenders, like the Vitamix, are a nice luxury, but you can do everything "good enough" with the fusion blade and an ordinary inexpensive blender, though it takes a little longer.

Food Processor – There is a mini processor for Oster blenders, but for grating and slicing, a 6-10 cup inexpensive food processor is best.

Inexpensive units are available in any department or "big box" store. Expensive units don't necessarily last longer. Manufacturing technology has evolved to the point that even inexpensive products are quite good.

Juicers – Any inexpensive citrus juicer will work for citrus fruits – manual or electric. For juicing veggies, including greens, the best type of juicer is a slow-speed auger (screw-type) juicer. Juicer technology is changing to include juicing leafy greens. For low cost and good quality juice, we use a manual juicer (Tribest Z-510 Z Star). We don't have a big family so we don't need a motorized juicer. Motorized juicers are much more expensive, but worth it if you juice a lot (Examples: Tribest SoloStar III, Omega NC800, Samson 9004, Omega 8006). Vertical auger juicers take up less counter space, can produce higher quality juice, but require more cleaning and are less time-proven (Examples: Tribest Slowstar, Kuvings Silent Upright, Omega VRT 330/350, Fagor Slow Juicer). The Champion juicer is popular, but won't juice leafy greens. I don't recommend it as your only juicer. Avoid centrifugal juicers. They are inefficient and make low quality juice.

Strainers - For sprouting grains, beans, and seeds there are plastic strainer lids that screw onto wide mouth mason jars. Stainless steel kitchen strainers are also useful, with fine or coarse mesh screens. You can also strain with cheesecloth.

Dehydrator - The best way to preserve foods for long-term storage is with a low-temperature dehydrator. Properly dried foods preserve more nutrients, take up less space, are lighter, and travel well. To dehydrate foods without destroying nutritional value you need a dehydrator with accurate temperature controls. In addition to drying racks, many units come with thin, plastic, non-stick sheets you can put on top of the racks. Both are quite useful. An example of a good temperature controlled dehydrator is the Excalibur brand. This type of dryer is for food preparation.

For preserving large amounts of produce (everything ripening at once), a much larger solar dehydrator is a better choice, but you need to build it, perhaps with the help of a friend. There are plans available, yet there are things to look out for and ways to improve existing designs if you so choose. The design should protect food from insects and exposure to light, which destroys some nutrients. The sun should heat indirectly, not directly shine on the food. The ideal dryer would have heat storage so it continues drying after sunset.

Food purists, which should be all of us, are concerned with safety and preserving enzyme nutrition. Here are some facts that we know. If food is dried at temperatures that are too low, it can promote the growth of mold or pathogenic bacteria. Enzymes are destroyed at high temperatures. When food is moist, the highest safe temperature is 117°F. When food is dried, enzymes become dormant and can withstand temperatures to 140°F.

Air temperature control is usually accomplished by air flow control using an adjustable vent or fan. A thermostat can control fan speed or vent position to maintain temperature. Passive gas-pressure devices with pistons can also control vents. The simplest design, though not as efficient, would be to set the vent control manually for the worst case, a high of 117°F.

The temperature of food when it is still wet should not rise above 117°F for any length of time. When food is dry, it can withstand higher temperatures without destroying enzymes. Research shows that enzymes are destroyed at 118° and above. Some enzymes are more stable than others. 105° F is considered the ideal maximum wet food temperature to preserve the highest quality, but wet foods generally stay up to 20° cooler than the air drying temperature due to the effects of evaporation. It's considered acceptable to initially set the air drying temperature at 105° plus a maximum of 20° = 125°F until the food is dry on the surface, which usually happens within a hour or two.

Search *indirect solar dehydrator* (without quotes), for solar design ideas.

Storage Jars and Bulk Containers - Dry foods can be stored in glass jars with screw tops. Use large jars for storing seeds, grains and legumes. Shelled nuts are best stored in the fridge. Mason jars with plastics strainer lids are great for sprouting. Small jars are used for spices. Small mason jars, sometimes called "jelly" jars, with the standard top, can be used with an Oster blender. Natural food stores also sell bulk herbs and spices and it's very cost effective to purchase modest amounts. Store in small jars. For large volumes of bulk foods such as grains and legumes, five gallon buckets with snap on lids work well. Put a few bay leaves in on top to prevent problems with pests. It's wise to keep a selection of various seeds, plus grains and beans, on hand. In case of natural disasters, you could live comfortably for weeks.

Crock Pot - Since your diet may not be 100% raw, you may want a crock pot for cooking beans and grains. For automated cooking, crockpots can be connected to appliance or light timers to turn on and off at predetermined times. You can load a crockpot before bed and have a whole meal ready to take for lunch at work in a widemouth thermos. If you don't process grains and beans through fermentation, at least soak and drain the soak water before cooking to minimize anti-nutrients.

Using Bulk Foods - What foods, herbs, and spices to keep on hand? How to save money on purchases? These and other subjects plus intricate methods of food preparation are addressed by many wonderful "cook" books. There are starter ideas in the Resources Chapter.

Learn how to use herbs and spices and prepare foods by looking at recipes. You don't need to follow recipes exactly. You can substitute different ingredients and different herbs and spices. Just get a sense of the amounts used. Soon you'll be able to make up your own recipes using what you have on hand. With a little practice you can use your hand for most of your measurements. I have an extensive list of foods, herbs, and spices listed in the Resources Chapter at the end of the book.

For healing purposes, very simple meals such as green smoothies or soups can do miracles. When you don't feel well, simple is best. Here are the basics:

Simple Recipes for Restoring Health
Green Smoothies
1. Water, a cup or more as needed
2. Orange or other citrus (plus other juicy fruit if desired)
3. Mild Dark Greens, enough to make a large salad
4. Handful of Soaked Almonds and/or Seeds
5. Powdered Greens (if you can afford them)
6. Powdered Kelp or Dulse, a Tbsp or more for trace minerals
7. Herbs and Spices to taste
8. Blend in a high speed blender

Green Soups
1. Dark Greens, enough to make a large salad
2. Other Fresh Vegetables
3. Almonds or other Nuts and/or seeds (soaked)
4. Powdered Kelp or Dulse, Tbsp or more
5. Lemon Juice and Olive Oil to taste (or Avocado and Lemon)
6. Two Tomatoes, if you like a tomato base
7. Salt, Herbs, and Spices to taste
8. Blend in a high speed blender

Green Slaws
Same as green soup but add cabbage and process in a food processor until it has the consistency of cole slaw. Vary veggies, herbs, and spices for variety.

Salads

Salads may include: lettuce (including romaine, bib, Boston, red leaf, green ice), arugula, radicchio, endive, frisée, watercress, celery, spinach, cucumbers, tomatoes, broccoli, cauliflower, peppers, radishes, kohlrabi, snow peas, carrots, beets, cabbage, fruits (both dried and fresh) such as apples, raisins, apricots, etc., and all kinds of sprouts.

Enjoy Your Food, Enjoy What You Eat!

No matter what you eat, enjoy it. You make your meal doubly troublesome if you eat something that's not ideal and then berate yourself. If you are going to go off your healthy diet, ENJOY IT. The joy is important. It will help make the best use of the food. Conversely, eating even the best food in an unhappy state reduces the value of the food. The ideal is to eat the most delicious, life-enhancing foods, and be in a joyous mood when you do.

You Choose

Some of the most important decisions you make every day are what you put in your mouth. In general, your daily habits determine your health or lack of it. The more consistent you are, the better. The payoff for a well-chosen life is joy, peace, health, and a profound conscious awakening. I've tried to communicate the benefits of making such healthy choices.

It's not possible to express in words the benefits of a body that is strong, slim, flexible, and pain-free, with senses fully alive to the beauty all around us. I invite you to continue to explore this new, incredible experience of life by using this information. You now have more practical, useful information about diet, health, and nutrition than the vast majority of the world's population, including many graduate "nutritionists" who learned from outdated texts. Put it to practical use!

Help guide your friends and family if they show interest. Be careful not to force your knowledge on others. Entice them into better health choices through your own personal demonstration of health, joy, and attractive personal presence – as well as delectable dishes.

Action Plan - Chapter 6, Diet and Nutritional Healthcare

1. Read this book with others in your household and discuss it.
2. Decide together on a plan to improve the health of your family.
3. Construct a positive image of yourself in your mind's eye, see yourself smiling and willing to change. Remember your goals. Run your positive mental movies often.

sure your body is sufficiently clean on the inside, with the proper pH, you can absorb nutrition. Purchase pH paper and test the pH of everyone in your family. If you currently suffer from any serious disease or illness, quickly change the pH of your body. Quickly adopt the natural diet.

5. Let go of your old diet "religion," and return to the natural human diet. Start with least one or two days a week. Add a day each week.

6. Throw out all your processed, unhealthy foods. Feed all meat products to friendly animals. Throwing them out will deter you from purchasing them in the future. Here's the list to throw out: meat, eggs, conventional dairy products, sugar (hummingbirds can handle white sugar, but not powdered or other sugars), processed refined table salt, all white flour products, all alcohol products, all nicotine products, all caffeine products, all soft drinks, your microwave oven, all hydrogenated oils, anything with additives such as artificial flavors, colors, sweeteners, or preservatives.

7. Create a shopping list for the 7 food groups: fruits, melons, vegetables, nuts, seeds, grains, and legumes.

8. Start eating more fresh fruit salads and vegetable salads. You can live very healthy on gourmet salads embellished with a variety of nuts, seeds, and sprouts. It's the perfect way to lose extra weight, because you can eat all you want. Make green smoothies and raw vegetable soups.

9. Pick up a few raw food recipe books or get raw recipes from the Internet. Change the recipes that include steroidal onions/garlic/green chilies.

10. Begin working with the principle of choosing long term happiness instead of short term gratification. Make choices for present AND future health.

11. Purchase the mineral supplements you need to restore major, minor, and trace minerals.

12. Purchase probiotics or make your own sauerkraut at home. Experiment with making sourdough bread and dosas.

13. Order seeds, start some gardens – a greens garden, a vegetable garden, a vine crops garden: berries, grapes, etc. Plant fruit and nut trees. Start bokashi food recycling. Integrate probiotics into your soil and garden. Expand your gardening knowledge with the resources listed.

14. Buy herbs and spices, and begin experimenting with them. Review the Resources Chapter for more ideas.

15. Purchase kitchen accessories as needed or desired: Knives, blender, food processor, juicer, strainers, dehydrator, storage jars, crockpot, etc.

Chapter 7
Natural Healthcare for Infectious Disease
Freeing Yourself from Deadly Invaders

When your body is free of invaders – worms, flukes, bacteria, yeasts, molds, viruses, and so forth – it functions with great ease and comfort. You can't be comfortable with worms, flukes, and other invading pathogens crawling around inside you – critters that think YOU are food! When they're gone, life is good. No more bloating, no more weakness, no more threats to your health and wellbeing. Your body rests in serene peace. You sleep easily through the night. Your vim and vigor return. The war for the conquest of your body is over.

When your body suffers from invasions of pathogens, it's difficult to be healthy. Invasions happen when your body is overwhelmed with more than it can cope with. Then measures need to be taken. I include several classic approaches in this section.

How To Know If You Have Parasites
There is no need for a parasite diagnosis. You don't have to know which pathogens, specifically, are invading. It isn't necessary. If you've been eating the typical Western diet, you can be sure that you have them. If you're frequently weak, if you run a fever, if you're often down with colds and flus, you have them. If you're overweight, you have them. There are over 8000 pathogens that invade the human body. Tests can be done on blood and fecal wastes, but usually these tests only screen for about 40 or so, and they're notoriously inaccurate. Why bother? It's much easier, simpler, and cheaper to do pathogen cleanses, which rid the body of them all. It's not worth testing. Do a parasite cleanse on a regular basis, perhaps once or twice a year, depending upon your exposures. Keep your diet pure and your body free of congestion.

The Causes of Invasion
Have you ever watched bugs devour a garden? They especially go for weak plants. Strong healthy plants fend off attacks. In nature, bugs eliminate the weak plants so the strong ones, with the healthiest characteristics, survive. When a tree falls in the forest it becomes acidic. Nature recognizes that it's time to recycle the fallen log and sends all manner of recyclers to do the job.

If your pH is acidic, nature thinks it's time to recycle YOUR body. Invaders attack your body when 1) there's good food for them, 2) life-force conditions are low, and 3) your body is acidic. If you don't want to be food for parasites, you have to change the environment that attracts them. Change the acidic pH to alkaline and increase oxygen levels through deep breathing. The food that parasites want is the congestion, phlegm, and cesspool like conditions that develop from 1) years of poor diet, 2) lack of internal cleansing, and 3) congestion-causing habits, such as lack of exercise. If you follow the guidelines on diet, nutrition, toxicity, and congestion, it will be difficult for these invaders to come back. Do it to avoid the *Invasion of the Body Snatchers!* (old sci-fi movie)

Infectious Disease – Types of Invading Pathogens

Different types of pathogens invade and flourish in an unhealthy body. The approach to eliminate them varies with the type. They fall into these categories: 1) Multi-cellular parasites (flukes, worms, etc.), 2) single-cell parasites such as bacteria, 3) viruses, 4) fungi, 5) molds, and 6) yeasts. In nature's plan, they are the recyclers. You don't want your body to be recycled until *after* you've left it. Once you change the environment of your body and remove their source of food (by changing diet/nutrition, toxicity, congestion) you are no longer recognized as a suitable host, so they flee. The discussions below describe how to help them leave, but it won't be permanent if your diet remains conducive to an unhealthy internal environment, and if congestion remains in your body. You must change the environment and remove the food supply that allows them to flourish. You have to make conditions unsuitable.

1) Multi-Cellular Parasites

Multi-cellular parasites such as worms and flukes can grow to be quite large, even to several pounds. Tapeworms can grow to 30 feet inside your intestines. Masses of worms the size of your fist can exist in your bowels. Liver flukes, some an inch or more long can exist by the dozens, even hundreds, inside your liver. Intestinal flukes likewise can make a home in your bowels.

In times past, every society had some method of dealing with parasites. Castor bean oil, kim chi, hot chili peppers, noxious herbs (wormwood, chaparral, etc.) were all used. The idea was to make the environment unfavorable for parasites. We're told to worm our dogs and cats, but we never think to worm ourselves! All indigenous societies had some form of purification on an annual basis, often including fasting. Some health systems, such as Ayurveda, recommend a cleansing ritual as many as 4 to 6 times per year.

How frequently you need to deal with parasites depends upon the climate where you live, your state of health, and your potential exposures. If you're exposed to tropical conditions, pets, or children (who often carry "bugs"), you'll need to do a parasite program more frequently. Herbal parasite programs are now available. They are quite good at dealing with the larger multi-cellular parasites. You should do an herbal parasite cleanse at least annually.

The best herbal programs have these ingredients as a minimum: Black walnut (hull, seed, and tincture), wormwood (there's a reason for this name!), clove, grapefruit seed, and pumpkin seed. The American Indians used chaparral. In Ayurveda, Neem bark and leaves have been used. Haritaki is another valuable Ayurvedic herb. Check with your local health food store for recommendations. Your choice of product could have more ingredients, but these are the minimum. Purchase an herbal product and follow the directions. Herbal parasite cleanses are a little hard on the body because they're noxious. They create noxious conditions in the bowels and blood stream to make conditions lousy for parasites. Limit the length of time you use the product to the product guidelines. These are harsh, but necessary herbs. Afterwards, use probiotics such as homemade sauerkraut.

2) Bacteria

Infectious diseases are often caused by bacteria. Bacteria are single-cell organisms that set up house in your body when conditions are favorable. For years the fight against infectious diseases has been waged by the medical profession through antibiotics. It's one of the things the medical system learned to do well, but there's a problem. Antibiotics kill good bacteria in the digestive tract along with the bad bacteria in the body. Plus, many antibiotics have lost their effectiveness against deadly bacteria. There are strains of staph and pneumonia that can no longer be combated with drugs. Other infectious bacteria are developing super strains that are resistant to all known drugs.

This is a dangerous situation. Plagues have killed vast populations of weak individuals. The world's population is weak now, but it's nothing compared to the Middle Ages, which lacked even basic sanitation. Yet, we've created super strains of invaders. The best defense against bacteria is a strong immune system.

There are new tools to destroy bacteria that are virtually unknown to medical science. Many kinds of bacteria are eliminated with herbs like the ones used for multi-cellular parasites. Essential oils like lavender and tea tree have antibacterial and antiviral action. These essential oils can be misted and inhaled to combat lung and sinus infections. Tea Tree oil was used by the Australian aborigines quite successfully for all kinds of infections. Thieves' oil was used by the gypsies during the plagues of the Middle Ages. Such oils originally appeared in ancient sacred texts, including the Bible. See the discussion later on essential oils for formulas and recommendations.

Colloidal Silver

Silver has been used throughout history as a protective agent. It's the reason silverware exists! Ancient Egyptians lined their drinking vessels with it. Pioneers put silver dollars in milk to keep it from spoiling. Wealthy children were "born with a silver spoon in their mouth." Sucking on the silver spoon saved them from the diseases of the poor. Silver has a long tradition of very successful uses. It disables the respiratory functions of pathogenic single-cell organisms and viruses. It appears to have no significant effect on healthy bacteria in the gut and no effect on human cells. Still, it's a good idea to get probiotics frequently from lactic acid products such as sauerkraut, yogurt, and other fermented foods. These products encourage the good bacteria in the gut that your life depends upon.

Colloidal silver is one of the best antibacterial choices today. A colloid is a suspension of particles so fine they will never settle out. They're invisible. The ideal colloidal silver should have a particle size of less than .015 microns and a concentration of about 5-10 parts per million. The smaller the particle size, the better it works.

Large concentrations cause agglomeration into larger particles, which are ineffective. If greater antibacterial action is needed, take larger quantities of a low concentration product. There has been no problem taking even 16 ounces daily for short periods as you would normally do with commercial antibiotics. Lately, there's been confusion about colloidal silver versus silver compounds. Silver compounds have high concentrations of silver and can turn the skin a blue-gray color. This has never happened with ultra-fine colloids in low concentrations, it would require drinking a gallon a day for years to cause argyria. I have used modest amounts for over 20 years without any problems. Beware of the volumes of misinformation on the Internet with regard to argyria and colloidal silver. Even if someone developed argyria due to a wrong choice of silver colloid, it can be, and has been, reversed with vitamin E and selenium supplements.

The best thing about colloidal silver is its effectiveness. No single-cell disease-causing pathogen has ever been discovered that survives in the presence of silver. Over 650 have been tested. Colloidal silver was the antibiotic of choice before modern antibiotics were invented. It was used by the very wealthy in the 1930's, when a very time-consuming method of production was initially developed. It was prohibitively expensive, unaffordable for the masses because of the laborious, mechanical production process. It cost over $100/oz back then. Today, you can make your own colloidal silver easily using an electro-sintering process. Colloidal silver is used as an anti-cancer treatment, a treatment for every kind of virus and bacteria, and is considered the best treatment for infections that often accompany severe burns. In recent times, the Russians developed a microfine silver capsule that could be ingested in the case of biological warfare. It was their antidote for all biological weapons.

Making Colloidal Silver

To make colloidal silver, suspend two .999 pure silver strips or wires about an inch apart in 16 ounces of distilled, ozonated, water. Then connect 30V DC across them for 20-23 minutes. All commercially bottled water is ozonated. NEVER use sterling silver, it's poisonous. Use only .999 pure silver. Get pure silver from a silversmith, jewelry supply, or precious metals supply. (Note: Pure silver coins are .999 pure silver, and in an emergency could be used.)

There are simple ways to suspend the silver electrodes in water. Clamp them between two popsicle sticks or chopsticks, about an inch apart. Hold together with rubber bands. Make sure the silver electrodes don't touch. They should protrude perhaps a quarter inch above the sticks so you can clip wires to them. The bottom of the electrodes dangle in the water.

Apply 30 volts DC to the silver electrodes using "alligator clips," that you can get from an electronics store. Three 9-volt batteries can be snapped together, one to another in series, to give 27-30 volts. Two batteries will sit side by side with one opposite in the middle snapping them all in a line. Two remaining battery terminals will be exposed at each end of the series.

Connect a wire from the two remaining battery terminals to the tops of the two silver electrodes to energize the electrodes. Leave connected for 20-23 minutes, or until the current builds up to 2 milliamps. You can measure current with a digital multimeter if you have one. Find someone to help you if you want to play with a meter, but meters are not required.

After about 15 minutes, you'll see a yellowish-brown mist sintering off one of the silver electrodes. The mist or cloud of silver gradually disappears into the surrounding water. The other electrode turns black.

After 20-23 minutes, disconnect the battery and remove the silver electrodes from the water. Filter the resulting colloid to remove any large black flakes (particles of silver hydride). The black flakes are undesirable but easily filtered out with a coffee filter or paper towel. Prepare for the next batch by wiping the electrodes clean with a paper towel. If the silver becomes too tarnished, use a kitchen scour pad periodically for more thorough cleaning.

Overnight, the colloid may turn a very light yellow, which is OK. Dark yellow, orange, red, or gray is no good. Those colors indicate high concentrations and large ineffective particles. Colloidal silver is photosensitive to light and MUST be stored in a dark brown bottle, or kept in the dark. A reasonable dose is 1-2 tsp or tbsp, even up to 2-4 oz, 3-4 times per day. Start minimal. You don't need to mix it with anything. Use a plastic spoon, or perhaps a paper or ceramic cup. Never use metal utensils with colloidal silver because it neutralizes the electrical charge. You can buy ready-made units to make colloidal silver on the Internet. They should not be too expensive, after all, you can make your own for less than $10. Colloidal silver can be purchased at natural food stores, but it's expensive, about $20-30 for 4-16 ounces. You can make it yourself for the cost of distilled water, about a dollar per gallon, 128 ounces.

Uses of Colloidal Silver in Developing Countries

Colloidal silver is the most useful antibiotic for developing countries. It could prevent blindness from infections at birth. It can be applied directly in the eyes with an eyedropper for all eye infections. It could also wipe out malaria. Two to three tablespoons purifies a gallon of water of all pathogens in six minutes, eliminating all waterborne diseases, a perennial problem in the tropics. Every community, every family should know how to make it.

Gold and other Colloids

The Platinum Group of metals as well as other trace minerals have valuable biological effects. Gold colloid wicks mercury and fluorides from the body. This works by a G-protein process. Gold colloids also help with emotional healing. Gold colloid is made similarly to silver but at a lower voltage, about 12-15 volts, because gold is softer than silver. Gold was also originally valued for its health effects.

3) Viruses

Some infectious diseases are caused by viruses. Viruses are a problem with the medical industry because they have few ways to combat them. Flu, herpes, AIDS, Lupus, Epstein-Barr virus, and many others are considered incurable by medical means. However, researchers claim four ways to eliminate viruses: essential oils, herbs, colloidal silver, and electrocution. Many essential oils such as tea tree and lavender, among others, have antiviral action as well as antibacterial action. Herbs such as thyme, oregano, and sage are also antiviral. Consult herbal and essential oil references or consultants if you want to pursue this approach. A good reference is Valerie Ann Worwood's *Complete Book of Essential Oils and Aromatherapy*. Colloidal silver, described earlier, has been proven to be highly antiviral and antibacterial, so it's a good choice for colds and flu. It can wipe out the flu within a few hours. There is a developing field known as electro-medicine.

Electro "Medicine"

The field of electro-medicine is an amazing research area. If you do an Internet search, you will turn up many exotic, interesting, and sometimes bizarre devices. It is a field with a lot of promise. The electrocution approach to pathogen elimination or physiological enhancement is somewhat technical. If you want to use it, find someone who understands electrical lingo to help out. You might get help from ham radio clubs, community colleges, engineering societies at universities, etc. This approach works well with viruses and many bacteria. The theory behind this approach is that it takes a lot of electrical power to kill a person, but the human body is huge compared to a virus or bacteria.

Viruses in the blood can be eliminated or disabled with currents as low as 100 to 500 micro amperes (millionths of an ampere). Currents as high as 3-5 ma (milliamps) have been used. Blood purification devices have been designed with simple conductive-rubber or cloth/saltwater pads that attach to wrists or ankles. Most are built with simple alternating square waves, which are either bi-phase or mono-phase (one direction only). The best units are bi-phase where the current actually reverses direction to prevent the possibility of electrolysis of the blood. Very low-frequency devices are by far the best (under 20 Hz).

Devices in the kilohertz range or higher disturb the human system and give false radionic readings of success (i.e. Hulda Clark's system). Resonance systems, such as the Rife system also work. They destroy pathogens by vibrating them to pieces through resonance, but you must apply very specific frequencies for each pathogen, an unnecessary bother. Applying low-frequency current through the skin is more effective at frequencies well under 20 cycles per second. It's usually not worth the expense and complexity of a pathogen-specific resonance approach.

Wave forms should also be modified. Square waves, with their rapid impulse, disturb the nervous system. A better approach is to use a ramped wave such as a truncated, peak-limited sine wave or other slower ramp. If you're looking for units to experiment with or for research, check the Internet or have someone with technical skill construct one. Someday in the future, every family will have an electrical "zapper" device to minimize the threat of infection. (Note: Mild salt solution or colloidal silver improves skin conduction with all devices.) This approach of electrocution was used by the ancient Egyptians and recently revived by Robert C. Beck, Ph.D. (Bob Beck) former Dean of Physics, UCLA.

Note that there are many kinds of "medically approved" electro-therapeutic devices on the market that generally come under the umbrella name of TENS, transcutaneous electrical nerve stimulation. There are also microcurrent devices for pain reduction and wound healing. These kinds of devices will not work for this application because they operate in the wrong frequency range, the wrong power range, and use a square waveform, which is not the ideal waveform.

At the turn of the 19th century, Nikola Tesla researched and patented many electro-therapeutic inventions that demonstrated incredible health-promoting effects. Dr. Tesla is the amazing genius who invented the electrical generation and distribution system that we still use today. He is also the inventor of radio. His patents should be resurrected and studied. There are many people today doing experimentation. An in-depth Internet search may reveal new developments in this field that use various intensities, waveforms, and frequencies for healthcare.

4, 5, 6) Fungi, Molds, & Yeasts

Anyone with an acidic pH is prone to yeast infections. Yeast, fungus, and mold are invasive recyclers that attack and attempt to decompose the whole body. It's similar to what happens to weak plants in the garden and rotting logs in the woods. Symptoms mimic many serious diseases. It puts a heavy burden on the body and compromises the immune system. These problems can be eliminated by a diet that changes the pH of the body to an alkaline state, discussed previously. Yeasts, such as candida albicans, prefer an acidic environment. When the whole body is acidic, these yeasts set up shop everywhere. The only permanent solution is to change the body's pH.

However, in the short term, fungal yeasts such as candida are eliminated in a few days, with high concentrations of cellulase enzyme. Fungi, mold, and yeast have cellulose content in their cell wall, unlike animal (human) cells. Cellulase enzymes in high concentrations simply digests them. Ordinary digestive enzymes have perhaps 80 to 100 CU's of cellulase enzyme and are not effective.

To eliminate candida and other fungal yeasts, you need specialized products that contain 100,000 to 200,000 or more CU's of cellulase enzyme – a thousand times the concentration of ordinary digestive enzymes. A few days on such a product and the problem is cleared for the moment. Re-exposure, however, is guaranteed because these yeasts are everywhere. If your body pH is still acidic and the colon wall is compromised (excessively permeable), the problem will easily reoccur. To completely eliminate the problem, an alkaline body pH is required. Also, a healthy intestinal wall must be rebuilt through a healthy diet. Ask the personnel in your health food store for recommended products. If you can't find them locally, check the Internet for suppliers. Two common products are Candex and Yeast Away.

There are herbs and other products that can destroy fungi, mold, and yeasts. These products also work, but are not as gentle. When they kill off these pathogens, additional toxic byproducts are added to your system. It would be better to avoid those kinds of products.

To keep candida at bay, you will have to adhere to a very strict diet. You will need to avoid all products with white sugar or simple carbohydrates like breads, pastries, and other "refined," processed foods. This is a good idea for the rest of your life anyway, so you may as well start now (if you haven't already). You must eat very low on the "junk food" index. There is also the glycemic index, a rating of how quickly foods are converted into sugar. The little "yeasties" love sugar. So does cancer.

As discussed extensively in the chapter on healing through diet and nutrition, the Glycemic Index assigns a number to how foods covert into glucose sugar in the body – from a high of 100+, to 20's and 30's for some foods. In my experience, if you follow the natural healthcare dietary recommendations, your body pH will rise, you will heal more rapidly, and all invaders will be a thing of the past.

ential Oils

Essential oils have amazing healing properties. One of the most powerful blends of oils is Thieves' Oil. During the plagues of the middle ages, gypsies who knew the formula for Thieves' Oil, would douse it on a handkerchief, cover their mouth and nose, and enter the homes of the wealthy to steal valuables and even rob jewelry off the plague-dead bodies. Thieves' Oil is a combination of oils: clove, lemon, cinnamon, eucalyptus, and rosemary. Today a better oil would include lavender and tea tree. This protection might be a good practice today in hospitals, which now harbor the world's most dangerous bacteria and viruses. Proportions shown below are just one example, and could be varied for particular uses or liking. Classically, Thieves' Oil contained only the oils in the left column. A better version might include oils in the right column.

Classic Thieves Oil		Possible Additions	
Clove	3 drops	Lavender	5-10 drops
Lemon	5 drops	Tea Tree	10 drops
Cinnamon	5 drops	Peppermint	1 drop
Eucalyptus	4 drops	Red Thyme	3 drops
Rosemary	5 drops		

Add these essential oils to about 10 ml of a carrier oil such as sweet almond, jojoba, olive, or coconut. A few drops of this oil, applied to the gums with an eyedropper, has quickly reduced the pain and swelling from an abscessed tooth. In some cases it has completely reversed tooth abscesses and saved the tooth. For this purpose, lavender and tea tree can be used without dilution.

Like the gypsies, a few drops of these essential oils can be put on a handkerchief, held over the nose and mouth, and breathed into the sinuses and lungs. This can often rapidly stop colds, flu's, and other respiratory conditions. They may even cure respiratory tuberculosis which is not treatable by other means. Colloidal silver can also be misted and breathed into the sinuses and lungs. Both essential oils and colloidal silver can be used with nebulizers.

Ayurvedic Oil Mouth Rinse

For thousands of years Ayurveda, the science of health from ancient India, prescribed many methods for maintaining and preserving health. The classic mouthwash to preserve the health of your gums and teeth is simply a small amount of sesame oil swished around the teeth for 5-10 minutes, more if you have gum or dental problems. This practice creates healthy teeth and gums by drawing bacteria and toxins from tissues. One addition to improve the method is to add a few drops of essential oils. For 4 oz of oil, add 5 drops of lavender, 3 drops of tea tree, 3 drops of lemon, and 2 drops of peppermint. As you learn about essential oils you can make other mixes that appeal to you.

Healing using physical approaches is not the only approach to natural healthcare. We heal on other levels beyond the physical. In a later chapter I introduce the concept of energy healing. Non-physical approaches to natural healthcare create their healing effects by enhancing your body's ability to heal itself. For example, increasing life force energy changes your biochemistry to produce powerful healing hormones. It reduces damaging thoughts and emotions. It empowers your body to heal itself by boosting the endocrine system and immune system. It helps to promote constructive thoughts, emotions, and increased consciousness. This is the topic of a later chapter.

Action Plan - Chapter 7, Natural Healthcare for Infectious Disease

1. If you have others in your household, read this information together and discuss it. Decide together on a plan to remove parasites, it's better to do the cleanses together. Put it on your family calendar.
2. If you have a cat, dog, or other pet, purchase parasite products from a vet or pet supply for them and do a parasite cleanse for the whole household.
3. Purchase a cellulase enzyme product for candida and start using it right away. After 3-5 days on cellulase enzymes, begin an herbal parasite cleanse along with colloidal silver.
4. Learn to make colloidal silver.
5. The herbal cleanse will last a minimum of 15 days. As you complete the cleanse (during the last week), make sauerkraut or purchase pro-biotic supplements to reestablish intestinal flora. Start to reestablish healthy flora on the last day. Make your own sauerkraut. Purchase a few of the essential oils listed. At the minimum, get lavender and tea tree essential oils to have on hand.

Now you know how to remove invading parasites and prevent their recurrence. You may never have serious colds, flu's, headaches, and a thousand other ills again, certainly not for long, since you now know how to get rid of them. You have the knowledge and power to help your body heal virtually all diseases. You're on your way to a gloriously healthy body. As you purify, detox, and eliminate pathogens from your body, also remember your self image work. See yourself getting healthy and making healthy choices. Nurture positive qualities in yourself. Be strong in your resolution to rebuild your health and renew your life. You change your life by changing your self image and making new healthy choices.

Chapter 8
Physical Fitness and Natural Healthcare
Exercise for Health, Beauty, and Energy

Understanding Exercise
What to Expect

When you do the exercises described in this section, you'll get an attractive, slim, well-toned body. You'll be flexible, light, and strong. You'll move with grace and efficiency. You'll have more energy, sleep less, and feel great about your looks. Also, being in shape boosts your self esteem, adds to your longevity, and keeps you healthy at any age. People who are in shape get fewer injuries and everyone, especially women, suffer less from osteoporosis and brittle bones. Obviously, exercise is essential for its contributions to a healthy heart. No health program can be complete without focusing on physical fitness and encouraging daily habits for maintaining the body.

This is a short chapter. So much has been written on exercise, I won't belabor the point. I only want to introduce some ideas you may not be aware of and suggest a few simple exercises for health maintenance. Be aware that there is an incredible amount of hype in the exercise field. Just find some simple exercises, routines, and activities that you enjoy.

Exercise Fundamentals

Some moderate exercise is needed initially to get your body in shape, then a minimum to keep it in shape. I don't subscribe to the theory "no pain, no gain," only modest exercise is necessary for health. According to Ayurveda, you should never push yourself beyond 50% of capacity. That 50% will grow over time. In the future, your moderate exercise could be double or triple what you can do now. Don't push yourself to the limits. You run the risk of an injury that could set you back for weeks. Don't risk it.

Do exercises you enjoy and can do regularly, especially ones that don't require good weather. I suggest exercises that require no equipment, (or a very minimum) so you can do them anywhere, anytime. My recommended dynamic tension-resistance exercises are simple and effective.

Five Kinds of Exercise

Different exercises accomplish different results. Most people don't want a freaky, muscle-bound look. They just want to be lean and strong with stamina, energy, and flexibility suitable for a normal life. Muscle-laden body builders often have little flexibility, a weak heart, and are not usually very healthy. There are five basic kinds of exercises for different goals, 1) Lymphatic 2) Stamina 3) Strength 4) Flexibility and 5) Coordination. The exercises I recommend don't require any weights or special equipment. Some exercises, like Pilates and Yoga, develop several goals at once: strength, flexibility, and coordination.

Lymphatic Exercise - Bouncing and Wild Shaking

I mentioned this exercise when I discussed purification in the chapter on physical approaches to health. I'll cover it in more detail here. As mentioned earlier, the lymph system is the drainage system of the body. It's HUGE, about 5 times the size of the circulatory system, but it doesn't have a pump. It operates with differential (alternating) pressure and one-way valves. Lymphatic exercise moves lymph fluid to clean up your body. Every time you move, you squish lymph fluid along the lymph channels, sending wastes back to the liver to be purified and recycled. Without this cleansing, you would quickly die. This is why exercise is so important, especially for sedentary workers.

All movement causes lymph flow. Stretching, bending, squeezing, massaging, in fact, any movement, but the best of all is bouncing. Bouncing alternates extra pressure at the bottom of the bounce (compression) with weightlessness (release) at the top. It exercises tissues you can't even reach, like inside your brain and internal organs inside your chest. The best bouncing exercise requires little effort, so that metabolic waste products don't build up. I've mentioned it before, but it's worth adding a few pointers here.

Procedure: Lightly bounce on your toes or lightly jog in place. Emphasize jostling your body. Breathe deeply with each bounce. If you begin to tire, bounce less and breathe more. Take a deep breath as you go up and exhale as you come down – deep, rapid breathing synchronized with each bounce. If you get lightheaded while breathing with every bounce, take a breath every other bounce.

You don't need equipment to do this, but if you have a rebounder (a mini trampoline), it's easier to get a good bounce with little effort. Ideally, spread your lymphatic exercise throughout the day, perhaps 2-5 minutes, 3-5 times

a day. Even if you can only do mornings and evenings, it's very benefici\
Everyone should bounce daily. It has incredible benefits. It's reported tha\
this exercise alone completely cured cases of multiple sclerosis. If you can't
bounce yourself, another person can bounce you on a rebounder. You just sit
and the other person bounces as they normally would. Start lightly.
Gradually work up to a normal workout. You don't need a rebounder to get
the bouncing effect. You could do jumping jacks, though it's more strenuous.

Even just shaking your body helps to wake up the energy flows in your
body and produces some lymphatic cleansing. Just shake wildly from the
tips of your fingers to your toes. You can even jostle or shake your body
while seated. Shaking wakes up the nadis, the thousands of energy points
distributed throughout your body.

Stamina Exercise

Stamina exercises like running, aerobics, or vigorous sports like basketball
or volleyball, will get your heart rate up and keep it there for a while. Unlike
lymphatic exercise, it's tiring. Jumping jacks or jumping rope can be a light
lymphatic exercise if done gently, or an aerobic exercise if done vigorously.
Stamina exercises put more demands on your body, increasing your blood
flow and heart rate.

There are many exercises to choose from: jogging, running, various
sports, or even dance-step workouts in classes with personal trainers.
Repetitive dance steps often involve bending, high-step marches, jumps,
punches, lunges, kicks, squats, and twists, often to musical accompaniment.
If you want pre-programmed exercises, there are DVD's, Internet sites with
videos, even apps for phones and tablets. You can borrow DVDs from your
library, or rent them from online vendors to see what you like. Internet sites
have examples to choose from. Then buy one or more to use regularly. Some
people rotate between several aerobic programs for variety. Or simply write
down the exercises you like most and put on your favorite upbeat music.

Whether you do jumping jacks, programmed dance exercises, or one of
the vigorous martial arts routines doesn't matter. These routines generally
involve repetition of various sets of exercises with or without weights. You
can make up your own. There is a prescribed sequence for any program of
stamina exercises 1) warm-up, 2) start up, 3) build up, 4) maintaining, 5)
slow down, 6) cool down, and 7) rest. Most people find that 15-20 minutes, 3
days a week is adequate to keep in shape. *Suggestions:* 1) Jumping Jacks, 2)
Punches, 3) Squats, 4) Kicks, 5) Lunges 6) High Steps, 7) Jog in place.

Strength Exercises

When most people think of strength exercise, they think of weightlifting. Weightlifting is one option, but it has drawbacks. It requires a set of weights or sophisticated resistance equipment. People often overdo it. Mistakes can cause injuries. It requires substantial space in your home, or subscription to a weight training facility. Because it's not convenient, people often drop out. There are better options. The best choices for developing strength are: bodyweight exercises, and dynamic tension-resistance exercises.

Body-Weight Exercise

Rather than using external weights, you can use your own body weight as resistance. Depending upon the angle of your body or the leverage applied, you can control how much of your body weight you want to resist. This has distinct advantages. There is less danger of injury. It's totally portable and requires very little space. Some common examples are push-ups, pull-ups, sit-ups, leg raises while lying down, and squats. An example of changing the resistance by changing the angle is doing push-ups from your knees rather than from your feet. It makes it easier to get started. If you are interested in bodyweight exercise an Internet search provides lots of material. Pilates and yoga both incorporate some bodyweight exercises.

Dynamic Tension-Resistance Exercise

Dynamic tension-resistance or self-resistance exercise uses muscle resistance instead of gravity. Isometrics also uses tension-resistance, but it's static and is not as valuable as tension-resistance with movement. With the dynamic method, opposing muscles resist each other as you move dynamically. For example, to strengthen your biceps you can do curls by pushing down on your right hand with your left hand and moving dynamically up-and-down. One advantage of the system is that it's much safer because you can always release the muscle tension before hurting yourself. This idea was developed and promoted by the famous Charles Atlas program from the early 20th century. He also included bodyweight exercises in his program. I have a chart of dynamic tension-resistance exercises that you can download from my website for free. Once you understand the principle, you can create many exercises on your own.

Flexibility and Coordination Exercise

There are also exercises for developing flexibility and coordination. The primary system is the fantastic system of yoga asanas, or postures, from the Vedic tradition. It is thousands of years old and is the most widely practiced system on Earth. Yoga asanas fall into two categories: floor postures and standing postures. An example of standing postures is the famous Sun Salutation, known in the original Sanskrit language as Surya Namaskara. An Internet search of the words "Sun Salutation" will turn up many graphic examples of the 12 postures. You simply flow through the 12 postures in a continuous sequence from beginning to end, then repeat.

There are also floor postures that have tremendous value. I have a one-page set of floor postures that you can download from my website for free. Yoga is one of the safest, most powerful, most effective systems for physical development. It develops flexibility, coordination, and also provides lymphatic benefits. It can also be used to develop stamina or strength depending upon the methods used. If you only did one kind of exercise I would recommend yoga asanas. If you want to go deep into the study of yoga, get authentic teachings from the ancient texts. The two best books are the *Hatha Yoga Pradipika* translated by Swami Muktibodhananda, and *A Systematic Course in the Ancient Tantric Techniques of Yoga and Kriya* by Swami Satyananda Saraswati. Both are published by the Yoga Publications Trust in Bihar, India.

Another well-known exercise that is excellent for developing coordination is T'ai Chi Ch'uan, usually shortened to Tai Chi. It is one of the many martial arts systems from Korea, China, and Japan. Tai Chi is characterized by its slow, deliberate, delicate movements. You may be attracted to other martial arts exercises.

How to Learn and Practice Exercise Routines

Any of these exercises can be learned from Internet sites, books, downloadable charts, online videos, neighborhood classes, personal instruction, and apps for smartphones and tablets. Choose one or more exercise types and find a source of instruction that appeals to you. One very important aspect of exercise that is not well known is that your mental and emotional state is reinforced when you exercise. Your mental and emotional state becomes more deeply embedded. Therefore, it's vitally important to be in a good mental and emotional mood. It helps to put on beautiful music and consciously choose your mental/emotional state through suggestion, visualization, and samyama as described in upcoming chapters.

Action Plan - Chapter 8, Physical Fitness and Healthcare

1. Grab your calendar or your scheduler. If you don't schedule your exercise, you won't find time to do it. It doesn't happen by itself. You must commit to a regular schedule. Decide what time each day of the week to do

your exercise and put it in your scheduler now, while you're thinking about it.

2. Download the exercise charts from my web site. Yoga, Pilates, and Dynamic Tension-Resistance charts are available for free. Laminate them if you like. Put them where you'll do your exercises. Do some kind of exercise every day: a bouncing/breathing exercise, a mild aerobic routine, a mix of exercises from the charts. Mix and match as you like. You don't have to do every type of exercise every day. Choose exercises you like to do and find an instruction method to learn the exercises you feel attracted to.

3. If your floor is not cushy, get an exercise mat. They're inexpensive, often around $10. Or use an area rug. If the rug is thin or slips and slides, put a non-slip pad underneath. I simply use an open space of carpeted floor. The bottom line is: Create a space that you enjoy for doing your exercises. Avoid the unnecessary commercialization that has overtaken the exercise field. You don't need fancy equipment, fancy clothing, or anything else.

4. If you want motivation, create positive images in your mind of how you'll look and feel when you follow through with your exercise routines. See yourself doing them and see your body changing. Make them more fun with music. Always exercise while in a good mental and emotional mood. Use techniques to change your mood if necessary.

5. If you like video instruction, find videos that you like and put them on your shopping list. There are many good ones. Or find videos online. Find a style, personality, music genre, and routine that works for you. Get exercise apps for your smart phone or tablet, or simply print out charts and keep them handy.

You now have simple and practical ways to build fitness. Fitness is not difficult, it just has to be scheduled. Use daily exercise to rebuild your physical body into the attractive, graceful body you were meant to have. Be gentle when starting your routine, but be consistent. Slowly work up to more difficult exercises. Remember, you don't have to look like a body builder, but you do want to be trim, fit, strong, flexible, and coordinated. Use your mind to create the images of the new you. Changing your body is not only a physical challenge, it's a mental challenge as well. Be willing to accept a strong, well-proportioned body as the new you.

Chapter 9
Bio-Energy Healthcare
Reconnecting Bio-Circuits and Boosting Life Forces

What to Expect

When energies flow properly in your body you have incredible energy to accomplish your desires. The organs of your body will function at full capability. Health is enhanced. Your body maintains proper alignment and structure. Your vitality is abundant and you require less sleep. Your coordination, dexterity, sensory acuity, and other aspects of physical integration and performance are vastly enhanced. Your musical, athletic, and artistic talents are more easily maintained and developed. You realize that you are more than a physical body, and that the invisible aspects of your existence are as important as the physical. You are more sensitive to environmental factors and forces, but you are stronger and less damaged by deteriorating forces in the environment.

The Importance of Bio-Energy Healthcare

Bio-energy is the life force energy that sustains all of your bodily systems. Even if your physical body were perfect, you could still have health problems, or mental and emotional problems, because you are more than a physical body. You have a subtle energetic body that is impacted by physical trauma, destructive emotions, and mental stresses. The subtle bio-energy body is made of up three primary systems: 1) the *aura*, a field of energy that surrounds your body, 2) the *chakras*, energy vortexes that enter your body in many places and help to sustain it with life force, and 3) your *meridians* which circulate life force energy to different locations throughout your body.

Acupuncture and acupressure are two methods that balance the meridians to promote healing. Elimination of blockages and improved flow of life force energy enables your body to heal faster and better. The five primary ways to resolve energy imbalances are 1) increase life force energy in an area, 2) manipulate the meridians and their points directly using pressure, needles, or temperature, 3) alter breathing patterns, 4) apply yoga and kriya techniques to rebalance and energize, and 5) work with conscious awareness itself. I will describe how to use all of them.

Understanding Bio-Energy Healing

Bio-energy healthcare is based on life-force energy or bio-energy. Bio-energy is an altogether different kind of energy. As a former engineering physicist, I am aware of many kinds of energies and forces: heat, light, gravity, magnetism, EMF (radio waves), nuclear radiation, etc. One thing they have in common is that they obey the inverse square law. When you double the distance, the intensity diminishes by the square of the distance. The light from a candle won't help you find a lost object if it's 50 feet away. The farther you get away, the more faint it becomes. Life force energy is unlike the energies you are familiar with. It is intimately connected with life and it maintains its intensity wherever it is directed.

This energy has been used for thousands of years in practically every culture in the world. In India, it is called "prana," in China, "chi," in Japan, "ki," in Hawaii, "mana." It's even visible to some people. In Africa, villagers knew to ask for the shaman with the shining hands. Some people intuitively know how to use it for healing. Others learned through training. Yet, there is nothing special about it. It turns out that healing with bio-energy is a natural human ability that everyone already has.

You don't need to be born with special abilities. You can easily learn to use it. We can all learn to ride a bicycle, because balance is built into us. We can also learn bio-energy healing, because the ability is built in. We all have access to bio-energy, we can all learn to use it. You don't need to see it to use it anymore than you need to see electricity to use it. It's a simple skill. You just plug into it. You gather it and direct it exactly where you want it to go. It is a natural human skill.

In order to be a more powerful bio-energy healer, you need to gather more energy to work with. You don't want to use your own energy reserves and deplete yourself. You need to gather extra energy. When you have lots of energy gathered, you direct it using attention and intention. Let me explain.

A Simple and Powerful Method of Bio-Energy Healing

One way to gather life force energy is by breathing deeply and rapidly. When you're energized, you can then mentally direct the energy to where you want it. Even if you know nothing about healing, this simple technique can create miracles. Simply breathe deeply until you feel slightly lightheaded. Your system is then saturated with energy. Then place your attention on the area that needs healing. This is more powerful than you imagine. You can use this technique very easily to heal yourself of many conditions.

To begin, allow yourself to feel any physiological sensations and do NO try to escape them. Ordinarily, we're taught to run away from pain, to take painkillers. That's the wrong thing to do. The purpose of pain is to get your attention, if it doesn't get your attention, then the pain has to get worse to get your attention. If you allow your attention to go to the pain, the pain will subside and that area will be healed. Once any part of your body gets your attention it no longer needs to send intense pain signals. It knows you are cooperating by flooding the area with your attention.

Simply increase bio-energy by breathing deeply and then localize your attention on those places where you feel sensations of pain, tension, or other disturbance. It can cause dramatic healing. Just passively observe any pain or other disturbing sensations. Scan your body to locate points of sensitivity and pain. Also, locate places where you have difficulty feeling anything or difficulty keeping your awareness localized – places you are cut off from. There is often hidden pain in these areas.

When you find a place that needs attention, give it your gentle localized attention while breathing deeply. No need to concentrate, just place your attention there innocently, like a child. Breathe deeply, keeping your attention gently localized. Come back if you get distracted. Return again and again. If the pain moves to another location, then move your focus of attention to that new place. Follow the pain. This is a very powerful method of healing. You just have to cooperate with and nurture your body instead of opposing painful or disturbing sensations. To help you focus, you can even place your hands over the area that needs help.

Bio-Energy Healing Refinements

The simple technique I just described has been used for thousands of years. First flood your body with energy and then localize your awareness to where it's needed. This is the essence of all bio-energy healing, but there are many refinements that can add effectiveness. Refinements in the field of bio-energy healing have been developed by sages and healers around the world. These refinements center around 1) how you collect bio-energy, 2) how you direct it to where you want it to go, and 3) methods to increase the intensity or improve the quality of the energy. Some of the refinements can dramatically speed healing. In every case, this type of healing is thought to operate at very subtle levels, even quantum levels.

Using a variation of this technique to boost and direct energy, I have been able to accomplish extremely dramatic healing for such problems as degenerated joints, scoliosis, and cancer. Photos on my web site show how lifelong scoliosis was reversed in only one hour! Not all healing is so rapid, but it often can be. Headaches and minor pains often disappear in as little as 30 seconds. Major pains and discomforts commonly disappear in a few minutes. The technique is truly awesome. I have had phenomenal success with it. It's very easy to learn.

There is so much research yet to be done on how life-force energy transforms tissues so rapidly. I like to think of it as *energy nutrition*. Your body always wants to heal, and it knows how to heal, but it doesn't always have the resources. Bio-energy is an energetic resource that your body can use to heal itself or heal others. When healing happens, it's almost as if the human body is being redesigned on a molecular, subatomic, or quantum level, and then brought back to the physical state again. Bio-energy is a universal energy that is capable of upgrading human life in every conceivable way.

It appears to help every condition. I have seen dramatic healing of skeletal deformities, misalignments, infectious diseases, emotional imbalances, and more. It has even reversed the physical and mental deficiencies of Down's Syndrome if started early enough. In many cases, it appears to repair DNA. Massive infusions of life force energy have created and can create miracles, especially if started as soon as the problem is noticed. I cannot recommend this simple technique highly enough. Let's look at more methods and refinements for making practical use of it.

Streaming Energy – Heal Yourself First

A wonderful refinement developed by Bob Rasmusson is to heal yourself first by streaming energy through your own body. This development was popularized by Richard Gordon as Quantum Touch™. Essentially, the method involves breathing deeply while moving your awareness through your own body, then allowing the energy that flows with your attention to exit the palms of your hands. This creates intense energy at your hands. When you place your hands on someone, the presence of bio-energy is infused into the person receiving treatment. You also could think of bio-energy healing in terms of resonance. If you have two guitars, and you strum one of them, the strings on the other will resonate. Whether you think of bio-energy healthcare as an infusion of a higher energy *intensity*, or resonance to a higher *frequency* of energy, it is an energy that transforms and upgrades your physiology.

Let's start with the technique of moving energy through your body, because it's a wonderful and effective technique, then later I'll introduce more powerful techniques that I developed from my experience of healing over many years. Of course, nothing is new. These techniques are universal and eternal.

This method of streaming energy, unlike many other kinds of energy work, is easily learned. As you practice, you'll build confidence that it really does work. Let's learn it now.

How to Heal with Bio-Energy

You can use this basic technique on yourself and others. Although the focus of this book is on self-healing, there are three reasons why you should learn to heal others. 1) Many people have children who are too young and not yet able to learn self-healing techniques. You can help them to recover rapidly. 2) In emergencies, and at other times, people may be unconscious or incapacitated. They cannot help themselves. I have, on more than one occasion, prevented people from going into shock following auto accidents. 3) It powerfully reinforces the whole process of healing when you experience how bio-energy operates on others. This helps to develop tremendous confidence that bio-energy is real and that it has powerful healing effects. Whether you work on yourself or on others, you know from experience how bio-energy healthcare works.

The first step is to increase your bio-energy to a high level, so you have plenty of energy to work with. As I describe the steps, do them with me.

Always begin with deep breathing, that is, breathe more than you actually need. I call this *over-breathing*. Over-breathing means breathing 2-3 times more than you need, which gives you extra energy to work with. Breathe deeply enough that you began to get slightly lightheaded, then keep yourself at that highly oxygenated, highly energized level. Don't over-breathe so much that you hyperventilate. You don't want to get uncomfortable, become dizzy, or pass out, but you do want to continue breathing more than normal, enough to maintain a high energy level. Breathing more intensely is a basic method of collecting bio-energy to work with. There are other methods of collecting and directing energy that I'll introduce later.

The second step in bio-energy healing is to move the energy to where it's needed or wanted. The basic principle is that *thought directs energy*. Thought consists of *awareness, attention,* and *intention*. Awareness is the stuff of consciousness. Right now you are aware that you are awake, alive, and reading these words. Awareness is the self-luminous quality of being consciously aware. The more aware and conscious you are, the more powerful your thinking is. Attention is the focus of your awareness on a particular object, location, or idea. Intention is the desire for it to change in a particular way by giving it a direction, a purpose, an objective that you want to happen, either verbally – using words out loud, or silently, within your mind. We also think with pictures, with visualization. Visualization can be still pictures or moving pictures – mental video. We can set our intention either with words, visuals, or both.

Wherever you direct your thought, through awareness, attention, and intention, that's where the energy goes. You are going to first move your awareness through your own body. This provides you with a basic level of healing whether you are working on yourself or others. First, understand the process of moving awareness through your own body. Practice as I describe it. Bio-energy will automatically follow your awareness.

1) Localize your awareness just below your feet. This means, place your attention under your feet in the same way that you would focus on any part of your body to feel sensations. It's a simple thing. If I say put your attention on your left-hand, that's easy, isn't it? If I say put your attention on your right knee. That's easy, too. We can put our attention anywhere instantly. That's all there is to it. Just below your feet there is a reservoir of energy that we can tap into for healing.

2) Now, move your awareness, direct your attention, up into your feet, up through your legs, up through your torso, all the way to the top of your head. You're just making a gentle sweep, moving your awareness from just below your feet to the top of your head. Allow your awareness to encompass all the tissues of your body, all the way to the center of your bones. Also, allow your awareness to expand several inches or even a foot or more surrounding your body. This is a visualization. It's like sweeping a big bubble of awareness, your attention, from below your feet to the top of your head. You are moving your attention through the core of your body, all the way to the bone, *and* you are including the space surrounding your body.

The trick is to make sure you're not skipping any areas. Sometimes we're a little cut off from some regions of our own body. If you find yourself skipping over places, go back and practice moving through those areas slowly until you feel comfortable moving your awareness through your whole body.

Moving your awareness through your body like this heals your whole body first, which is a good idea, especially when you're working on others.

3) Now, from the top of your head, move your awareness down through your head and neck, across your shoulders, down your arms, and finally out the palms of your hands. You've made a complete sweep through your body from bottom to top, and then from the top, down and out your hands. Practice this sweep of awareness through your body for several minutes until it feels really comfortable and easy. You might even do several practice sessions over a few days to get really familiar with localizing and sweeping your awareness through your body.

Okay, you've charged your body with a lot of energy from breathing deeply, and you've learned how to sweep your awareness through your body. People find it's often easier and more effective to synchronize breathing with sweeping. As you breathe in, move your awareness from below your feet to the top of your head. As you breathe out, move your awareness from the top of your head down and out your hands. It's often good to breathe out more slowly, to give a longer time to flow the energy from your palms. Try it. Take four or five seconds to breathe in, and about the same time, or even a little longer, to breathe out. Practice for a while until it becomes really easy. I call this "streaming energy."

If you're a little bit sensitive, you can feel this energy as a kind of pressure. Some people also feel it as electrical tingling, or as heat or coolness. People sense bio-energy in different ways.

See if you can sense the energy. Place your hands about 6 to 8 inches apart and start breathing and sweeping awareness through your body and streaming the energy out of your palms. Within a minute or so, if you move your hands towards each other, back and forth, you can feel a kind of pressure between them. You have created an invisible ball of energy between your hands. For most people it's invisible, yet there are some people who can see this bio-energy. It is this bio-energy that does the healing.

Now, all you have to do to heal yourself, or someone else, is to put this ball of energy where it's needed. That simply means that you sandwich the area between your hands. Just put your hands on each side of the affected area. If that's not possible then put your hands side-by-side. Try it on yourself or a friend. Ask around and find someone with a headache. Then put one hand on their forehead and one hand behind their head at the base of the skull. You can also put your hands on each side of the skull. Breathe deeply, and sweep your awareness through your own body, allow the energy to exit your palms. The energy will infuse into the other person. See what happens.

159

hin 30 seconds to a minute their headache will be gone. Migraine usually take a little longer, even several minutes.

orks with any other kind of pain such as muscle pain. Find some ᵕ with pain anywhere in their body. Ask them to rate their pain on a scale from 1 to 10, with 10 being the worst (find their starting point). Now, place your hands to surround the pain, then breathe, sweep your awareness as described, and stream the energy out of your hands. After a few minutes, ask them to rate the pain again. Usually, their pain will either be gone or much reduced. This is a wonderful help for children when they get hurt. You can usually heal their pain in just minutes. Children respond so quickly. Occasionally, the pain will increase for a little while before it decreases. If this happens, just stay with it for a little longer and the pain will subside.

Sensing Energy, Knowing When to Stop

When you're streaming bio-energy, you can often feel it tingling as it comes out of your palms. As mentioned before, people sense energy in different ways. For some people, it will feel tingly and electrical, others may feel it as heat or pressure. However you sense energy, it's okay. Actually, you don't even need to be able to sense it. Many people can't feel the energy at all, especially in the beginning, and yet they can do amazing healing. If you practice for awhile, the ability to sense it in some way will come. The advantage in sensing it is that you know when to stop. When they have taken all the energy they can use, the sensation stops because the flow stops.

When you first begin streaming bio-energy into an area, you may sense the energy moving right away. At other times it seems blocked and starts more slowly. Either way, just continue streaming the energy. It will stream out of your hands and create the desired healing effect. At some point the energy flow stops. Either their healing is finished or you may need to boost the energy to break through a barrier to restore the flow of energy. You boost the energy by breathing more intensely. When you sense the energy is no longer flowing and a boost doesn't help, you're done. They can't use any more bio-energy right now. If you can't sense the energy, you can just ask the person if the pain or problem is gone. That's another simple way to know you're done.

The only thing that can convince you that this kind of healing is real is to get experience. It's really simple, but it's really powerful. Practice working on friends and family. If you are a professional in the medical or healing arts, enjoy the profound power of healing this gives you. You may be able to heal in minutes what would otherwise take days, weeks, or months to heal. Of course, the first priority of healing is to heal yourself. If you choose to others, that's a choice only you can make. It's a wonderful service to re the pain in the world around you. People will be grateful for any help you can give. Certainly, healing within families is always appropriate. Every family will be far healthier and happier if there is at least one bio-energy healer to help other family members. Ultimately, every person, early in life, should take a few days to learn the art of healing. The more people who learn to heal themselves and others, the more the world will be beautifully transformed.

How Long Does It Take to Heal? How Long Should Sessions Be?

People always ask, "How long does it take to heal X?" "X" could be any condition. Another question is "How long should a healing session be?" No specific times can be given to heal any particular condition, because people are so different and the causes, even for the same condition, could be different. I have cured carpal tunnel syndrome with one five minute session. I have spent hours working on other conditions with only a 30 to 50% improvement. Sometimes people need more than just energy healing. If energy healing doesn't do the whole job, then there are other factors at work that need to be addressed – which is why this approach to natural healthcare addresses all five levels.

All we can do is infuse as much energy as possible into the area and allow their system to do the healing. We can also educate people about other levels of healing. For many people their diet needs to be addressed. The purpose of this book is to provide all this information. You might recommend this book to friends and associates. It will really help them.

Sessions can be any length of time. I can often structurally align someone's body in 1 to 2 minutes. Major help can be given in 5 to 10 minutes. I rarely work for more than 15 or 20 minutes on any condition. If I work on several conditions, I could spend an hour. I've tried different experiments streaming energy for long periods of time, up to three hours. What I found is that people cannot use that much energy all at once. Small doses are better. 10 to 15 minutes is reasonable. Two or three times a week is sufficient for most serious conditions. For life-threatening conditions, many people working together around the clock might be necessary. Many conditions are resolved in one session. Rarely do I need more than four or five sessions. Your "mileage" may vary.

Healing Reactions

Whenever there's something wrong and it's getting healed, there's often a reaction. That means, if a pain starts out at a 5 or 6, it could seem to climb to peak at 8 or 9 before it reduces and dissipates. It isn't really getting worse, but it feels like it. That's because we don't really know how much pain is really there until we go into it. Pain is often buried. Pain doesn't always peak higher before decreasing and dissipating, but sometimes it can. If the pain doesn't disappear completely, breathe more and continue. Sometimes all the pain won't disappear in one session, but it will usually be cut by two-thirds or at least in half. Oftentimes, it will disappear within a few hours after the session, or even overnight. Some people take longer than others to respond and there are often cases where multiple sessions may be necessary. Sometimes the pain will return, because a new layer of that condition requires healing. Sometimes people will recreate the problem by doing the things that caused it to begin with. This is why we all need to understand the primary causes on all five levels. We have to understand and change our habits that have been causing our problems all along.

Aligning the Body

One fundamental need in all approaches to natural healthcare is for the body to be aligned. Bodies don't work well if the skeletal structure is misaligned. One important thing to do at the beginning of any natural healthcare session is to align the body. Physical therapists and chiropractors have all kinds of ways to measure misalignments using various instruments. For many kinds of measurements they often use their hands as a handy measuring guide. Our eyes can see very subtle differences quite easily.

Aligning the skeletal structure often requires aligning only two primary locations, the lower skull region at the top of the spine and the hips at the lower end of the spine. It's best to align people while they're standing so that gravity exerts its natural effects.

To check the alignment of the skull, measure the occipital ridge at the back and bottom of the skull. Place both your thumbs under the ridge at the base of the skull, each thumb about two inches from the cervical spine. Look carefully to see if one thumb is higher than the other. Note how much. With a little practice, your eyes get very good at seeing differences of even 1/4 inch or less. Often this area is quite misaligned and is easy to see.

To correct the alignment of the occipital ridge and lower skull, keep your thumbs just under the ridge and spread your fingers wide, lightly touching
 of the skull with your palms hovering over the ear. Breathe and

162

stream energy out of your thumbs and fingertips, just as you would out of the palm of your hands. After 30 seconds to a minute of streaming energy, recheck the alignment. Amazing as it sounds, the cranial bones easily move into place. You have to experience this to believe it. Try it on several people until you become familiar with this alignment.

Aligning the hips is a similar process. You first measure to see how far the hips are out. Working from the back of the body, just under the ribs, find a soft space where there is no bone. Gently push into this area with your finger tips. Just below this soft gap below the ribs you will find the top of the hips. The hips for men and women are quite different. Men's hips are higher than you expect.

Make your hands flat and level like a board and place the tips of your fingers on top of each hip. Put your eyes level with your hands and without tilting your head, looking straight on, examine the height of the hips on each side to see if one is higher. Again, this is an easy measurement to make. One hip can often be over an inch higher than the other due to stress and muscle tension in the area.

If the hips are misaligned, you can easily align them. Sit behind the person on a chair or stool and place your thumbs near the base of the spine. Wrap your hands around the outer hips. Stream energy from your palms into the hips for a minute or so. Examine again. The hips will align easily. If they fail to align after a minute or two, the hips may be torqued or twisted. In that case, work on each hip separately with hands front to back on each hip. As you're working, people often have to adjust their standing posture to accommodate the new structural alignment. Later in this chapter I'll introduce another method to align the skeleton even faster. It's important that you learn to make these simple measurements. You can also measure the alignment of the shoulders and shoulder blades with this simple method of using your thumbs or hands as a gauge. Physical alignment is another powerful way to recognize the power of bio-energy healing.

After you have aligned the skeletal structure, then you can work on other areas of concern. Just ask them where the problem is and go there. Wherever there is pain, pressure, tension, or sensations, infuse that area with energy. If the pain or sensation moves to another place, go to where it is strongest. Keep working until there is no longer pain or sensation. If they know they have a weak organ, infuse that area with energy. This is how you work on yourself as well. Just have someone else measure your alignment. You can work on yourself or teach someone else how to help you. Bio-energy healing is so easy and so wonderful.

Cautions

You can never harm anybody with bio-energy. Their body will use all the energy it can get and when it can't use any more, it simply won't accept it. The only caution is that when you start healing people and begin to experience healing miracles, you may begin to think that you are a great healer. Of course, everyone is a great healer, but actually, it's the energy that does the healing. If you think you are doing the healing, then you may become egoistic. If ego is involved, then it's possible to take on the karma of the one being healed. You don't want to do that. As you are streaming energy, it's best to be in the no-mind state. In a later chapter, I'll explain states of consciousness and states of mind. Just be simple, like a child. Enjoy the miraculous effects of the energy as it heals. It's awe inspiring.

There is also a deeper aspect to healing. Understand that people have physical or other problems for many reasons. Sometimes the problem itself is the only way they can learn a lesson they're trying to learn. In that case, it would not be appropriate to take that lesson away from them. So one aspect of healing is getting people to discover what it is they are trying to learn. Of course, if we are compassionate, then we think we should try to fix everybody. But our fixing could cause other problems if we are preventing people from learning and growing. So, whether you are working with yourself or others, examine the deeper issues involved and try to learn the deeper lessons.

This will be explained in more detail in a later chapter about patterns and mental healing. In every case, you always want people to grow and learn by helping them to see the deeper causes of their conditions. If you can help them in this way, they won't have to re-create a similar problem to learn what they need to learn. Oftentimes, fortunately, as a person heals they internally process the deeper causes and reasons and they are able to grasp the lessons on their own. Sometimes you can help, but not everyone is open to getting to the root causes of their problems.

Other Sources of Energy

There are other ways to gather energy. We began our healing procedure with sweeping awareness through our own body, but we can bring energy to us in other ways, just using the power of intention. The sky is full of tremendous energy. Think of how much energy is in the wind and lightning. The sun is constantly infusing energy into the atmosphere. You can use sky energy just through attention and intention. See the sky energy streaming into your body as a sparkling golden light. Then you can stream it from your hands or fingers to wherever you want it to go. You can also stream energy directly from the source to the person you are working on, and to yourself at the same time if you like. The Earth itself is also bursting with energy. Many people consider the sun, the planets, and especially mother Earth to be conscious energies. Regardless of your beliefs, there is no doubt that planet Earth, with its electrically-charged sky and life-charged surface, ionosphere, northern lights, lightning, winds, and oceans is full of energy. You can utilize all these Earth energies to assist in healing.

You can also draw energy from trees. You can stream energy from any or all these energy sources and then utilize it for healing purposes. Usually, you won't need any more energy than these Earth sources can provide, but if you do need more energy you can draw it directly from the sun. The sun has lots of energy! It's also a warming energy. If you want cooling energy you can draw it from the moon. It's fun to experiment. Just be light and receptive to possibilities. Later, when I talk about consciousness, quantum mechanics, and the mind, I'll introduce other options. Life is much more amazing than we know.

Emotional States Can Boost Healing

The emotional state that you are in can inhibit or boost healing. I always tell people to stream healing energy in the same way a devoted mother goes to her crying child, with loving, caring attention. Be in a state of loving compassion. Pure, innocent, compassionate love is the best emotional state to be in for healing ourselves or others. Be innocent like a child and compassionate like a loving mother.

Another effective emotional state is gratitude. If we don't happen to feel very loving and compassionate, we can always find something to be grateful for. Gratitude is a wonderful state to cultivate. There are other emotional states that you could use. Anything that puts you into a high, pure, light, transcendent, and caring space will work.

Other Ways to Stream Energy

I explained streaming energy out of your palms and your fingers. But that's not the only way. One extraordinary way to stream energy is to stream energy directly from your heart. You can even stream it from both your hands and heart at the same time. This is a much more powerful method than streaming energy only from your hands. Streaming energy from your heart is natural. Just visualize it going where you want it to go. You could think of it as a sparkling golden-white light beaming to where it is needed.

Distance Healing

Bio-energy is not like the energy of classical physics. As I mentioned, ordinary forms of energy like light, electromagnetic radiation, and sound, all dissipate rapidly with distance, since they radiate in all directions. They actually decrease in intensity with the square of the distance. Bio-energy is not like that. It goes exactly where it's directed, so distance doesn't matter.

One way to heal at a distance is to create a ball of energy between your hands and simply imagine the person, or the part of the body you want healed, between your hands. Another way is to envision the energy from your hands or your heart streaming directly to where it is needed. Visualization is a powerful technique to direct energy. Awareness, attention, and intention direct bio-energy to where you want it. Visualization is one method of focusing your attention. Practice distance healing on friends, family, and animals. Animals often respond quickly to bio-energy healing, as do children. Distance healing can be as effective or even more effective than hands-on healing. I often heal crying children while waiting in line at stores. Nobody knows how it happens, but I'm sure the parents feel relieved!

Multiple Healers

You get faster results when more people work together on a single person. Everyone in your family can become a bio-energy healer. Whoever needs help can get help from everyone. Just have them read this section of the book. Many people working together have even reversed stage-four cancer. Even celebrities like Dr. Oz have said that energy medicine is the future of medicine – but it's not really medicine. Its healing, the energy basis of natural healthcare. The world view of what is possible is expanding. There will come a time when we look back upon the medical world as it is now and realize how far back in the dark ages it was in many ways.

Energizing Food, Water, and Plants

In addition to healing people and animals with energy, you can also stream energy into food, water, and plants. When food and water are energized, they are healthier to consume. Energizing plants helps them to grow more abundantly and makes cut flowers last longer.

Advanced Healing Techniques

Some people feel that crystals can amplify bio-energy for this kind of work. In this method, bio-energy is streamed through a quartz crystal or other crystal. Hold the crystal in your palm and stream energy through the crystal just as you would if you were using your palm or fingers. I have experienced this phenomenon and find that sometimes crystals really can help. It's interesting, but of course, it's not necessary.

It's possible to heal multiple conditions at the same time or multiple people at the same time. All you need to do is visualize a streamer going to each condition and to each person from a central point. For instance, you can visualize a golden glowing ball of light in front of you. Then, by sending energy from your heart into that iridescent orb of light, see the energy going to each healing location through golden-light energy streamers. It happens just as you set it up. The universe is intelligent. It will happen just as you intend it to happen.

You can even radiate compassionate, loving energy to the whole world or any part of the world that needs help. Send energy from your heart to wherever it's needed. It's more powerful than you can imagine and it's one practical thing you can do to help the planet.

Primordial Structures: Primordial Skeleton and Primordial Brain

The three most complex bones in the body are the *sphenoid bone*, the *temporal bone,* and the *occipital bone*. They are among the first bones to be created before we are born. I call these bones, the cradle of the brain. These three bones make up the lower frontal part of the skull behind the eyes and behind the mouth. They form the lower frontal skull (sphenoid), the lower sides of the skull (temporal), and the bottom and lower back of the skull (occipital). These three bones exert significant control over your whole skeletal structure. They house and protect the primordial central and lower brain – the cradle of the brain.

The central brain is the most powerful and extraordinary part of the brain. It contains amazing structures that will be covered in a later chapter. The central brain and lower part of the brain, including the cerebellum at the lower back of the brain, control the physiological functions of the body. The cerebellum contains more cells than all the other parts of the brain combined.

The important thing to understand is that by streaming energy into these three bones and into the primordial brain, the whole body can be brought into alignment and balance. The whole skeletal structure will become aligned, including the spine and hips, and all the physiological processes of the body will come into balance. If you stream energy from the heart into this region, remarkable healing takes place. Search the Internet for images of these three bone structures, so that you will know what you are working on. Also, search the Internet for images of the brain, so you can see the various parts. There are many images to look at, more than I could ever include in a book.

In addition to streaming energy into these three bones, and into the lower and midbrain, you can also stream energy into the brain stem, the whole spine, and the hips. In this way, you are energizing the whole primordial structure of the body. You are energizing the whole nervous system and nervous system pathways to all the organs of the body. Of course, you can always energize any of the organs of the body individually. It would be a good idea to learn the positions of the endocrine system and all the various organs of the body. There are many graphical resources on the Internet. If you know of any organ that is weak, you can stream energy into that organ.

Psychic Surgery

Psychic surgery is an energetic form of surgery. There are three kinds. To understand this, you first need to realize that everything is energy. If you study quantum physics, you learn that matter is not what you think it is. In school, we all learned about molecules and atoms and the components of atoms – electrons, protons, and neutrons. As the understanding of the physical world deepened through greater research, physicists discovered that protons, electrons, and neutrons were not the fundamental building blocks. They are made out of even finer subatomic particles, of which many have been discovered and still others postulated. They include quarks, muons, neutrinos, mesons, photons, gluons, bosons, and more.

As physicists delved even deeper into the structure of reality, they found that particles were not really particles, but simply congealed forms of energy. Even so, the space between "particles" is vast empty space, similar to the space between the planets in our solar system. Planets are tiny compared to the space between them. Likewise, the space between energy-particles of matter is also vast. This allows us to see through some forms of solid matter. We can see through glass for instance, even though it's "solid." How "solid" matter actually appears or reacts, and which of it's characteristics change, depends upon the frequency with which it vibrates. This vibration can be altered by consciousness and bio-energy.

Classic Psychic Surgery

The first form of psychic surgery is the real thing. It's extremely rare. There are some people, specially trained in the Philippines and perhaps elsewhere, who have the ability to reach inside the body with their hand and remove unwanted material. What makes this possible is that they have developed the ability to alter the structure of matter and to alter the structure of their own body. I have met only one such person and have no contact information. I have not learned it and can't teach it. It would require extensive training. I mention it because it exists. It's related to the supernormal abilities that some yogis develop and that some founders of different religions expressed.

Placebo Psychic Surgery

The second form of psychic surgery is a fake form of the first. But that doesn't mean it doesn't work. The so-called surgeon pretends to do the surgery and reveals some tissue, like the gizzard of a chicken, and tells the patient that he has removed the offending problem. He is like a magician using sleight-of-hand. The way it actually works is through the placebo effect. As part of clinical trials, medical researchers found that giving a pill to someone, even if it was inert, often cured people just as well, or even better than an actual drug, but without side effects. Oftentimes the placebo effect was more powerful, more effective, than "real" medicine. In trials, medical placebo surgery by M.D.'s was shown to be as effective as the real thing. Belief can have a powerful effect on us. If we believe that we are healed, we can actually be healed. Essentially, this is mind over matter. The placebo effect should not be discounted. It is often at least 30% successful, even up to 60-75% successful or more. The placebo effect is likely the basis of much of the faith-based healing experienced in religious circles. As Hippocrates, the father of Western medicine said, "The mind is the great healer."

The way the placebo effect works is that belief alters body chemistry and creates healing effects. Everyone is familiar with the concept of how thoughts create emotions and sometimes powerful hormonal changes (e.g. infatuation). Through powerful impactful thoughts or beliefs, positive changes in body chemistry can regulate and enhance the healing process. I don't recommend that you use this technique on anyone. In our sophisticated society, people could be offended if they found that you were using what they might interpret as deception. It's better to explain to them what the placebo effect is, how powerful it is, and how they can consciously use it by reprogramming their own belief patterns. You can decide what you want to believe. You can use mental conviction to heal yourself. This is particularly true when you understand the nature of quantum physics and the nature of reality. As described earlier, thought directs energy and is capable of reprogramming body chemistry. Life force energy is the bridge between thought and matter.

Etheric Psychic Surgery

This is a method of psychic surgery that you can use and practice on yourself and others. You already understand that you are more than a physical body. You have an energy body (etheric body) as well, sometimes referred to as the etheric double. You can operate on this body through visualization and intention just as you do with your physical body.

When there is a physical problem in the body, there is also a problem with the corresponding etheric component of the body. You can do surgery on this etheric component using your own etheric body. Simply reach into the other person's body using your etheric hand to grab and remove the etheric component of the problem. When that part of the body no longer has the etheric, bio-energy support, the physical problem withers away. This is all done with visualization. You can either remove the offending component, or you can energize the area with such intense life energy that the offending tissue is no longer compatible, which brings about a correction. Basically, if there is extra unwanted tissue, you remove it. If the body tissue is supposed to be there, but is not functioning properly, you want to transmute or energize it. Restore the etheric complement to its perfection.

Be aware that you do not want to take on anyone else's problems. When you are helping someone, ideally, you want to be in the no-mind, or egoless state, which is explained in the chapter on mental healing. The state of compassion or gratitude is also good. Remember, if you are working on another person, they somehow *created* this problem. You want to help them to understand how they created it and what the lesson is they wanted to learn. If you just take the problem away without them learning what they need to learn, it could be a disservice. Always help people to heal on all five levels.

The same is true with your own healing. This is a fundamental concept that makes this form of natural healthcare extraordinary – every regenerative method adds to greater healing potential. We don't depend upon a single technique. Several methods working together creates a synergistic effect. Let's say that a particular technique could heal 20% of the problem. If you add another technique with 20% potential, then together, because of synergy, you may have a 50% or 60% success. Add a few more regenerative techniques on more levels and you could have a strong 100%. I used this approach to heal a problem with my wife when her inner ear filled with fluid and she couldn't hear from her right ear. By combining several techniques together, including the etheric surgery, her problem was resolved completely when nothing else could help. There were not even any good medical alternatives.

Comparing Approaches

There is a tendency in both society and the medical world, to think that techniques like etheric surgery are just hocus-pocus, fake, and useless. Yet visualization and energy techniques have enjoyed tremendous success worldwide, especially when combined with other regenerative methods. At trade fairs and expos I used to set up a booth to demonstrate bio-energy healing and would heal over 100 people per day of their long standing problems. This is nothing special, anyone can do it if they know how to stream bio-energy to where it's needed.

There is also a tendency in society to think that if the natural methods don't work, we always have the medical solution as a backup. We think that allopathic medicine is *real* medicine, real healthcare.

What many people don't know or realize is how much of a failure the medical system is. There was an intensive cancer study into the effectiveness of chemotherapy for adults. It lasted over 12 years and was reported in the Journal of Clinical Oncology. The study demonstrated that chemotherapy was a failure 97% of the time. Why is it still used? It makes a lot of money and they have nothing else to offer. Even worse, because allopathic medicine uses primarily destructive methods, it creates much bigger problems when they combine therapies. They do get a synergy effect, but negatively. Combine three options with 20% potential, and you may get 5% success because of the destructive nature of most allopathic techniques.

Remember, all healing is really self-healing, and it requires a transformation on many levels – physical, bio-energetic, emotional, mental, and consciousness. The more levels you work on, and the more regenerative methods you apply, the more powerful the healing potential will be.

Teach Natural Healthcare for Self Empowerment

Bio-energy healing is a wonderful skill and it's possible to help so many people, but there's something even better – teaching people how to heal themselves. We've all grown up in a culture where we are taught to be powerless, to run to experts whenever we need help. When you heal other people, in a way, you are teaching them to be powerless, to rely on someone else instead of themselves. It's okay to heal people, but as soon as possible, you want to empower them to heal themselves. Give them their power back.

No one is powerless. We all have the power to heal ourselves and to heal others. As an initial compassionate offering to others, it's good to do healing. It teaches them that bio-energy is real and that healing is possible. Once they know that, encourage them to take their power back and learn to heal themselves. Pay it forward. We can multiply the number of healers and heal the whole world.

How do we go about healing ourselves? Everything you've learned about healing so far applies to you also. Start with paying attention to the sensations of pain or tension in your body. Learn to listen to your body and discover the underlying causes of your problems. Then go to work.

1) First rate your pain, sensation, or condition on a scale from 1 to 10, with 10 being the worst. This gives you a starting point. Often when you are healed, you even forget how much pain you were in originally. If you rate it first, you will have a scale to measure how much transformation has taken place.

2) Build up the bio-energy to work with by over-breathing and/or streaming energy from any of the sources described earlier.

3) Align and energize your primordial structure. Stream energy from your heart (you can also use your hands for areas that are easy to reach) – A) Stream energy into your central and lower brain. B) Stream energy into the bones that make up the cradle of the brain C) Stream energy into the brainstem and spine D) Stream energy into the hips. No matter what your condition, or what you want to work on, it's valuable to do this basic alignment and energizing of your whole structure.

4) Scan your body for sensations of pain or tension. The original pain or tension may be gone or may have changed in some way. Re-scan to find the area of greatest pain or sensation. Start streaming energy into that location. If it's comfortable to reach with your hands, you can place your hands on the affected area. You can work with your etheric hands. Otherwise, use distance healing on yourself. Visualize the affected area inside a ball of energy between your hands. You can also stream energy from your heart to anywhere in your body. Heart energy is so nurturing, so powerful, so effective. You can use it in lieu of all other techniques. Remember, bio-energy is not a dead energy, it is alive. It carries with it the intelligence behind all life. You don't have to be particularly precise. It is your attention

and intention which directs the energy. The energy knows what to do to carry out your intention.

5) As you work, you can feel the transformation in the affected region. You may also be able to sense the transfer of energy. When energy is no longer flowing, you can either boost the energy by breathing more deeply (to break through to a new level), or stop streaming the energy, if the condition is sufficiently healed. Remember, you can draw from many sources of energy.

You are more powerful than you realize. Bio-energy healing is a way to restore your mind and body and reclaim your original power. Continue to work on any area of weakness until it is made strong.

Summary of Bio-Energy Healing

1) First learn bio-energy healing by working with others. Practice with a partner and learn together. Listen carefully and discover the needs of the person you are working with. (All the lessons you learn will also apply to your self healing.)

2) Have them rate their condition on a scale from 1 to 10, either as pain level, sensation of tension/pressure, or degree of disability it causes, 10 being the worst. Explain to them how pain is a cry from their body for their loving attention, and for them to willingly go into that place while breathing deeply. Explain how the pain can temporarily increase before it dissipates and goes away. It can also move to a new area, and if it does, they should tell you where the pain is now most intense so you can help there.

3) Gather the energy you need for healing through breathing, visualization, and intention. Allow the energy to fill your body.

4) Infuse yourself with loving emotions of compassion, gratitude, or another high transcendent state. Be in the no-mind, silent-mind state.

5) Stream the energy into the affected area from your palms, fingers, and/ or heart. On every person, begin by streaming energy into the primordial structures. Check their body for alignment.

6) Check with them periodically to learn of their progress.

7) Continue to flood their body, or affected area, with energy.

8) Through gauging the sensation of energy flow and through intuition, determine if they have taken as much energy as their system will allow at this time. Try boosting the energy to see if you can break through to a new level of energy acceptance.

9) When their condition has been minimized, and energy stops flowing, end the session.

10) Listen with care to their story and discover the underlying lesson they are trying to learn. Help them to break through to a new understanding of themselves. Explain to them that the energy does the healing and they can easily learn to heal themselves and others.

11) Now apply all these lessons to yourself. Always begin with the primordial structures. Then work on each area that needs help, starting with the areas of greatest pain, sensation, or imbalance. Constantly use your intuition to refine how you work with yourself.

Bio-Energy Healing Using Acupressure and Marma Points

Another form of bio-energy healing works with the energy that flows along the meridians and the associated energy vortexes or points along these meridians. There are various points on the surface of the body that, when stimulated, create biochemical, hormonal, and neurochemical changes. They transform your inner pharmacy to dramatically accelerate healing. Point therapy is known in China as *Acupressure* and *Acupuncture* and as *Marma* therapy in India's system of healing known as Ayurveda. A limited version in the West is called Trigger Point therapy. Activating or clearing various points balances the energy forces in the body, refines the nervous system, enhances the endocrine system, and improves major organ systems, and ultimately heals the whole body.

The energy channels are called meridians. Numerous points lie along these meridians that control various areas and organs of the body. To balance the meridians, selected points are stimulated with heat, needles, or pressure. An acupuncturist may use needles or heat, but pressure is a do-it-yourself method that is wonderfully effective. Plus, it costs nothing! It's easy to locate the points that need work because the points where energy is excessive or blocked are sensitive to pressure. That's nature's way of telling you of problem areas. Using your own sensitivity offers opportunities to heal points and meridians that are not even known or charted.

Pressing, Squeezing, Tapping, Patting, Slapping, Rapping, Thumping, Pounding, Digging

There are many different techniques for working with the points and meridians. If these points are massaged, pressed, or lightly pounded with your fingertips, knuckles, or hand, or even with a massaging device, it breaks up the congestion. The amount of pressure used in pressing or squeezing can range as high to 10-15 pounds and can be held for 5-10 seconds, a minute, or longer. Tapping or lightly patting a point can be done for 30 seconds to 20 minutes or more. Slapping creates a slight stinging sensation similar to the use of acupuncture needles. When thumping or pounding, you should hear a decided thud sound. It also has lymphatic benefits. Digging means to probe deeply into a knotted, congested point to break up the congestion.

None of these techniques should leave physical marks or bruises behind, perhaps a little redness only. Some of the Classical Chinese Medicine techniques such as Paida are overly intense. I consider them to be too intense, even brutal. Although such techniques can work, they often leave broken capillaries and patches of blood under the skin, which they claim is beneficial and therapeutic. Those areas do clear over time, but I don't recommend such harsh techniques. They are not necessary. In this book's introduction I described the experience of an elderly woman who simply used a modest patting technique for an extended period of 30 minutes, a few times a day. She practiced this technique at the elbows, behind the knees, and on GV-14 (at the C7 vertebra). She also practiced a unique body-opening stretching exercise – lying down with arms over her head, and one leg lifted vertically, resting against a support (alternating left/right). She eliminated her cataracts and other visual problems by lightly patting her closed eyes. Such a simple regimen, consistently followed for months, produced the miraculous results.

One of the interesting things about natural healthcare, as opposed to the medical approach, is that although some techniques work slower, they are more thorough. Plus, they actually work. Oftentimes, the way to create success with natural healthcare is simply persistence. Simple techniques such as acupressure can have dramatically positive and curative effects. Combining several techniques works even better.

Acupressure – A Great Do-It-Yourself Technique

Even if you know nothing about acupressure, marma therapy, meridians, or trigger point therapy, you can still be extremely effective. Your body is always telling you where to work through pressure sensitivity. You know what needs work better than anyone, because you can feel it.

The beauty of this system is that you don't have to know anything. All you have to do is scan your body using pressure. Simply press with modest force using your fingers or any blunt instrument. I've often used smooth seashells or river rocks as natural blunt massagers. A pencil eraser works for small areas. Golf balls work as rollers to locate sensitive areas. Give yourself a nice shiatsu acupressure massage using two tennis balls stuffed in a thin sock or nylon hosiery. Lie down with them positioned on each side of your spine. With a little practice, you can move up and down and side to side to work the points along your spine. Many natural food stores and bath & body boutiques in local malls have foot rollers, handheld pressure rollers, and various shapes of blunt tools for massage/acupressure. Massage stores carry various body-work tools. Look for a store in your area.

One popular self-massage and acupressure tool for hard-to-reach areas is the Backnobber, a large S-curved device with blunt ends. It's excellent for working on your own back and neck. An Internet search will locate many sellers of this and other massage/acupressure tools if you can't find a local source. Even the curved end of an ordinary old-fashioned walking cane or umbrella cane can be used for the neck and shoulders when nothing else is available. Find your own collection of tools and go to work. It can bring amazing relief from both tension and pain, and also helps to restore your inner pharmacy.

Pressure scan your whole body. When you find a place that hurts a little, work on that specific location with any of the techniques mentioned, to "work out" the blockage in that area. Draw a simple gingerbread man outline to map your body, front and back. Mark the places of sensitivity to remind you of what needs work. As part of your daily regimen, *press, squeeze, tap, pat, slap, rap, thump, pound, or dig* into these points to keep them clear. When a location is no longer sensitive when pressed, then the blockage has been released. If you bruise easily, be gentle. Work up to using more substantial methods. If you are ever injured or bruised in an accident and start to develop black and blue marks, or a sprained muscle, repeated gentle squeezing can often reverse the injury from turning into a bruise. Gentle squeezing repetition can often clear the problem within 5-15 minutes. You can also stream energy into any location that needs help.

When you scan for pressure sensitivity, don't be surprised to find many locations that need work. Most people have lots of stress and energy imbalances. If you are interested in learning more about the locations of the meridians and acupuncture points, an inexpensive chart can be purchased from http://www.permacharts.com. Search their site for "acupuncture" to locate the chart. Sometimes college bookstores have these charts. They also have summary charts on a few alternative health subjects such as homeopathy and herbs that may be of interest. The study of acupuncture or marma therapy is a discipline in itself. But you don't need to study in order to derive the benefits when working on yourself. Let your body be your guide.

If you want to go deeper and learn what various points do, portable devices like cell phones and tablets now have apps for acupuncture/ acupressure points.

Remember, you don't really need to know anything, just work on the sensitive points of your body. Eventually, all the blocks will be released.

Reflexology

Have you ever wondered why a foot massage feels so good? It's because it heals your body. Your body says, "More! I like this!" Reflexology is like a heavy-duty foot massage, essentially a form of acupressure, but its focus is the feet. It goes deeper than superficial massage. Maps of the organs of your body exist on your feet, hands, ears, face, scalp, tongue, and lips. These maps contain a microcosm of your whole body and are used in Chinese medicine and Ayurveda as integral parts of those healing systems. Pressure applied to small areas on each of these "maps" reflex to other parts of the body breaking up energy imbalances. Feet and hands are very effective.

As with acupressure therapy, when you press certain points, they may be quite sensitive. With foot reflexology, sometimes there is a sharp jarring pain as the area reacts to the pressure. These painful spots are often congested with uric acid crystals and must be worked until the crystals disappear, even if it hurts a bit. You don't have to do it all at once, in fact it's rarely possible. Work to your level of tolerance. Pain is especially noticeable underneath the toes, and at their tips. Uric acid crystals build up in these locations and block nerve and meridian energy. Breaking up these deposits improves the flow, and while it may hurt somewhat to break up these points of congestion, you will feel a sense of peace and balance following the session for several days to follow. Some people like to do foot and hand massage every few days or at least weekly. Teaming up with a partner is a great way to share time together and help each other.

Colorful laminated reflexology charts and wallet-sized cards can be purchased from http://www.innerlightresources.com and at many health food stores. I've included a simple chart on the website that you can download.

Percussive Massage

Working with pressure, as we did with acupressure, is also something of a massage technique which has lymphatic as well as acupressure benefits. The percussive methods have tremendous value, but they can be tiring for long treatment times. There are electrical percussive massagers with many different features on the market. These devices have one or two hard rubber pounding elements that create a strong percussive massage. They are driven by an electric motor so that you don't have to work so hard. They can be really effective in moving lymph fluid and working on acupressure or marma points. They can really soothe many aches and pains from built up tension. The cheaper ones can bog down easily, so if you can afford it, purchase a strong unit. Test them out before purchasing.

Bio-Energy Healing Using the Breath

Various methods of conscious breathing can bring about extraordinary healing. In India, these breathing patterns are termed pranayama and are part of the yogic system of development, but breathing patterns have been used in every culture. In general, breathing techniques begin with vigorous breathing to infuse greater oxygen and life force into your body and often proceed to quieter, gentler techniques as a prelude to deep meditation, contemplation, or affirmation techniques. Deep breathing gives your system more power for healing. Below are some common techniques used in the yogic system.

Deep, Rapid Breathing

Begin with deep, somewhat rapid breathing until you feel slightly lightheaded. By breathing double or triple your normal breath, what I term over-breathing, you charge your system. Then level off to maintain that level of life-force (pranic) charge. Many diseases exist because of a lack of oxygen. Cancer, for instance, flourishes in a low oxygen environment. Charging the body regularly is valuable and should be done several times daily if your health is compromised. It alkalizes the pH of your body and improves many other factors.

Alternate Nostril Breathing

Ordinarily, we don't sense how much air enters through the left or right nostril. Most people think that, unless congested, air enters equally. Not so. Although we usually don't think about such things, the nature of your breath makes a huge difference in your clarity of mind and your physical and mental vitality. Special tissues in the nostrils precisely regulate airflow through the sinus cavities to manage brain and endocrine functions.

We know from brain studies that the left and right hemispheres of the brain control different functions. The left brain, for instance, is considered more logic and time oriented, while the right brain is considered to be non-linear, artistic, and timeless. When you breathe favoring one nostril, that side of the brain is stimulated accordingly. You can balance your brain's energy functions by regulating this flow.

Forms of Alternate Nostril Breathing

All forms of alternate nostril breathing use the right thumb to press and close the right nostril and the right ring finger (or ring and middle) to cover the left nostril.

1st Method: Inhale one side, switch, exhale, inhale, switch. (Switch when you're full of air) You can start more rapidly and then slow down, or just use long slow breaths.

2nd Method: Breathe in on one side, switch, exhale, switch, inhale – Same side inhalation with opposite side exhalation. After 3 breaths, reverse the process so you're breathing in on the other side. If you want to reinforce more fire in your system, continue breathing in on the right side only. This is the sun side and it can help burn away toxins and mucus. If you are overly fiery, you can breathe in on the left side, the cooling side, the moon side, and exhale on the right.

3rd Method: Breathe in and out on one side for a few breaths, switch, repeat (Same side inhale and exhale).

Generally, method 1 brings great peace, calm, and balance to mind and body. Methods 2 and 3 can be used to accentuate either hemisphere of the brain and promote heating or cooling effects. Experiment to see what helps you the most.

Ultra-Slow Breathing

If you slow your breathing down to an ultra slow level, your mind will become serene. Your mind follows your breath. Breathe in very slowly to a desired count, then breathe out to the same count. Start with 5 or 6 seconds and work up to ten seconds or more for gradually inhaling and exhaling. After being charged up with deep breathing, ultra-slow breathing really slows down the brain chatter and brings tremendous peace, If practiced for several minutes it leads to deep meditation, deep silence.

Sigh Breathing

Sigh breathing, extended exhalation, is another powerful breathing technique. Every time you breathe out, simply give a big long sigh and let yourself "melt" or unravel. Let go of all the ways you hold on physically, mentally, and emotionally. Let go of all muscle tension and effort of any kind, even the effort to think. Completely let go of control. Then just innocently observe the reactions, as if from a distance. Often what happens is a release reaction, as you are no longer "holding the lid on." These reactions can be physical, emotional, or other cathartic releases. Huge blocks of stress can be released this way. This gentle release process is a very safe and is an extraordinarily effective de-stressor. I'll come back to these breathing techniques when I talk about meditation. You can start using these techniques now, though.

Kumbhaka - Your Own Hyperbaric Oxygen Chamber

Sufficient oxygen and prana can have a powerful influence on healing. Medical centers often use hyperbaric oxygen chambers where you breathe pure oxygen under pressure. You can create your own high oxygen environment just by holding your breath for a little while after deep breathing. It's a powerful technique, so be gentle and don't overdo it. Breathe deeply for 7 breaths then hold for about 10 seconds, then exhale. Repeat up to a dozen times or more. It's better to repeat short sessions several times a day than to do long sessions less frequently. You can also hold the air out to improve the expulsion of undesirable gases. If you have strong reactions to holding your breath in or out, reduce the time and intensity until such reactions are minimal. Or discontinue the practice for a while as you practice other methods. Then come back to it.

10-Point Bio-Energy Tune Up – Basic Energy Methods

The following 10-point energy tune up incorporates several methods to heal and keep your energy body functioning normally. These are not the only methods, but they're a useful set to use daily or a few times a week. The set can be done in about 15-20 minutes. These can be used in addition to the bio-energy healing methods referred to earlier.

1) **Cook's Hookups** – Increases and balances meridian energy flow. Procedure: Put your left leg up with your foot on the right knee. Place the right hand, with palm down over the left ankle. Reach over and place the palm of your left hand centered on the ball of the left foot. Breathe deeply and hold this circuit for about a minute. You know you have it correct if your arms are crossed. Then switch and do the other side.

2) **Cross Crawl** – Stand and march in place for a minute or two. As each knee comes up, touch it with your opposite hand or wrist. Arms cross over the body. This crossing over motion has the effect of reminding the left brain to "talk" to the right side of the body and vice versa. When the brain tries to control the same side, poor coordination results, similar to the way dyslexia affects eye/brain coordination. The cross crawl can help correct many long-

standing problems associated with mind-body coordination. These first two exercises are drawn from a discipline called educational kinesiology, which includes many kinds of exercises for helping children and others overcome dyslexia and similar energy/coordination problems. For children, the exercises are often called "brain gyms." It's not a panacea, but it can be useful.

3) **Triple Thumps** – These next three techniques have the effect of balancing the meridians in the upper part of the body. Many energy-work practitioners use them. They also comes from acupressure, which itself was derived from the Indian energy healing system for awakening the "nadis." With moderate to substantial pressure, pound the following points with an audible thumping sound, using the tips of your fingers or knuckles.

Collar Bone: Locate the hollow where the two collarbones come together at the base of the neck. An inch below the hollow and 1 1/2 inches toward the outside, locate two small hollows (indentations) just below the collarbone. They are often a little sensitive to pressure. Pound these two points with the fingers of both hands for 30 seconds to a minute.

Thymus: About half way between the hollow of the throat and the end of the sternum (breast plate) is the thymus. Pound this area for 30 seconds to a minute with either hand.

Bottom Ribs: Half way between the sternum and each side of your body, on the bottom rib directly below the nipple, are the locations to activate. Pound, or thump these two points for 30 seconds to a minute.

4) **Neurolymphatic Rub** – In the upper quadrant of the chest, near the shoulder, about a hand width below the outer collarbone, is a neurolymphatic point. One on each side. Rub, or deeply massage this point. You will know where it is because it's sensitive for those who need work in this area. Activating this point will help the lymph system drain properly.

5) **Upward Flow** – This procedure is much like zipping up a winter coat. Place your hands in front of the base of the spine (at the pubic bone) and sweep both hands in an upward motion, staying in contact with the body, to a point just under your lower lip. Repeat a few more times bringing your hands to the outside and down by your side to the starting point, then again upward. This motion has the effect of bringing upward flowing energy to the body and can help you recover from fatigue. You can even do this process mentally, similar to the way you moved energy from your feet to your head when learning bio-energy healing. Use the mental version any time you feel

tired or out of sorts. This strengthens the central meridian and also flows energy up the spine to the primordial brain. Use it as a quick "pick me up" any time of day. Repeat several times in a row until you feel the energizing effect. You can mentally set this upward flow to continue on its own, just by your intention. See it properly maintaining itself.

6) **Sigh Breathing** – This technique, mentioned earlier, is amazingly powerful, though simple. Every time you breathe out, give a big long sigh. As you do, let go of everything, at least for a moment. Let go of all muscle tension, all cares, all intentions, all expectations, just drop everything. Be completely empty just for a moment. When you do, you will feel the tension melt away. Sometimes you will notice big blocks of stress quickly release. Keep this sigh breathing going for at least a minute or so and you will experience a release throughout your whole mind and body.

7) **Holding Fingers** – Nearly a hundred years ago in Japan, a man named Jiro Murai rediscovered an ancient healing art drawn in part from the ancient Kojiki records. His body was wracked with disease. With no resources at his disposal, he was left to die. All he could do was lie down, fast, and wait to die. He had heard of an ancient technique, which is simply holding each finger, one at a time – just wrapping your palm around the end of each finger, just behind the nail. He tried it. After 6 days of fasting and doing this technique, his body heated up and all diseases were immediately purged from his body. He expanded the method to include numerous ways of unblocking energy by holding points on the body. He named the healing system Jin Shin Jytsu. In this system there are 26 primary body points, but much of the healing can be activated simply by holding the fingers as Jiro Murai did. The palm, as we know from many systems, is energized. By simply folding your palm around each finger, one at a time, you reinvigorate the whole body by activating the meridians that begin at the tips of the fingers. You can do this anywhere, anytime.

8) **Awareness Bath** – Thought directs energy, so thought can be used to bring about energetic effects in the body. When you localize your attention in any part of your body, it brings a healing influence. Procedure: 1) Move your awareness or attention from the top of your head slowly down through your body, then back up to the head. It's as if you were passing a hoop or ball of awareness from head to toe and back. Let your awareness move slowly and note any areas of anomaly – extra sensation or lack of ability to sense any part of your body. Spend more time in areas of anomaly – excess, deficit, or inconsistency. 2) Make a tall hoop, as tall as your body, but instead of

moving top-bottom-top, as you just did, move it left and right. Start in the center with a hoop as tall as your body. Move it from the center of your body to the left side, then over to the right side and back to center. Slowly pass it back and forth from left to right. Finish in the center. 3) Now move the hoop of awareness front to back. Start at the center, move to the front of your body, then to the back of your body, then back to center. Allow your awareness in each motion to extend a couple of feet beyond the boundaries of the body as well. End the practices with your awareness at the top of your head and keep your awareness there throughout the day.

9) **Chakra Energizing and Purification** – There are energy vortexes, called chakras (pronounced with a hard ch not sh), which feed energy into the body. There are hundreds of them like miniature tornados. There are 7 large primary centers that meet along the spine (see chart). They are actually quite complex structures. If you could see subtle energy, you would see that the chakras are different colors. Search the Internet for IMAGES of the chakras for both front view and side views if you a curious about them.

#	Location	Name	Color	Emotions that Lock / Unlock
7	Crown of Head	Sahasrāra	Violet	Discontentment / Gratitude & Contentment
6	Between Eyebrows	Ājñā	Indigo	Seriousness, Egotism, Arrogance / Innocence, Simplicity, Unselfishness
5	Throat	Vishuddhi	Blue	Comparison, Jealousy / Realizing your Uniqueness
4	Heart	Anāhata	Green	Craving Love & Attention / Selfless Love w/o Expectation
3	Navel	Manipūraka	Yellow	Worry, Anxiety / Awareness, Non-Resistance, Letting Go
2	2-3" Below Navel	Swādhishthāna	Orange	Fear, Fear of Death / Acceptance of Death, Knowledge of Death
1	Base of Spine	Mūlādhāra	Red	Fantasy, Expectation / Welcoming and Accepting Reality

The 7 chakras are connected with the endocrine system. Each one also controls an emotional aspect of yourself. The chakras range in size from as small as a coat button to the size of a cart wheel, depending upon how closed or open it is. Note the colors and positions of the chakras in the chart.

The 7th chakra, violet, enters into the top of the head. The 1st chakara, red, comes up from the bottom entering into the base of the spine. The other five (numbers 2-6, orange through indigo) are roughly horizontal. They enter the body along the spine with a pair of vortexes opening up in front of and behind the body. The points of the funnels touch the spine.

The only important thing to know for our purposes now is that you can activate and purify your chakras by your intention, by flooding them with bio-energy and consciously energizing them.

Techniques: Using visualization, consciously flood each of these chakras with your awareness, starting from the bottom (#1). Spend a minute or so with each. Move up to the next, one at a time, until you reach the top. Visualize them as energized, relaxed, and open. Have the intention that each is in perfect harmony with your life purpose. Another method is to see each chakra bathed in a ball of brilliant light. Visualize each chakra as pure, energized, and radiating bliss. Always complete working with all seven chakras – never leave it half done. You can then visualize the whole spine immersed in brilliant light.

10) **Acupressure Tune-Up** – Continue clearing any of your previously found acupressure hotspots.

Summary

Now you have many practical ways to heal yourself, and to heal others using bio-energy to enhance the energies of your body. Take the time you need to practice these techniques and enrich your life and the lives of others. These methods are a primary energetic defense against illness and a powerful way to regenerate your health and the health of others. Keeping your energetic body functioning smoothly helps you stay alert, energetic, and focused.

Action Plan - Chapter 9, Bio-Energy Healing

1. Grab your calendar and schedule the techniques you want to use.
2. Trade healing sessions with family members. Schedule them.
3. Schedule time to experiment with breath and energy techniques. When tense, use deep breathing techniques.
4. Practice bio-energy healing by streaming energy through your body and out the palms of your hands.
5. Practice bio-energy healing by streaming energy from your heart.
6. Practice aligning people's skeletal structure and eliminating their pains and headaches.
7. Be aware of the cautions of healing others.
8. Practice collecting healing energy from other natural sources.
9. Practice culturing emotional states to boost healing.

10. Practice distance healing. Especially work on animals. Stream energy to crying children while waiting in line. It often helps.

11. Practice advanced healing on multiple people, multiple conditions, or both. You can even radiate compassion or love from the heart to the whole world, or any part of the world that needs compassionate support.

12. Practice advanced healing on the *primordial structures*. Search the Internet for images of the sphenoid bone, the temporal bone, the occipital bone, and the brain so that you know what you are working on.

13. Practice acupressure, reflexology, and percussive massage.

14. Practice healing with various breathing techniques. 1) Deep, Rapid Breathing, 2) Alternate Nostril Breathing, 3) Ultra-Slow Breathing, 4) Sigh Breathing, 5) Holding Breath In and Out.

15. Put the 10-Step Energy Tune-Up on your daily or weekly agenda. Make a reminder. 1) Cook's Hookups, 2) Cross Crawl, 3) Triple Thumps, 4) Neurolymphatic Rub, 5) Upward Flow, 6) Sigh Breathing, 7) Holding Fingers, 8) Awareness Bath, 9) Chakra Energizing, Opening, Purifying, 10) Acupressure Tuneup

Chapter 10
Emotional Healthcare

Healing Painful Emotions and Emotional Traumas

A Guide to Restoring Peace and Creating Enthusiasm for Life

What to Expect

When you heal your emotional body you will have peace. You become lighter in spirit. You carry yourself in the world with dignity and grace. You have compassion for those who are still gripped by harsh emotional realities. You feel in command of yourself and your life. Emotions no longer dictate your responses to others or towards yourself. You enjoy a sublime life of fulfillment and inner joy. Yet, you have access to any emotional state that is required by any situation. You have freedom of heart. Mental acuity will increase and you will see the connections between destructive mental habits and the emotional states they create.

Emotions and Their Impact

Emotional stress causes an overload on your system. When you can't handle an emotion, it gets stored in your system for future review. As long as these emotions are embedded in your physiology, they continue to reduce the quality of your life. They accelerate aging. They severely affect your relationships. Emotions affect the health of both your mind and body.

When you hear sad news you have physical reactions. You slump over, you may cry. Your immune system is depressed. Driven "Type A" personalities often have heart attacks. Cancer is often a product of depression, among several other causes that weaken the body. People who are addicted obviously have deep cravings, strong emotional attachments. All these emotions cause endocrine changes that chemically alter the body. Diseases, both physical and mental, flourish because of negative emotional states. It makes sense to address your emotional life and take steps to reverse destructive emotions.

Negative emotions are not stopped either by opposing them or unconsciously venting them. Neither suppression nor indulgence works. This has been very hard for western doctors, psychologist, and psychiatrist to understand. Most talk therapy approaches to emotional healthcare try to uncover suppressed emotions in order to "release" them. While some intellectual understanding may result, and some release can take place, the process, more often, usually renews the experience, re-infecting the emotional body. People are sometimes in therapy for years. They understand their condition completely, but they still have it. There are better ways.

Ordinarily, we resist feeling painful or negative emotions like anger, hate, frustration, anxiety, addictions, and cravings. We have been taught to suppress these types of emotions, because they are "bad." The conservative, religious, moralist types of people condemn these kinds of emotions. We are all taught to be good, and we always try to be good people. So, in order to be good, we suppress the "bad stuff." The problem is, suppressing emotions doesn't work.

Commercial interests, on the other hand, always try to get you to indulge in your emotions. They have a financial incentive to get you addicted to whatever they're selling. Their sales pitch usually includes sex, food, alcohol, nicotine, caffeine, or drugs. The problem is, indulgence also doesn't work. You can never find fulfillment by either resisting pain or indulging in pleasures.

Commercial interests are often extremely devious. For instance, in some countries with strong moral leanings, tobacco companies would secretly go in and tell the priests to tell their followers not to smoke cigarettes. They knew from psychological studies, that if they could get people to resist smoking, to suppress, they would soon become addicted. Soon millions of people were addicted to cigarettes. The same method works when you say, don't do drugs. The "Say No to Drugs" campaign has no doubt created many addicts, because it puts the idea of drugs "do drugs" in their awareness. It's a proven principle that we don't hear the words "no" and "don't."

The same is true with addiction to sex. We have all seen news stories of priests and preachers, who because of their suppression and denial of sexual cravings, drove the addiction deeper, often to the point of perversion.

The reason that resisting and suppressing emotions, or venting and expressing emotions doesn't work is that they are resisted or indulged in unconsciously, without full awareness. It's an unconscious pattern that is instilled in us in our youth. When you try to push away unwanted emotions, they are impressed deeper into your system. Emotions are actually stored in your muscles and biochemistry. The same is true with indulgence. Any method that tries to subdue or release emotions without conscious awareness, fails to release them. There is a third alternative.

The third alternative is to consciously and passively watch emotio without reacting. The interesting thing about conscious awareness is is automatically healing. We don't have to do anything else, the simp consciously observing, directly heals emotional pain and suffering. I'll explain in a minute.

Emotions can be positive or negative. Positive emotions such as enthusiasm and inspiration are the driving force behind all accomplishment. Without them, in an emotionless state, we have no purpose to life, no expression of life force. That means you can't heal emotional causes of disease by becoming emotionless. You would have a dry life.

Negative emotions restrict the expression of life and prevent you from becoming who you are meant to be. Negative emotions are actually "wake up" calls as to what is happening in your life. They are a kind of barometer. When your life is off track, negative emotions are a corrective force, an indicator that makes you stop and take notice of the situation. Negative emotions tell you that you have an unresolved situation in your life and that you need to go about life differently. Ultimately, you heal negative emotions by completing them. That includes releasing the charge they hold and finding the lesson you were trying to learn. Usually a lesson is connected with some form of love and realization of oneness. Unresolved emotional turmoil is connected to ego and your sense of separation. You are required by life to heal your emotional baggage in order to have the "juice" to engage in life more abundantly.

Below are several ways to approach emotional healing that don't entail either suppression or indulgence. They also don't involve talk therapy, guilt trips, condemnation, or other unnecessary and ineffective pursuits.

Healing Negative Emotions

The the most powerful method to heal negative emotions is to willingly and consciously feel both the physical and emotional pain but observe them from the perspective of the innermost observer. Let me explain.

Emotional pain is stored in your body physically, biochemically, and psychologically. Rather than engaging the psychological aspect – all the negative chatter and stories behind your pain – you can directly release the emotional pain by allowing yourself to consciously and willingly feel and consciously observe the *physical and emotional sensations* where the emotion is stored. This is similar to the way we go about healing physical pain. Breathe deeply and flood your attention into your physical body where you feel the emotional pain or disturbance is manifesting physically as a pressure, pain, tightening, gnawing, churning, convulsing, twisting, heavy, or wrenching sensation. Where you feel physical intensity is where it's stored. Be bold. Be courageous. When you turn your attention towards it physically, your emotional pain shrinks. Generally, the pain will be in your belly or in your heart, but sometimes in the throat or somewhere along the trunk of the body. Avoid unconsciously wallowing in the psychological aspect. That just feeds it more when you become attached to it. The unenlightened mind likes to keep you in drama. Don't let it. Return to feeling. If the incident comes to mind, it's OK, but watch it from the place of the innermost observer. Don't brood or wallow in it or let it dominate.

Procedure: 1) Close your eyes. When you close your eyes, you will immediately experience some degree of peace. That's because when you close your eyes there is an immediate expansion of consciousness. In that expansion, our usual pains are smaller by comparison. Closing your eyes will also prevent you from acting out your negative emotions.

2) Breathe deeply. Breathe two or three times your normal rate. Breathe deeply until you become slightly lightheaded. At that point your body will be charged with energy.

3) Now, scan your body. When you are in an emotional upheaval, there will always be a physical disturbance of pain, pressure, or some other uncomfortable sensation.

4) Allow yourself to feel it physically. Consciously observe it as an impartial observer. Continue to stay with it. Keep your awareness localized in that place. Sensations may increase first before they subside. Continue to breathe, feel, and observe impartially. The secret to observing impartially, is to recognize that there is a space inside you that is the pure observer. In every experience there are three things going on 1) the object of observation, 2) the process of observing through one of your senses, and 3) the pure observer in the background, behind the scenes, that is always watching. That pure observer is your pure consciousness, pure awareness, and it is a place of power and intelligence that has the power to heal everything. So the secret is to let go of the dominance of the object, move back within yourself to allow the pure observer to become dominant as you focus on the physical expressions of the emotional pain.

5) Follow the pain. Often the pain will move to another place. When it does, follow it with your awareness. If you have pain in more than one area, stay with whichever pain is the most intense. Stay with it until it subsides. If

the new location is more intense, go there. Keep chasing the pain until it diminishes and dissipates.

6) Emotional pain, like physical pain, tries to control you and make you run away. When you run away, it chases you and looms larger than it really is. When you turn and face it directly, it shrinks away from you. There is nothing that can withstand the light of your conscious awareness.

This technique has extraordinary power and can even bring people who are hysterical or psychotic back to normal consciousness within minutes. This same technique also works with addictions. Allow yourself to feel the craving physically. Breathe and saturate the region with your awareness. Later, I'll describe more techniques for getting rid of addictions.

Understand, just by localizing your awareness to an area physically, healing power is directed to that place and the emotions behind it are healed. This is extraordinarily powerful. As you heal, you will often receive tremendous insights as to how your emotional pains were originally created. I'll explain more about these insights in the chapter on mental healing.

Mirror Work

This technique comes from more than one enlightened source. People sometimes wonder, "How can I discover the hidden, unconscious part of myself that is controlling me? How can I be free of the powerful hidden emotions that are messing with me?" Mirror work is one way to do that. Here's the method:

1) Whenever you are faced with an emotional upheaval in your life, sit in front of a full-length mirror, or at least one large enough to see your whole body while seated.

2) The person in the mirror is the hidden, unconscious, incomplete part of you. When you do the process with the person in the mirror, the hidden emotions come to the surface to be recognized. As you recognize the emotions and their causes with awareness, you restore the person in the mirror and restore integration with the person in front of the mirror. You bring completion to yourself, inside and out.

3) Connect with the person in the mirror. Look directly into the eyes of the person in the mirror.

4) Recall incidents and situations in your life where you experienced low-level energy and emotions such as anger, guilt, frustration, powerlessness, and agitation. These are areas of incompletion, in some form, that are affecting you in the present moment.

191

5) Take responsibility for liberating yourself from this incompletion that you have kept alive within yourself.

6) Relive those incidents and situations consciously, with full awareness. Talk aloud with the person in the mirror, look into the eyes. It's important to talk out loud. Talk about what happened, talk about how you felt. Speak your mind, speak your heart. Keep talking. Don't stop talking. Talking out loud will take you deeper into healing. New things will start coming out that you had forgotten. Keep talking. Allow any emotions to surface. All negative emotions are okay. Feel what you feel and keep talking. Each time you feel something or recall a new incident related to it, observe it with awareness, from the place of the pure observer, and keep talking. Huge volumes of negative emotions will come purging out of you. Don't worry, you are perfectly safe. If you need to cry or yell, it's okay. If your body shakes, it's okay. Stay with it.

7) Continue re-living the incidents and situations and keep talking more and more. Keep talking and looking into the eyes of the person in the mirror until you experience being free of the low-level emotions inside you. When you no longer feel an emotional charge. When you can recall those events without reactions, the negative, destructive emotions have been cleared. You may find yourself laughing.

8) Repeat this process each time you are stuck with low-level emotions related to yourself or others. This also works for all kinds of negativities, including phobias, any situation that is emotionally charged with fear, anxiety, frustration, anger, powerlessness, etc.

This is a very powerful process that can free you from many lifelong emotional barriers. Just be a little courageous to face these hidden aspects of yourself. It isn't difficult. You just have to summon your courage and do it. Although it may be uncomfortable while you do it, the benefits are more than worth it. After you've done this work with a mirror several times, you can try without a mirror. A mirror is always helpful.

Healing Your Relationships

The only way to heal your relationships is to eliminate the emotional baggage you have been carrying for years. The two techniques just presented for healing negative emotions by retracing your past emotional traumas is the only way to bring fulfillment to your relationships. You must bring them to resolution, to completion, so they no longer have an emotional charge. This is how you heal all your relationships. If you are in a relationship, first begin working on yourself. Heal yourself. Then you will find your relationships are totally changed. As you heal yourself, you will discover that all of your relationship difficulties were not just due to the other person, they had causation within yourself as well. As you heal yourself, your relationships will change. Then the people in your life may be interested in healing their own emotional pain. There is no way to have healthy, happy relationships when either you or they have a backlog of unresolved emotional traumas.

Tapping Acupressure Points

One interesting approach to dissipate unwanted emotions, especially phobias, is to unlock how they are stored in the energy body. This involves a simple acupressure technique that originates in ancient 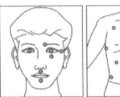 cultures, but was revived recently by psychologists. It involves tapping specific acupuncture points. You can experiment, since tapping various points does no harm if they don't resolve the imbalance. In this process, first bring the emotional situation to mind and then tap the points until the emotional intensity subsides. Points include: the inside edge of the eyebrow, the outside edge of the eye, under the eye, just under the nose, under the lip, and several points on the chest as shown (see diagrams). Then, squeeze your fingertips and toes which activates the meridians from their end points. A simple and rather complete system is to tap all these points working from top to bottom, then squeeze each fingertip, including the thumb.

Thought Replacement

Emotions follow thoughts. Change your thoughts and your emotions change. Most people wallow in emotions and believe they are a victim and cannot change the emotion. If you shift your focus of thought, your emotions WILL change. It's like turning on a light in the midst of darkness. Your inner state is the product of programming, it's software. You have the ability to reprogram it just by deciding to and then doing it.

1) The first step is to recognize the negative emotion consciously. Face that emotion, do not suppress it. Often, negative emotions come to you because you have developed a well-rehearsed habit of returning to them again and again. Depression itself is nothing but a highly reinforced habit.

2) Consciously realize that it is no longer serving you. It is not what you want.

3) Decide you are not going to fulfill it, you are going to drop it,

4) Replace it with something you do want,

5) You will need to do this each time the emotion surfaces.

When you stop feeding that emotion, it will begin to dissipate, and over time, it will no longer bother you. What you feed, grows, what you starve, dies.

If you focus on something beautiful, then beautiful emotions follow. A good plan is to have several beautiful thoughts always ready. Whenever your old emotions begin to infect you, decide not to feed them. Understand that it is no longer serving you. Bring in the new thought or thoughts without any attempt to push away the unwanted thought and emotion. Simply replace them. It takes no more energy to think a new thought that it takes to think the old thought. No force or willpower is required.

Bringing in a new element is often very effective, but you only have about 15 seconds from the time a negative intrusion begins. You must catch it and nip it in the bud. Once you start tumbling down, the weight of your negative emotions will pull you down more rapidly. If you allow yourself to fall into old patterns of negative thinking, it takes more work to climb out.

Your brain is like a computer that will accept any instructions you dictate, and it follows them. If you choose to allow and follow negative thought patterns, your brain thinks that's what you really want! When you give your consent to it, when you allow it, when you support it, it takes hold of you. The fact that it leads to suffering is an unfortunate result that is simply the product of a poor decision. If you want a different emotional state, you must choose different thoughts, make different decisions. You are the only one with the power to choose your thoughts. If you exercise that power in a sloppy way, you will reap those consequences. If you exercise that power in an intelligent way, you will reap beautiful consequences.

One way to take the power out of negative thoughts and emotions is to follow them to their logical conclusion. Whenever they arise, ask yourself, "What will be the inevitable consequence of following this line of thinking, of indulging in this emotion?" Examine the end product. Is that what you want? If not, you can see that those thoughts and emotions have no utility, no usefulness in your life. They are not going to help you. Just recognizing the futility and uselessness of pursuing such thoughts and emotions takes their power away. There is no reason to support it. When you realize the thought and emotion is illegitimate, illogical, and self-destructive, it makes it virtually impossible to support it.

The problem is, most of us choose our thoughts unconsciously. The secret is to watch your thoughts like a hawk while being in the innermost space of the pure observer. Do not continue to follow or act on any thoughts that you don't want to nurture. Pretend you are living under a wish-fulfilling tree and that every thought you think is going to come true. This is actually the case. The universe is always trying to bring you what you want and responds as though the thoughts you think are really what you want! If you don't want it, replace it with what you do want.

Old habits die with the repetition of a new habit. The new quality of thought must become your natural state. Then your computer-brain accepts the new environment of lightness, sweetness, and constructive thinking. You reprogram your brain through repetition of the thoughts you want and by clearing out the old programs that were controlling you. You can choose any thought you want. Think of three uplifting thoughts that you can use to replace your old negative conditioning. Use them quickly when you sense you're heading into dangerous territory. One could be a beautiful scene in nature, another could be the face of a young child or a loved one, another could be a beautiful flower. Think of anything that is beautiful and uplifting to you and it will work.

Or, you could just have a glass of water! You can't have two thoughts at the same time. As soon as you think of having a glass of water, the old negative thought is gone. It has been replaced. You could also substitute the opposite version of the negative thought you are having. Any new thought will work to replace the negative thought you had. Just don't follow a negative trend of thought. Replace it. Use this method in conjunction with the "Say-See-Feel-Do" method presented in the chapter on Mental Healthcare. Don't just change the thought you say in your head. See it, feel it, and act on it. In the Mental Healthcare chapter I explain the different kinds of thoughts – verbal (language), visual (images), and emotional (feelings). For now, just change to a new thought of any kind – verbal, visual, or feeling.

Attitude Shifting

It's possible to see your situation from another vantage point. See it in another context, perhaps from the other person's point of view. Pretend you're visiting a wise counselor and ask the counselor about the situation. You may think your situation is dire until you see how other people in the world live with so much less than you have. Many times they are very happy, even with very little. Life happens. We are all part of a circumstance. You may not be able to instantly change your circumstances, but misery is a choice. Happiness is also a choice. A new perspective can be totally refreshing and give you the courage to feel and act differently. You can always find something to be grateful for.

Learn the Lesson

What is it you are trying to learn from a painful experience? Learn the lesson quickly, and learn it well, so you don't have to repeat it. Behind every emotion stored in your body is an experience that once held a lesson for you. It's not the particular experience that is so important, it's the lesson. All experiences eventually result in knowledge. It's tragic to have to repeat painful experiences over and over, because you didn't "get it." Have you noticed that you meet the same kinds of people, have the same kinds of bosses, have new partners with different names, but with the same personality faults? Focus on learning. Grow. You may confront your fears and move through or away from situations, but you can never escape until you learn what you wanted to learn from them. You are here on planet Earth to learn and grow.

It's even faster to learn from the mistakes of others, so you don't have to go through so much pain yourself. Observe the choices that others make, i.e. your friends, family, and neighbors. See the consequences of their choices. Read biographies. Study history and the ancient teachings. There are many wonderful stories that teach the consequences of making poor choices and the lessons learned. You don't have to learn everything the hard way. Make it easy on yourself by gaining knowledge and culturing a pure heart.

Healing Emotions with Light, Sound, and Nature

Many conditions, like depression, can be addressed in the short term, by simply shining a specific color of light on the skin. The skin is known to have receptor cells much like the brain. Doctors already use phototherapy with premature newborn babies. They often have a weak liver, causing jaundice that can have severe consequences, even death. These babies are routinely saved by shining a blue light on their skin. I am constantly amazed that doctors never pursued what other spectrums of light can do.

Various colors of light activate skin cells in different ways. They can produce the neurochemistry necessary to resolve emotions. For instance, depression is easily lifted by shining a yellow light on as much skin as possible. A simple yellow "bug light" placed in a common arm lamp will do. An hour or so a day will reverse depression within a few days in most cases, a week or two, maximum. Still, you want to look at the other methods of emotional healing to clear the condition permanently.

Particularly, learn as much as you can from the experience that triggered the emotion. There is a related method that also works. It may stretch your belief system and our current science, but it really does work. Water can carry light information. Interestingly, if you shine the light on water and drink the water, it will have a similar effect as shining the light on the skin. The same neurological chemicals are produced. Try it. Yellow light for depression. Blue light for agitation. Green for physical healing. Magenta for emotional balance. For more information on healing with light, read "Let There Be Light" by Darius Dinshah. It's helpful for conditions of all types, not just emotional health.

Pulsed Light and Sound Therapy

Many addictive patterns and other negative states can be resolved by pulsing light into the eyes and sound into the ears. Specially designed light and sound units with frequency and pattern controls are available for this purpose. These systems operate by entraining the brain into altered states in which deep healing takes place. Alpha and Theta brain wave states are known to have amazing healing properties. Drug and alcohol addictions have been quickly and painlessly resolved with such systems. Studies show roughly a 90-95% success rate, as compared with talk therapy or programs like Alcoholics Anonymous that consistently have less than a 5-10% success rate when examined after a year or more. Search the Internet for "light and sound machine" to find sources for these devices. Brain entrainment can also be accomplished just with pulsed sound. You can find apps for portable devices like smartphones and tablets that work quite well and cost only a few dollars. Just put on your earbuds, run the app, and select the brainwave state you want in order to heal negative patterns and addictions.

The Failure of Talk Therapy And Willpower Programs

Understand that willpower and talk therapy programs (like most 12 step programs), foster strong dependencies and negative programming. For instance, clients are taught to believe they are addicts forever. They think of themselves as permanently weak, flawed, and powerless, and then integrate such negative programming into the structure of their self image. This is not a good thought to put into someone's head. It's best to avoid such negative conditioning. This is why the long term success rates of such programs are so incredibly low, practically a total failure. The underlying low self image and the embedded traumas have not been transformed. Nor have the structural state and brainwave patterns been changed. Every approach given here works and is more successful than such limited superficial therapies.

Music for Emotional Nourishment

Music, with a rhythm of about 60 beats per minute, has a settling effect on the brain/mind. Music soothes the heart and soul. If there is also variety of frequency, especially sparkling highs with complex overtones, the effect is even more wonderful. Whenever you feel overwhelmed, put on some beautiful music. Classical music by Bach, Vivaldi, Telemann, or some delightful progressive jazz, or classical Indian sitar music, can all produce the effect. Any high, transcendent music will work.

Be careful not to put on music just because you like it. It may not structurally have positive characteristics. When tests were done to determine the effects of musical genres – country/western, blues, rock & roll, many forms of jazz, acid rock, and similar "dark" music – they all produced negative effects. The darkest, heaviest, harshest music had the worst effects. Music that is light, joyful, clear, sweet, expansive, and richly textured has the best effects.

Being In Nature

Nature walks can have a very beneficial effect on your emotional state. When you are outside, you are away from the triggers that normally affect you. Also, natural settings, like forests, creeks, springs, rivers, and the ocean have very soothing and healing effects. It's worthwhile to schedule nature walks. Many of the most successful people in the world take frequent walks just to settle themselves, and often find innovative solutions to problems or have insights into new inventions. Schedule nature walks in your calendar. Otherwise, you get pressed for time and forget to take the time to be in natural settings. It's too easy to put it off.

Meditation

Deep meditation heals all levels of life, including emotions, but only if it's practiced correctly to produce a deep experience. Powerful methods of meditation are covered later, when I talk about consciousness.

Symbols In Your Life

You are always being guided. The symbols and events that arise in your life hold lessons for you. It's been said that planet Earth is a big "university" where we come to learn how to be whole and how to love. The unbounded consciousness that is behind all phenomena guides us with hints and symbols. Anything that stands out to you as you are experiencing it, is something to pay attention to. If a particular kind of experience occurs two or three times in a row, it's really time to pay attention.

For instance, you may be studying in school or working with colleagues in an office. You are confronted by people who keep telling you the same thing, but you avoid listening because you don't want to hear it. In such circumstances, they are giving you feedback on something you need to hear. Listen. When you get the same recommendations from several people in a row, listen. When the same ideas turn up in conversations, the media, magazines, or anything that catches your interest, or if you find yourself particularly resistant, that means it's time to listen. What is it you are trying to learn?

The important thing is to learn not to react unconsciously, but to contemplate the deeper causes and try a new response, either from intuition or logical analysis of the situation. Your quiet inner voice is your best guide. Use it to learn how to interpret your symbols. In order to clearly tap into your inner voice, place your attention above your head and quietly ask to be in touch with the part of you that is all-knowing. Ask the question, listen for the first response. It usually comes before you can even finish asking the question. It comes without any kind of "charge" on it. It's neutral, simple, just the truth. Pay attention. Be grateful. You don't have to be particularly religious or spiritual to use this technique. You can think of it as a kind of communing with your own higher spirit. The information presented earlier on intuition will be of value in discovering your needs and solutions.

Forgiveness

Forgiveness does not mean approval. It simply means you do not choose to be enmeshed any longer. You will be able to forgive more easily after you learn the lessons connected with an experience. Examine the situation. Learn as much as you can. Forgiveness applies to forgiving yourself, also. Forgive and move on. Forgiveness does not mean condoning the situation, rather it removes the power of that situation to control you.

There is peace in letting go of situations that you cannot change or control. If there is something that needs to be changed and you have the power to change it, then change it. You have the power to change things through the decisions you make and the upgraded self image that you bring into the decision-making process. Through your inner wisdom you can know what needs to be changed, what needs to be accepted, and what needs to be forgiven.

Give It Up

You are never alone. You can always turn something over to a higher power, whatever you consider that to be, to resolve situations for you that you can't resolve yourself. Always do your best with every aspect of life that awaits you. If you can't resolve something after giving it your best shot, turn it over. Realize that you are part of a grand cosmic scheme. Give it to Creator to work it out for you. Sometimes we get stuck after trying everything, but grace is always available. Be willing to accept grace. Religious belief is not required. The reality exists, whether you believe in it or not. Whether you resolve things yourself or get help, remember that you are still responsible. Asking for help does not absolve you of responsibility. Also, don't let the idea that you don't yet know how to resolve an issue lead you to believe that you are powerless. Ask for help from a place of power – to know more, to understand more, to become more powerful, to be more competent.

Be open to higher sources of help. Humans are not the most advanced form of life. Non-physical beings, which are beyond our present knowing, manage things to help us move forward. Allow them to do their work. Accept the help. One technique is to make a "God or Goddess Box." Write your problem on a piece of paper and put it in the box. Then if you start thinking of it again, remember that you gave it to The Divine to take care of. This concrete method can be a good reminder system. Like mailing a letter, once it's mailed, you know it will be received and taken care of on the other end. Be aware of when it's time to do your part, to complete your responsibility.

Non-Resistance

Non-resistance is one of the most powerful techniques for living your life. It should not be confused with acceptance. Acceptance carries with it a subtle sense of powerlessness, fate, and inevitability. Acceptance is often an endorsement of the inability to change things – excuses. It leads to inaction. For practically all people, the first emotional response to events in life is usually opposition or acquiescence, acceptance, mostly opposition followed by acceptance. Both habits are destructive and keep your mind and emotions continuously in drama. You can never see life as it is when your initial reaction to life events is either to oppose or acquiesce. Your first encounter with every life event should be non-resistance. Just experience life as it is without any judgement. Place yourself in the middle between the two polarities of opposing or accepting.

When you are in the middle, you can see clearly, without judgement. Then you have the power to decide what to do, "Do I want to oppose, change, or accept this thing that is happening?" It's time to discriminate, to wisely judge the most appropriate response. Sometimes opposition is necessary. You may have to fight for your beliefs, be courageous, stand up for yourself, not allow wrongdoing to persist. You then need to decide the right way to oppose, the effective way to oppose. Direct confrontation may not be best, or it may be necessary. Use intuition and discrimination to guide you.

You may decide to change the game entirely. Bring in a new response or new approach. How can you upgrade or change the situation to make the problem disappear? This is where creativity comes into play. By being creative and taking action you solve the problem on a different level. This is how your imagination, willpower, and personal skills can be powerfully expressed. This option is rarely discussed or promoted. Society is so polarized. We're constantly being told to oppose or endorse one side or the other. Creative transformation of situations requires more from us than either opposition or acceptance. Creative responses require our genius, our new ideas, our inventiveness, our enthusiasm, the ability to think outside the box. This approach almost always leads to the best solution to any problem.

Finally, after looking at the first two options, i.e. you decide that opposition is not going to work and you cannot arrive at any creative way to change the situation, then comes the last option of acceptance. If you really can't change something, only then is acceptance appropriate. At this point, acceptance becomes a powerful technique to keep your mind and emotions out of drama. There are indeed things that you have no control over, which you cannot change. If you *can* change something, then do it. But if it really isn't possible, then to be continually frustrated by it is not helpful. In those cases, acceptance is the most appropriate choice.

For instance, you may not be in a position to influence the direction of governments, or other large institutions, because you are not in positions of power. If there is a way to voice your opinions, you should do it. Then let go and choose to change situations directly in your life – where you *do* have some measure of influence. Change the things you can through opposition or creativity, and last (and also least), accept the things you cannot change. Certainly, we all can radiate the energy of love to change those conditions indirectly that we can't change directly. As you expand your consciousness, you will be able to have greater influence and greater power to change things. Your creative options will explode.

Let's take an example. We know that pesticides are destroying our soils worldwide. They destroy the microbial life that make plants strong and healthy. They destroy wildlife. They poison our air and water. They sometimes cause physical deformities. There are powerful companies making billions promoting them and have huge resources behind them. What to do? We could change our buying habits and not support them. We could start our own garden. We could try to oppose them by organizing rallies, marches, demonstrations, etc. These are all good things to do, but has that done anything to stop them? These powerful companies just buy more lobbyist to get around any opposition. Who can compete with all that money? Do we just accept that nothing can be done? No!

In the 1970's, the expansion of the organic food movement contributed a positive, creative approach. It has been successful in making pesticide-laden products less attractive in the market. Scientific research shows organic is better for food quality, soils, people, and wildlife – a very positive development that came about through hard work and innovation. An even more creative approach, happening worldwide today, is demonstrating to farmers how natural farming methods can be even more productive than the pesticide approach promoted by big business. The agricultural poison companies neglected to mention to farmers that their soil would be destroyed, and to produce large crops in the future, massive amounts of expensive fertilizers would be required (sold by the same companies), and even then, would yield progressively less product over time.

Demonstrating that organic methods are more profitable and sustainable required innovation and commitment. Now farmers are listening. They never wanted to deal with poisons and neurotoxins, or destroy their soils in the first place. They just didn't have a healthy alternative to losing their crops. The more creative solution was to show them they didn't have to compromise. This example shows how creativity is more powerful than either opposition or acceptance. This book is an example of a creative approach to the current healthcare debacle. Eliminate the need for huge medical expenses through low-cost, no-cost healthcare. Eventually, truth and word of mouth will win out over big money.

Change Emotions by Activating Higher Brain Functions

Many negative patterns are held in the newer, less developed parts of the brain, the cortex. All problems associated with darkness disappear when a light is turned on. Likewise, the problems you encounter in life are often the result of the inability to see, think, and feel on a higher level. You can change your sensitivities and patterns by activating higher brain functions. It's said that we use less than 10% of our capacities. One way of activating higher functioning is to put your attention, intention, and imagination into the part of the brain responsible for higher functions, the central or mid-brain, and also to bring light into the newer cortex areas that need healing. Let me explain.

There are two glands on each side of the head about 1 inch inside the temple known as the amygdala. (It's called the temple for a reason). If you place your attention in this part of the brain it activates the amygdala, and increases higher functions of the brain. Other locations to activate higher cognitive, intuitive, and sensory functions are 1) the area between the eyebrows, 2) the center of the head in the region of the pineal and pituitary glands, 3) at the crown of the head, and 4) about 18 inches above your head. Your attention in these areas brings life force to them and energizes them. You can use your imagination to activate them by imagining swirling energy, joy, beautiful golden-white light, or any uplifting visualization you care to use. This is a practice that you can do many times a day.

It's also helpful to bring light into the whole brain. Any area of the brain where you place your attention, and infuse it with love, joy, appreciation, or other positive, constructive visualizations is helpful. Primarily, it is the presence of your awareness in these regions that is the activating force. I'll include more on these ideas in upcoming chapters.

Gratitude Journal

This technique has been promoted by many people for centuries. Every day, write down 5 things you are grateful for. When you appreciate the blessings you do have, more will come. When you focus on negatives, negative conditions will come. Regardless of your situation, you have a choice as to where and how you focus your attention. You must learn to use your mind and heart and not let them run rampant. You are the one to choose. Choose to focus on the things that you want to manifest and be thankful, even for little things.

Emotional Nourishment

There are other ways to nurture yourself that positively affect your emotions. For example, musical or artistic expression can have positive effects on your emotional state. Simple light play. Interact with people who you love and love you. Be around young children and experience their joy and innocence. Join in their play. Go for walks with people. Have picnics. Find activities that energize you or create peace and calm. Devotional activities are always a good choice. Directing your awareness towards enlightened or higher beings who have mastered the human journey will bring that quality of energy into your life.

Addictions

Several techniques have already been mentioned in other sections about addictions. Addictions stay with you because you have cultured them, either by indulging or suppressing them unconsciously. Watch someone smoke a cigarette. You'll notice that they don't even recognize what they're doing and they are not enjoying it anymore. It has become an unconscious, addictive habit.

One way to eliminate addictions, is to make them conscious. For instance, if you are addicted to smoking, just smoke a cigarette totally consciously. Feel the cravings physiologically and emotionally. Watch yourself as you search for a lighter and a cigarette. Notice your frenzy to light the cigarette. Feel totally what it feels like to inhale. Feel what it feels like when the smoke enters your lungs. Sense what smoking is doing to your mind and your body. Experience totally, with full awareness, what it feels like to exhale, what it looks like to others, what it does to the environment, what it does to your clothing. Experience the whole process of smoking a cigarette from beginning to end without shame or judgement. Just intensely experience the reality of it. If you do this with every cigarette you smoke, for even a few cigarettes, the addiction will become repulsive and simply drop away. You will understand it, fulfill it, and no longer be interested. Avoid shame and blame, they do not serve you. Just be with the direct experience.

This method of healing addictions with cigarettes works with all addictions. No addiction can stay in your system when it is repeated consciously. Your whole system will react and throw it out. Any behavior that is not good for you will simply disappear.

Cathartic Emotional Meditations

There are unusual meditations to release deeply embedded emotions. One such technique, used by early Christians, but no longer currently taught or correctly practiced, is called Glossolalia. The Sufis later adopted it, improved it, and call it Gibberish. In the East, this ancient technique is known as the Manipuraka Shuddhi Kriya, a cathartic technique to purify the third chakra, which is locked by stress, worry, anxiety, and negative mental patterns.

This 30 minute technique bypasses the usual mental processes and roots out worries and anxieties in their most elemental form.

Worries, negativity, and suppressions are held like a weight in your navel area. Do you feel heaviness, a tightness, or a churning in that area? With this technique, you act out your suppressions with nonsensical vocalization and demonstrative actions, but no actual words in any language that you know! Using words with meaning to you, only has a superficial effect, which doesn't help much. During the process, don't use any language or words you recognize. Go to the core of your deepest suppressions and purge them out of your system as sounds. You can make vocal sounds of any sort, like animal noises, nonsense sounds, any type of vocalization.

Purging with nonsensical sounds unblocks your unconscious suppressions and allows more negativities to dissolve. Typical psychoanalytic sessions, in which patients talk to an analysts or even throw things around for catharsis, only tap into superficial layers. Only 10% of your stress will be released. Processes such as hypnosis are not under your control. This technique is a superconscious process in which you retain awareness while cleansing yourself. It is completely under your control. It should always be practiced on an empty stomach, and at least four hours before sleep. It is an entirely safe process, but highly cathartic and often dramatic.

Instructions (from the Life Bliss Foundation):

Step 1 (20 minutes) You can use a 20 minute timer to alert you.

Choose a place where you will be alone and no one will hear or bother you. Stand with your feet slightly apart and your eyes closed. For a minute, concentrate on the manipuraka area (navel region). All your worries and suppressed negativity will start rising up into your conscious mind. Just experience this tension and stress inside, as it is. Now, visualize yourself in some situation of conflict. Imagine that you're fighting hard with someone. Talk to him – but use a language that you don't know! Just use nonsense sounds. If anyone hears you, they should not make any sense of it. Try to convey your problem, your pain, to the other person. But they don't listen or agree with you! How do you feel? Angry? Throw out your anger at them!

Express all the turmoil inside you as sounds. Do NOT use words in any language you know. If you use words, only familiar, recent emotions surface. Words only give rise to more words, without actually releasing the emotions beneath them. Shout absolute gibberish. Only this will open up your unconscious. Only this will bring up the deeply hidden emotions. Continue the process, recall all the painful incidents of your life.

Visualize the people involved and feel the emotions from those incidents. Become completely immersed in them. Be aware of nothing else. If tears come, let them come! Don't stop yourself. Scream, wail, cry, throw your arms and legs about, roll on the ground if you feel like it. Create as much active catharsis as possible! Once you start, you will find so much more will come out. You may feel like vomiting. Keep a sick bag ready! Nothing to worry about, it's a sign that your system is getting cleansed and balanced, that's all. Do the technique sincerely – this is your chance to get rid of a whole lifetime of suppressions. Go into the meditation completely.

Step 2 (10 minutes): Stop Abruptly!

Now, simply sit in silence and bring your awareness to your manipuraka chakra, the navel region. You will feel a tremendous coolness and lightness in that area. During this silence, just be a witness to your thoughts. Do not suppress them, pursue them, or act on them. Just let them flow within the deep silence of your being.

Repeat this meditation every day for 21 days or until you feel you have nothing left inside to throw out. From the very first day, you will find a change, a great peace blossoming in your inner being. Enjoy the peace!

Bio-Energy Healing for the Brain and the Heart

We covered bio-energy healing in a previous chapter. It combines breath, intention, attention, consciousness, and more. It can be used for emotional healing as well as physical problems. To heal the brain, you can stream energy into the head using your hands, or stream energy from your heart to your head. Stream energy into any location where you feel the physical aspect of emotional pain. It will heal the negative emotion and the physical manifestations of it.

How Emotions are Created - The Mind and Thoughts...

Emotions are created by your thoughts. Mind and emotions are intimately related. A much more profound solution to healing your emotions (and your body), must necessarily deal with managing your mental space, which is the subject of the next chapter.

Next Steps

Review this chapter and select the methods that you want to use. Schedule these in your calendar so you get them done. The ones you cannot do immediately, put into some reminder system to jog your memory later.

It's especially important to forgive yourself, and forgive anyone who needs to be forgiven. You don't necessarily have to visit or talk with them, but if it's appropriate, go ahead. "I forgive you" is a powerful thought, a powerful phrase. If you feel that you wronged someone else, say, "I'm sor please forgive me." These are two of the most powerful phrases in the English language. When you forgive, you are forgiven. These ideas will be taken further in the chapter on mental healing.

Avoid falling back into old patterns by nipping them in the bud. Stay on top of it.

Avoid getting tired. If you need rest, then rest. Take 10-15 minute naps when you can. Go to bed early. Sleep in on weekends. Build your energy reserves. Avoid the tendency to over schedule. When you are overwhelmed with too much to handle, it's harder to manage your emotional life.

You now have extremely powerful and practical ways to resolve emotions without having to "dump them" on someone else. When you use these methods, you will take your power back and be in control of your life. Take the time you need for your emotional healthcare. Work consistently with yourself. Do NOT berate yourself. Your self talk is VERY significant and it should always be constructive. Constantly build a beautiful self image. The methods in this chapter are listed below in short form, so that you can put them into your calendar or reminder system.

Action Plan - Chapter 10, Emotional Healing

1. Understand how you have been manipulated by suppression and indulgence of emotions.
2. From now on, consciously and willingly observe the localized, physical aspect of emotions in your body. Be willing to boldly and courageously feel these painful places, consciously and passively, without reacting. Let go of the psychological aspect, let go of old stories. Feel the physical aspect of emotions in your body. Emotions are healed by impartially observing the physical manifestation with conscious awareness, conscious attention. Keep your attention localized until it dissipates.
3. To heal painful emotions: 1) Close your eyes, 2) Breathe deeply, 3) Scan your body and find the physical disturbance, 4) Allow yourself to feel it physically, 5) Follow the pain until it dissipates.
4. Do Mirror Work: 1) Sit in front of a mirror. 2) The one in the mirror is the hidden, unconscious, incomplete you, 3) Look directly into the eyes of the one in the mirror, 4) Recall emotionally painful incidents and situations such as anger, guilt, frustration, etc., 5) Take responsibility for liberating yourself from these incompletions you have held within yourself, 6) Consciously re-live those incidents and situations with full awareness. Talk aloud with the person in the mirror, looking in the eyes, 7) Repeat reliving

those painful incidents while continually talking again and again until you feel free of the emotional charge whenever you recall those events, 8) Repeat this process any time you are stuck with low-level emotions.

5. Experiment with tapping acupressure points when you have intense emotions. You can tap in sequence or any points you like, perhaps the ones nearest the disturbance.

6. Thought Replacement - Don't feed what you don't want. Do feed what you do want. 1) Recognize your emotions consciously, don't suppress them. 2) With each negative emotion, consciously realize that it does not serve you, 3) Decide you are not going to fulfill it, 4) Now replace it with a thought you want to encourage. Feed what you want. 5) Repeat the process each time this emotion surfaces. What you feed grows, what you starve dies. When you introduce a new thought, Say it, See it, Feel it, and Do it. "Say-See-Feel-Do."

7. Attitude Shifting – See your situation in a different context, another vantage point. Find something to be grateful for.

8. Learn the lesson.

9. Use continuous light color therapy. Yellow light for depression. Blue for agitation. Green for physical healing. Magenta for emotional balance. Locate colored gels at a theatrical supply. Water energized by colored drinking glasses also works.

10. Use pulsed light and sound therapy. Research and locate a device you would like to work with, or use pulsed sound therapy provided by any of the applications for computers, smart phones, or tablets.

11. Put on beautiful, high, transcendent music.

12. Be in nature.

13. Practice meditation.

14. Review the symbols in your life. Understand how you are being guided.

15. Practice forgiveness.

16. After you have done your best, give it over to the Creator to work it out for you. Accept the grace, be grateful, and continue to pay attention not to repeat mistakes. Stay in your power.

17. Practice non-resistance to every event in your life as your initial response. Then decide "What to do?" Do you oppose, change, or accept the situation? Use your wisdom and discrimination. Use your creative talents to change the situation. If opposition or change it not possible, you can always radiate love to change things indirectly. Otherwise, accept it and let it go.

18. Activate higher brain functions by infusing energy into specific regions of the brain and into the whole brain.

19. Keep a gratitude journal.

20. Find activities that provide emotional nourishment for you. Devotional activities are always a good choice.
21. Be a conscious witness of your addictive behaviors. They will become repulsive and drop by themselves.
22. Use cathartic emotional meditations, such as the Manipuraka Shuddhi Kriya.
23. Stream bio-energy into the brain, heart or any other area where emotions create physical sensations. Especially send energy from your heart to those areas. Bio-energy heals.

Chapter 11
Mental Healthcare

Healing and Eliminating Mental Stress

A Guide to Restoring Right Use of Mind

What to Expect

Your mind can either serve you or become your inner dictator – driving you into chaos, even madness. Your choice. When you make your mind your servant, then your life becomes powerful, loving, intelligent, and joyful. You become a positive force in the world. If your mind is not under your control, you become its victim. Your life is destroyed. In fact, all the world's problems are due to the misuse of the mind, and that situation itself is due to lousy education, lack of knowledge.

Unfortunately, none of our institutions, whether educational, religious, or corporate, have taught us how to regain control of our mind. The most important knowledge in the universe is not being provided. If we had received the instruction we needed, our society would not be living with antidepressants, painkillers, psychotropic drugs, sexual excess, alcohol, stimulants, and "recreational" drugs. It is pure insanity to allow a civilization to develop this way. Our leaders should be ashamed – but of course they themselves are rarely better off. It has been the blind leading the blind for centuries.

At one time, due to my own poor education, I thought it really didn't matter what you thought, it was your actions that count. I was wrong. Your thoughts and your intentions are as important as your actions. In fact, the thoughts you think repeatedly, will eventually be acted out. Garbage in, garbage out.

Garbage In, Garbage Out

There's an expression in the computer programming community, "garbage in, garbage out." Whether you're looking at the quality of the programming or the data, you can't get anything out better than what you put in. The human brain is an extraordinary and very sophisticated biocomputer. It's very sensitive and reacts badly to bad programming. Years of nutritional abuse and high stress creates flawed circuitry. Brain chemistry and functions are severely affected by "garbage." You need to be careful of what you put into your biocomputer, whether from your own inner dialogue, your own thoughts, or from outside influences.

Choose Your Experiences Carefully - Disconnect Your TV

Your brain monitors every experience. Whatever you put in, it will try to use. It will try to fulfill. Everything you put in gets programmed into your system. Intense images get programmed more deeply. The current state of television programming is mostly violence, fear, and lust, 98% pure garbage. Do you really want to put stupid programs into your system? Your best bet is to simply disconnect your TV. Turn it off. The problem is, once you let something in, you can't get rid of it. It's there forever, permanently. If the garbage comes in unconsciously, then it unconsciously takes control of you. Save your cable TV expense and dramatically improve your life by eliminating psychological garbage from your life. Turn off your TV. You can replace it with better things.

If you learn how to search the Internet effectively, you can find much better information and much better inspiration than you could ever get from television – you can find quality input to help you fulfill your dreams and goals. The same is true for all other media sources as well. Be selective. You don't have time for everything. When you ingest garbage, you're spending your time and your life for it. Really, you lose doubly. You lose once by putting trash into your system and lose again by missing out on high quality input you could have had for that same time expenditure.

All media can be dangerous. Video games are another source of tension-producing imagery and sound. Why would you allow such stress-inducing experiences into your life? It is just an unconscious choice. Video game producers and movie producers thrive on getting you addicted to adrenaline. It is destructive drama. These adrenaline stimulants simply waste your life energy for no constructive purpose.

Be aware of how you are being manipulated by the media industry and make better choices. Read good books by the wisest authors you can discover. Seek out mentors who have self control and are intelligent and loving. Leave the worst parts of our society behind. Don't feed them and don't let them feed you. You and your family have a choice – to nurture yourselves with the best of what this world has to offer or to get mired by the worst that society has to offer. If you follow the herd mentality, you will end up with the rest of the herd.

In ages past, stories were the traditional method to teach us the wisdom of life. They formed the basis of civilization and culture. The classic fables and scriptures from all traditions are examples. Stories are incredibly powerful. They're captivating and draw us in. The brain/mind is programmed for curiosity and a desire to know. When we read the words, "Once upon a time," we are ready to be guided into an adventure, to dive into the story with anticipation. We don't realize that stories can be dangerous. Stories are too powerful to be chosen without careful selection. Stories can create enlightened masters or terrorists. They can evoke compassion or revenge. We must be very careful of the media that we allow into our lives and the stories they tell. Whoever controls the stories controls the civilization. The journalistic and commercial media often use stories to control us, to make us fearful and powerless. Be aware and learn to carefully discriminate when choosing the sources and stories for your mental inputs, your knowledge sources. Learn to read between the lines. Now, with the Internet and access to the world's literature, you can control your own stories. Avoid wasting your time and your life. Find the best literature and media to nurture your mind.

Mind: Best Friend or Worst Enemy?

Your brain/mind is either your best friend or your worst enemy. It depends on how you program it. The problem is, if you're already an adult, it has already been negatively programmed for you by your parents, teachers, the media, and later, your own unconscious self-dialogue. Now you have to deal with it. One way is to recognize that your brain/mind is goal-seeking/problem-solving. It is curious. If you don't give it a direction, a goal, it will create problems, because it's already been programmed to operate negatively. Of course, that will force you to grow, but it's a very inefficient method. So at least set goals. Goal setting will give your mind something constructive to do while you refine and improve its ability to function positively. As you develop yourself consciously and mentally, you gain the ability to live in fulfillment continuously. Then you will find yourself in a positive flow without the need to manage your mind with goal setting. In the meantime, create goals and pursue them enthusiastically. Enjoy the journey itself. Be careful not to get too serious about your goals. Seriousness is another mental disease.

In the Western world especially, but actually the world over, no one is taught how to use their biocomputer effectively. People allow their mind to run wild; they allow it to run unconsciously. People don't realize that they *n*stantly programming their mind/brain into greater dysfunction from *n*e of childhood. Instead of becoming more creative and capable as we age, we are becoming more dysfunctional.

Watch Your Thoughts like a Hawk

You must get into the habit of watching your thoughts consciously, relentlessly, intensely, like a hawk. At every moment, you should know 1) what you are thinking, 2) why you are thinking it, and 3) the result you can expect from that trend of thought. Why are you thinking the thoughts you think? What do you expect from them? How are those thoughts going to help you, or help others? This should be the environment of your mind.

Most people don't even know what a thought is. They have so many racing unconscious thoughts that it's not easy to keep focus for more than a few seconds. If you want to prove this to yourself, sit and write down every thought that you have as fast as they come to you, like an automatic transcribing machine. No pauses, no editing. Set a timer. At the end of 10 minutes look a what you have written. You will be shocked. Really do this exercise! Do it now or put it on your list to do soon. You will see that your mind operates totally illogically jumping from one disconnected thought to another with no logical connection, just random association. Your mind is racing because it's out of control. You won't believe this is actually true until you do the exercise. Everyone tends to believe they are much more logical and mentally organized than they actually are. So the first step in working with your mind is to slow it down. It is NOT possible to slow it down by force, by effort, or by suppression. You can only do it by using techniques, especially in the beginning.

How to Slow Your Mind

The easiest way to slow your mind is to slow your breath. Your mind follows your breath. Try it now. Start breathing slowly to a count of 4-5 seconds in, 4-5 seconds out. After a minute or two, continue to slow your breathing more, perhaps 8-10 seconds in and out. Notice what happens! Feel your whole mind and body transform into a state of greater peace and silence. Whenever you are anxious, frustrated, or confused, the first thing you should do is slow your breath. Once you have a sense of the timing, you don't need to count. Counting is tedious. Five minutes of ultra-slow breathing can put you in a totally different state. You are more in control. There are many techniques and processes to regain control of your mind, but breath is the best place to start. I'll introduce additional techniques later.

Mental Patterns

We usually create and reinforce many destructive patterns of thought daily. Whenever you say to yourself, "I'll never get that done," or "I'm so stupid," you have just programmed yourself. You have just made a decision, you have just defined what you believe to be real or believe to be true for yourself. You create hundreds of self-fulfilling prophecies every day through your inner self talk. You create justifications and excuses to avoid seeing what is really going on. Your mental clarity gets squashed. If you try to stop this negative inner dialogue by force, it won't work. There's a better way. All you have to do is be aware, *consciously aware*, of every thought that you think. Your whole system will automatically recognize the uselessness of such thoughts and begin to weed them out.

Trying to suppress unwanted thoughts by forcing them to stop doesn't work. Unwanted negative thoughts are due to past conditionings, past decisions, and interpretations of reality that have now become unconscious patterns embedded inside you. The problem is that your brain/mind is like a wish-fulfilling tree. Everything your mind thinks, and that you give support to, give assent to, it tries to fulfill. This is how you limit your possibilities and structure a false reality that you believe exists. You have to be careful of what you allow or let pass, what you endorse. Watch carefully. But don't suppress. Whenever a negative pattern of thinking begins, recognize that it is not serving you and decide to cancel it. Then replace it with the opposite or something else that you want to be fulfilled.

Not only should you watch your thoughts and the decisions you make or the conclusions you draw, also observe the feelings that you use to reinforce them, to support them, to endorse them. Which of your thoughts are you supporting by giving emotional acceptance or the "will to fulfill" to? Which ones have intense greed or desire behind them? Which ones have aversion and avoidance towards them? On the other hand, which ones create lightness, ease, enthusiasm, and joy?

Observe your thoughts and emotions objectively, as though you are a bystander just watching – without reacting to them. Consciously watching your thoughts and emotions heals the underlying conditioning because you recognize how you are choosing to support destructive emotions and decisions. I'll explore this in depth a little later. It doesn't have to take a long time to regain control of your mind. Within 21 days your brain/mind will start following your new instructions. Continue the process of watching every thought that arises. It will take time to reduce the load of past conditionings, but it is not difficult.

You heal patterns by 1) shining the light of your intense conscious observation on them, 2) recognizing them, 3) dissolving the physiological aspect with life-force energy, 4) purging the emotional element by reliving past traumatic incidents dispassionately, dis-identified, until the intense emotions dissipate, 5) correcting poor mental decisions and interpretations of reality, and making new decisions and interpretations of reality. You heal physically, emotionally and mentally. Let's explore this process in depth.

Conditioned Mental Patterns

Mental patterns are a mental conditioning that defines the image of who you think you are. Right now, you're reading this in a language you know. That's because earlier you conditioned yourself to recognize this language. Likewise, everything you believe to be true and everything you believe to be real is nothing but conditioning, not truth. The beliefs you have right now about yourself and about "reality," you constructed based on past conditioning that you accepted as you grew up, plus fantasies you created later. It's just like the movie *The Matrix*. You don't live in the realm of reality, you live in a self-imposed illusion. You overcome this conditioning by no longer feeding it, and by purging it physiologically, emotionally, and mentally from your system with different techniques.

The technique that you used in the bio-energy chapter, where you focused your attention on physical pains and sensations, is one method of locating the traumas and patterns that were embedded in your system. You found the physical aspect of the induced trauma and flooded it with bio-energy to dissolve it with loving, life-force energy. In the emotional healthcare chapter, you located the emotional element by scanning your past history. You found the incidents that were emotionally charged, and relived them repeatedly from the perspective of the pure observer until the emotional charge dissipated. In this chapter on mental healing, I'll explain another method of locating and healing your deepest destructive mental patterns.

Greed and Fear

The fantasies and imaginations you have, the "realities" you create, are mostly based on greed and fear. Greed is based upon unfulfilled desire. It can be desire for anything – money, pleasure, power, food, sex, etc. This is the dominant orientation of most men. Likewise, fear is based upon aversion, reacting against something you don't want. Fear creates the desire for security, safety. This is the dominant orientation of most women. This is why you see young women marrying old men with money. Security is paramount.

When you don't get what you want, you are unhappy. When you get what you don't want, you are also unhappy. In your present state, happiness and unhappiness are based on circumstances that you can never fully control. You can't control the world. As a result, except for the few moments when you actually get something you want or avoid some pain that you don't want, you are in a state of constantly desiring or avoiding. All your time is spent searching for happiness or trying to avoid fear or unhappiness. Even if you get what you want, you live in fear of losing it. This means that the vast majority of the time you are unhappy – trying to fulfill yourself by chasing pleasure or avoiding pain. It's a state of continuous anticipation of pleasure or avoidance of pain based on projected fantasies, not actually living your life in this moment of reality. It is a projection, not real life.

This is called the state of bondage, the unenlightened state, the state of continuous pain. Is there a way out? The answer is, "Yes!" Once you recognize that you can never find fulfillment through the senses or through the mind, you begin to wake up and come out of the matrix. The first step is getting control of the senses and the mind.

Being in Reality

In order to get out of living in fantasies based on greed and fear, you have to shift your attitude and orientation towards reality. You have to choose to be in reality, as it is. You might not like it and you might want to escape. That's the usual reaction. But running away from reality doesn't lead you anywhere, it doesn't help you to heal. One of the most powerful tools in your arsenal is non-resistance – simply not resisting reality as it comes to you. Non-resistance was mentioned in the chapter on emotional healing. Now let's look at the mental side of non-resistance.

Non-resistance has both an emotional component and a mental component. We usually react emotionally and then try to justify our reactions mentally. Mentally, we always want to be right. No one likes to be proved wrong, so we defend our mental patterns by digging in our heels and mentally justifying our reactions. This assertion, "I am right, you are wrong" is a product of ego created by past conditioning. It's based upon your *interpretation* of reality and may not have anything to do with reality as it is. You can never know reality as it is when you are either resisting or accepting reality as it comes to you through your filters, your patterns. Non-resistance

217

neans being in the middle, neither opposing nor accepting. Just observing innocently, without prejudice or judgment.

You don't have to mentally accept reality as it appears to you. When you accept things, you turn off your mental creativity, your capacity to change them. You become powerless. It's as bad as opposing reality, which is another blind reaction. Non-resistance does not mean acceptance. Acceptance is really an endorsement of things as they are – acquiescence. Why would you want to accept something that may not be worthy of your endorsement? Likewise, why would you want to fight and oppose without seeing clearly who the enemy is? Or to see if there is any justification for your opposition?

The sequence of your experience should be first to observe reality objectively, as it is, without judgement and without reacting emotionally or mentally. Neutrality keeps you in your power. First see things as they are, without resistance of any kind, then decide what to do. As mentioned earlier, you have three choices: 1) intelligently oppose what you have discovered, 2) change the reality to something more worthy 3) accept it as it is, and contribute your efforts somewhere else. The rule is, don't react. Observe with full consciousness. Reserve judgement. Then assess and choose your options. Choose intelligent options and power them with your emotional "juice" – enthusiasm, courage, love, joy, compassion, and willpower. This is how to manifest your power and creativity to change your world.

When you can see things as they are and focus your conscious awareness on reality as it is, solutions become self evident. You don't have to struggle to find them. Your mind will operate differently when you can stay in reality, in this present moment. Your mind will become quieter and you will begin operating from a powerful place of intuition, operating beyond logic, beyond the ordinary mind.

Mind itself has no power except through its association with consciousness, which I will discuss in a later chapter. The more the mind is separated from consciousness and awareness, the more into fantasy it operates. Then you become dominated and attached to outer circumstances. The more it is connected to consciousness and awareness the more into reality it operates. It turns out that reality is more amazing than fantasy, and infinitely more powerful.

Here is a simple technique you can use when you catch yourself distracted by fantasy, non-reality – simply bring yourself back to this present moment. See and listen to what is right in front of you, right now. Be within your own presence, the presence of your own being. Do this over and over. Come back to the reality of this moment. Be present in your own presence. Your life will begin to become more powerful, more creative, more inspired, more useful to yourself and others – and especially, more fun. It will take a little time to get used to reality.

This doesn't mean that there is no place for imagination. Imagination is different from fantasy, non-reality. Use creativity, imagination, and visualization to solve real problems that exist now, to create a better future. That's a far different thing from wild fantasies that are not directed toward solving real-world situations. Creative problem solving, brainstorming, and exploring ideas connected with the real-world is a constructive use of the mind. Creative problem solving is also very different from positive thinking.

Why Positive Thinking Doesn't Work

You have probably been introduced to the idea of positive thinking. You may have tried it and found that it doesn't work. You are correct. It doesn't work. All the time you are trying to be positive, you are fighting against a negative that you believe exists. Trying to overpower the negative with a positive doesn't eliminate the negative. It hides underneath, laughing at you. It surfaces again. Positive thinking doesn't work until certain requirements are met. The main requirement is to come to terms with the negative. The negative is there because you programmed it, or at least allowed it. Now, you have to retract that programming. Simply suppressing negative thinking never works for long.

One way to eliminate negative thinking is to bring the negative thought to conscious awareness. You need to examine it consciously, understand it, and consciously decide that you are no longer going to fulfill this negative thought. You need to feel the negative emotion stored in the thought until it no longer has a charge on it, until it dissipates completely. This is how you reach completion with prior programming, with your negative patterns. Suppressing negativity by forcefully introducing positivity is just another method of suppression. The problem is that you believed all the books that talked about being positive and thought the problem was with you. It wasn't you. The books are wrong. Positive thinking doesn't work as it is presently promoted.

Getting to Completion

You absolutely must resolve your past decisions and interpretations of reality. Those decisions and interpretations are now controlling your life. When you honestly come to terms with your negativity programmed ns and interpretations, by recognizing them and deciding not to them, you have a clean slate again. The memory of it is there, the lesson is learned, but the charge on it that incessantly controlled you is released. Therefore, it no longer causes you to react. Also, the mental decisions that you chose and the interpretations of reality that you assumed to be true can be changed, updated. This is the state of completion.

In the chapter on emotional healthcare, I described a practice of going back in time to find the emotionally charged events that are the basis of controlling you and preventing you from being all that you can be. In this chapter on mental healthcare, you go back to those same kinds of events, but you also look at the mental decisions that you made throughout your past that continue to control you, that continue to define your reality in terms of what is possible for you.

Arriving at completion doesn't necessarily happen by simply deciding once. Your mind will test you. "Are you sure? You once told me you wanted this!" You will need to examine your negative conditioning several times, perhaps many times over the course of a few weeks, until the decision not to fulfill this negativity, not to fulfill a decision you made, takes hold. You complete your old patterns by 1) Retracing your past, 2) Finding incidents that changed your life, and 3) Examining those events where you mentally made a decision, where you programmed yourself, or accepted someone else's programming. As with bio-energy healing and emotional healing, there is the same amazing secret in doing this.

The secret to completion is in *how* you review and resolve your past intense experiences that caused your deep-seated patterns. The past needs to be relived and reviewed in a totally differently way from the usual methods of psychotherapy – 180° different from the usual methods. Ordinarily, with talk therapies, you review your past, but you do it unknowingly from a place of identification with the experience. When you re-experience the past in your mind and heart, the experience itself dominates. The experience is foremost in awareness and the experiencer is hidden in the background. Your awareness as you recall your memories, as you relive your past, is dominated by the objects of your experience. In that state, because you are identified with the experience, you simply re-infect yourself with it. That's why there is often so little progress with psychotherapy. There is another way.

Go into your past with deep attention while remaining in the present moment, but completely dis-identify with the experience. Go deeper within yourself and let go of the attachment to the scene you are watching. As you observe a past event in your memory, you relive the event, and recognize the emotional charge on it, you also recognize the mental decisions and interpretations of reality you chose to believe, but you do it while not being identified with it. You experience it from the perspective of the innermost observer. Be an impartial observer of both the emotional and mental content of the experience, as if you were watching it on video or peeking around the corner seeing yourself. Actually, you are watching from your Being, which is separate from your mind, emotions, and body. You are watching from your pure presence, your pure consciousness, the innermost observer of all the experiences of your life.

Let me explain this idea of association and dissociation a little deeper. Certainly, you have been to the movies. When you first sit down to watch an exciting movie, you realize that you are sitting in a movie theater and that you are safe and everything is okay. But after watching the movie for 10 or 15 minutes, you get drawn into the movie, you get attached to the storyline and the events that are happening. Soon you forget you are even sitting in the theater. When the hero goes over the cliff, you go over the cliff with him. Your heart is pounding with excitement, sometimes with fear and dread. You are captivated and trapped by the intensity of the movie. Later, when the movie ends and the lights come on, you once again realize who you are. You realize that you are sitting in the theater and you were always perfectly safe, though it didn't feel like it at the time. Now, your identity has been restored. You are back inside yourself, no longer dominated by the events. This realization of your self identity is the recognition of the conscious observer inside of you. When the outer experience dominates it takes you on a roller coaster ride of drama and chaos. When your inner self dominates, you are home again in joy, peace, and stability. The difference is the dominance of your perception, either with outer objects or with the pure inner observer at your innermost core.

In the chapter on emotional healing, I described one method of using a mirror in front of you. You look directly into the eyes of the person in the mirror. That person in the mirror is the hidden side of yourself. But you dissociate from the experience. You stay within yourself as the observer. This is the same process, but you can do it without the mirror. You are looking at memories.

Recall a life-altering, life-damaging event from your past. Go into your past and recall the experience moment by moment. Usually, whenever we have our attention on something, we identify with it. In this case, we have total attention, but we do not identify with the memories. That is the secret key. Do this process of reviewing your past life-changing events, even going back into your earliest childhood. Do this every night before bed for at least 21 minutes, up to an hour. Work through all your life events until you have no emotional charge on them and you correct the mental decisions, the choices you made, and the interpretations of reality you chose to believe.

You don't need to analyze the past or go into any blame or shame. That won't help. You are just re-experiencing it from the perspective of the pure consciousness that you are, from the place of being the pure witness, the pure observer. That process itself is very healing. When you can recall the event without any emotional reactions, and you correct the mental decisions and interpretations of reality you chose, it is healed. You are free from its negative influence in your life.

With emotional healthcare, you used a mirror and talked out loud to yourself while looking at your eyes. You saw your whole past with intense attention, but you dis-identified with it. This is the same process, but now you are discovering the mental component, the mental decisions and interpretations of life that you chose. You recognize them, cancel and correct them, and introduce updated, better decisions and interpretations.

When you are complete with a past incident, you may then want to contact others involved and offer or accept forgiveness as appropriate to the situation. You may want to explore the incident with them to get their experience of it. It may not have happened for the reasons you believe. First get complete with the memory of it, then follow up with people as recommended in the emotional healthcare chapter. It is difficult to have enough clarity to complete with other people first and then try heal the incompletion in yourself afterward. It won't work. Heal both your emotional and mental incompletions. Come to a total resolution within yourself. Then you will bring a beautiful state of completion with you when you interact with others. Ultimately, you want to have no reactions with any memories or any incidents from your past. Then you will be in a place of power, compassion, love, wisdom, and joy.

Once you reach completion with your negativity, you can introduce positive thoughts and concepts. This is when positive thinking and planning can be of value to you, and why positive thinking worked for some people but not for most people. It can only be useful and effective when you have completed your negative patterns. Then you can decide who you want to be and how you want to live. You can reprogram your biocomputer. Actually, being positive and enthusiastic is natural. It doesn't require a separate effort. Just look at the exuberance of young children. They don't have to force exuberance and joy on themselves. They don't have to try to be positive. Positivity and zest for life is not something you have to force on yourself. Just pick a worthy goal and dive into it. The enthusiasm will be there when the backlog of negativity has no emotional charge on it and no power of wrong decisions and wrong interpretations of reality behind it.

You complete and clear your past programming either by following through and supporting it to the point of fulfillment, or deciding consciously that you no longer want to pursue it, that you made a mistake – you don't want to support it anymore. In the case of negative programming, following through to fulfill it doesn't make sense. The only intelligent option is to decide that you made a mistake. At one time you wanted it. Now you don't. Sometimes, you do things just to learn lessons or you just didn't know any better.

All you really need to do to come out of all your dilemmas is to get to completion with your past negative programs. You will see that with this process, past memories lose their charge and no longer dominate and control you. You gain freedom. Life becomes more blissful, more exciting, more joyful. You will be able to welcome change and avoid boredom, depression, chaos, confusion, and instability.

Example: Here's a common experience that can explain the process in a practical way. For those people who drink alcohol, remember that at one time you wanted to show your strength by rebelling against authority. Or maybe you wanted to show you were an "adult." Or perhaps you thought you would look sophisticated and cool to drink like you saw in advertisements or movies. Or you just wanted to fit in with your friends. Everyone knows that drinking alcohol is a bad idea. It has no nutrition. It is a poison. It causes the death of cells, addiction, and untold suffering. It takes you out of reality, into delusion, illusion, and intoxication. It isn't a lack of knowledge that causes a person to drink. The choice to drink is made for a different reason, usually to assert yourself in some way. Or maybe you hated yourself and wanted to commit slow suicide. Maybe you wanted to escape reality by intoxicating yourself.

Whatever the reason, you forgot it. Now you are stuck with an unconscious habit or social addiction. At this point you don't want the habit, though at one time you did. To eliminate the negativity, you need to go back and look at the decision to drink alcohol and the reasons behind it. Briefly relive that timeframe consciously. Then you can decide that you no longer want to fulfill those reasons that you chose back then. By doing so, you reach a state of completion and the negative programming no longer asserts itself. You are relieved of that burden. Now you can decide to introduce a healthy habit. This is how you clear past mental decisions and interpretations of reality that originally created a negative mental pattern, in this case, an addiction.

Healing Your Deepest Patterns

Your deepest patterns were formed at a very early age, before you were seven years old. When you were born, you were centered in your pure self and your mind was not yet contaminated by patterns of restriction. You felt a sense of expansion and connection with everything that exists, an inner state of universality. Babies are completely open and capable of learning extremely rapidly, even mastering language within two or three years. But what happens as you begin to explore the world as a baby is that you meet obstacles and restrictions. Someone yells at you, someone takes a toy away that you wanted, you are not allowed to have something you are attracted to. Every time you are stopped, you learn to doubt that you can have what you want. Within just a few years you are confronted by obstacles and restrictions that add to your doubt that you can have what you want or be what you want to be.

When you can't get what you want you become angry and throw a tantrum. You begin to hate these limitations both outside yourself and inside yourself. Gradually this develops into self-hatred. As self-hatred becomes embedded, you conclude that you can never have what you want and that the future is going to be filled with limitations and impossibilities. You construct a mental state of acquiescence, of giving up, of self denial about ever having what you want in the future. This chain of events, creates your deepest embedded mental patterns of 1) self doubt, 2) self-hatred, and 3) self-denial of future possibilities. It leaves a deep mental scar, a pattern that is stored in your mind and body. These three fundamental patterns are your root patterns.

The first expression of these limitations in a child are the reactions often called "the terrible twos." That's when we begin to fight. We learn to say no. We become obstinate. We throw tantrums. We cry and yell. We do everything to express our anger and frustration. We even become obstinate and arrogant. We also become fearful, threatened, and confused. We don't understand what is happening. This is when the ego gets created, when you started feeling separate from everything and everyone. Now you feel lost and angry. This process of internalizing self doubt, self hatred, and self denial continues and often surfaces again around the 7th or 8th grade as your body changes into an adult body. We have difficulty coping with change because our belief in a positive future has already been crushed.

As time passes, because of this negative, restrictive mental set up, your projection towards the world creates a self-fulfilling prophecy. You don't believe life can be easy and full of possibilities, you end up creating an outer life that matches the circumstances of your inner life. Every time you meet with obstacles and restrictions it adds to your belief that you can't have what you want or be what you want to be. You lose trust in yourself and life.

Then we try to compensate. We try to forget about these original negative assumptions about life. We try to put on a good face and project out into the world that things are really better than we feel inside. We learn to smile and get by, but these inner negative patterns continue to control us and prevent us from being all that we want to be, in spite of our attempts to overshadow them with positive assertions and positive projections of ourselves to others and to the world.

These fundamental negative assumptions about life that we all carry need to be reversed if we are ever going to expand and rewrite our future life possibilities. This primal negativity that we took on, needs to be canceled.

Three methods have been introduced so far to undo your embedded negativity, they are:

1) Infuse the area of your body where stresses are stored with tremendous life force energy. Dissociate, observe the pains, pressures and other physical symptoms from the perspective of your innermost observer, pure self. Flood the area with loving compassionate energy – Bio-Energy Healthcare,

2) Starting with a recent emotional trauma, relive it objectivity by not reacting. Dissociate, observe the incident from the pure observer, the pure conscious self. Consciously relive the event until there is no longer any emotional reaction, until it dissipates – Emotional Healthcare,

3) Starting with a recent life trauma, relive it from the perspective of objectivity. Dissociate, observe the event and discover the mental decisions you made and the assumptions and interpretations about reality you concluded. Recognize how those decisions and assumptions no longer serve

your interests. Cancel them, and replace them with new decisions and new interpretations of reality – Mental Healthcare.

In each case, we are positioning ourselves in our innermost core as we do this work of clearing the patterns that have held us back.

Recent emotional traumas, and recent life traumas and life patterns are derived from earlier incidents. You need to clear the earlier incidents. Trace back even further, eventually arriving at a time very early in your childhood when these original root patterns of self doubt, self hatred, and self denial of a future possibilities took hold.

Creating A New Future For Yourself

You have the potential to completely rewrite your future. Up until now, whenever you tried to change directions, to make a new future, you were held back by these negative patterns. When you tried to be positive, some negative element would creep in and you would sabotage yourself. Every time this happened and you could not live up to your dream, you felt worse about yourself and added another layer of self-doubt, self-hatred, and self-denial. Now, you can put an end to this process of self-destruction and create a new reality, a new future for yourself. Here's how to do it.

- Write down a short statement of what you want in life. Pick only one desire during any one Mental Healthcare session. You can do another session for another desire later, or tomorrow. Keep it simple and focused. Choose only one desire at a time. That's plenty to work with.
- As you consider yourself having your desire, as you try to visualize your success, your mind will bring up objections and try to convince you that you can't have it and why you can't have it, why it will be very difficult. Your mind says, "How is this going to happen?" "It's not possible."
- Write down clearly every objection that arises in you. You will clear each one of them in the process that follows. Pick one to start. Bring it to mind and consider the objection, the doubt that is facing you.
- When you see or feel the self-doubt, self-hatred, and self-denial coming up, look back to when it started – when you first felt you were not qualified, not good enough to have it, when you first felt that you were not going to get what you want, that you could not have what you want.
- Feel the deep pain – when and where self doubt, self hatred, or self denial arose in you. You felt yourself sink, collapsing into powerlessness. This is when and how you gave up on yourself. Whenever this happened to you, you strengthened your self doubt, self hatred, and self denial. It may have been a small, seemingly insignificant event as a child – not

getting some candy you wanted. See how you collapsed, how you cried bitterly, in sorrow and anger, in frustration and pain.

- You decided you were not good enough to have it, somehow not worthy of it. Continue to relive this incident, observing it until it no long has the powerful emotional charge on you, you will be freed from your self doubt, hatred, and denial. When complete, see if there is an earlier incident.

- Go back and see how many times you collapsed, you imploded into self doubt, hatred, and denial. You lost self confidence, your self image was crushed. You were shaken. You tried to fight with it, but to no avail. You finally gave up and became disillusioned, crushed. Feel the pain of it.

- Consciously relive and complete each event by observing it until it's power over you dissipates, until the emotional pain subsides and no longer returns when you relive the event. You have purged the emotional trauma from your system. It is complete on the emotional level. Now for the mental level.

- Understand how you made certain decisions about yourself, how you acquiesced, how you gave up on yourself, how you took on the mantle of powerlessness. Understand the decisions you made, the interpretations of life, the assumptions about life you chose to believe. Cancel those decisions and reverse those life interpretations. Mentally affirm your new decisions and interpretations and affirm that you will adopt them.

- Introduce a new image of yourself based on your new decisions and new interpretations of life. Feel comfortable with your new reality. See this desire for yourself already manifested, as though it has already happened. It has happened for a long time now and you have accepted it and are comfortable with it. It is your reality.

- Do this process, with each objection that you wrote down. Trace every incident connected with that objection back to its original source. Completely clear each previous incident successively along the way of its emotional and mental patterns until you get to the original incident in your childhood. Complete all your self-doubt, self-hatred, and self-denial in this way. You will rise like a phoenix.

- Rewriting your future begins when you complete your self doubt, self hatred, and self denial. These three are the source of all your problems and everything inauspicious in you. These three are what destroyed your self image. They are what controlled your life.

- Work on this sincerely. Spend your time, energy, intelligence, and intention on clearing and completing these fundamental root patterns. Do this every day. Pick a new desire for yourself and clear the obstacles.

Your Daily Mental Life

In your daily life, if you carefully watch your thoughts with full conscious awareness, you will know what you are thinking, why you are thinking it, and what you hope to accomplish with that trend of thought. You will be able to catch yourself when you start to get off track. When that happens, you want to take action to upgrade your mental healthcare. As before –

1) First slow your breath to slow your mind, 2) While established in the present moment, look at the thought you just had that was taking you in a negative direction. 3) Trace back in time. Recall some incident that is the basis of this thought. *Consciously* relive the incident that is controlling you. 4) Dis-identify, dissociate from the incident and watch from the place of the innermost observer 5) Feel the emotion until it is clear, recognize the decisions you made and the interpretations of reality you bought into. 6) Consciously choose not to fulfill those past destructive decisions. Understand the decision you made back then is no longer serving you, 7) Cancel that choice, un-program that program – decide and declare that you are no longer going to fulfill that choice, and 8) Consciously choose to fulfill a worthy goal. In this way, you can prevent unconscious and disastrous thoughts that can ruin your life.

When you review past choices, stay out of guilt. In the past, you did not have the wisdom to make better choices. If you could have, you would have. Judging the past with updated wisdom doesn't help you. Just learn from your past. Cancel past destructive decisions. Keep the knowledge. Discard the guilt. Don't repeat past mistakes. If you feel drawn to repeat a destructive choice, complete it with a Mental Healthcare session.

Four Kinds of Choices

Whenever you make a choice, you only have four kinds of choices to choose from. They're based on only two categories: A choice that FEELS good (or allows you to avoid fear, pain, or things that challenge you), or a choice that IS good (constructive to your life purpose) – or their opposites. Here's your four choices: 1) Feels good, is good, 2) feels good, is bad, 3) feels bad, is good, 4) feels bad, is bad.

You don't have trouble with things that feel good and are also good for you, like nutritious food that you enjoy. Likewise, you also don't have trouble with things that feel bad and are actually bad for you like spoiled food, poison, death, or injuries. You naturally avoid those things. The problem is the other two groups. You often avoid things that feel bad, but are really good for you, such as healing herbs, exercise, fasting, or admitting mistakes. You may not like them, but you know they will help you in the end. The choices that cause the most trouble are things that feel good, but are bad for you. Some examples are addictive drugs, addictive foods, overeating, lying to others to protect yourself, or cheating to gain an advantage. It's helpful to see this chart so you can clearly recognize what you are choosing.

Here's a chart with examples:

	Feels Good (we indulge)	Feels Bad (we resist)
Is Good	Nutritious food, like some grapes or an apple	Bitter herbs, exercise, fasting, admitting mistakes, forgiving others
Is Bad	Addictive drugs, junk foods, overeating, lying to others, not keeping your word	Spoiled food, poison, death, injuries

Your life will work well when you make better decisions. These decisions should be based upon what feels good and is good for you, and what is good, even though it may not feel so good in the short term. Understanding the four choices can keep you out of a lot of trouble, but you can rise to an even higher level of life by following a few core principles.

The Four Noble Principles of Life

There are four fundamental noble principles for the correct use of your mind and for guiding your life in a constructive way. If these four noble principles are followed, then your life will work really well. If they are not followed, your life will become chaos.

Noble Principle #1 - Integrity

Integrity means keeping your word with yourself and with others and becoming complete within yourself, with others, and with all things. We frequently tell ourselves that we're going to do something, or we're NOT going to do something anymore, such as a bad habit. Then, at the first sign of difficulty, we abandon the commitment that we made to ourselves. This is a lack of integrity. We all do it from time to time, but the more you do it, the less control you have over your life. To the extent you keep making commitments to yourself that you don't honor, to that same extent you lose ol over yourself. The Universe doesn't trust you anymore and doesn't help you, because it knows you are not reliable. Why bother?

On the other hand, if you keep your commitments to yourself, then every aspect of your life is strengthened. The Universe then makes every attempt to support you in the directions you have chosen. It may sound strange to talk about the Universe supporting or not supporting you, but the reality is, you are not separate from everything else. It's like every point in space knows everything about you. It knows what you will do and what you won't do. If you are to regain the trust that the Universe has in you, then you must rebuild the trust that you have in yourself.

This same principle is true with your commitments to other people. If you continuously break your commitments, then that unreliable quality in you will be sensed by everybody you meet. If you wonder why people don't respond to you in the way you want them to, it may be that they sense your lack of integrity. When you begin to honor your commitments to others and to yourself, a new energy builds around you that signals to others that you are a reliable human being who can be trusted.

What does it mean to keep your commitments? It means you're really going to do the commitment with every fiber of your being. Do or die. That doesn't mean that you can't change your mind. If you make a commitment, and later realize it's a mistake, then you can decide to change the commitment. In that case what you tell yourself is, "I made this commitment. At the time I thought I could honor and fulfill it. I now realize it was a mistake and I'm not going to fulfill this commitment. I'm going to make another choice." So with yourself, whenever you make a commitment and realize you've made a mistake and you're NOT going to fulfill it, then you must consciously acknowledge that you're canceling it. Otherwise it becomes a drag on you.

The same is true if you make a commitment with someone else. Don't just say, "I'll call you," and not do it. Oftentimes you may think you're being nice by telling someone you're going to do something. You want to keep them happy by not saying "no" – but now, they're expecting you to do it. When you don't do things that you say you will do, if you don't fulfill your commitments, they feel let down. If you do it repeatedly, soon they don't trust you. In addition, as before, the Universe doesn't trust you and doesn't send you reliable people to work with. In the end, you are both damaging yourself and hurting others. When you lose integrity, you lose relationship to life itself. If you don't walk your talk, your life degrades into chaos. Carefully watch every thought and every commitment you make.

Noble Principle #2 - Authenticity

Authenticity means that when you say you'll do something, you will do it wholeheartedly and sincerely to the peak of your capacity. It means you will fulfill the commitment with excellence, using your full capability, not just lip service. It means responding to life from your highest self perception, your highest self projection towards others, and the highest expectation that others have of you towards them. Let me explain.

You respond to life in three ways: 1) from your *self identity*, self image, self perception 2) from your *projections,* your persona, what you show to the world, and 3) from the *expectations* of others. These three aspects of your responses to life need to be authentic. For example:

Let's say you make a commitment to yourself to lose weight. To fulfill that commitment, you decide you're going to eat fewer sweets, and you choose to eat one less cookie every week. From the integrity point of view, you are fulfilling your commitment. You are technically keeping a commitment to eat fewer sweets, but it's not authentic. Eating one less cookie isn't your best effort to lose weight. You are being inauthentic. Keeping the letter of your commitments without keeping the spirit of your commitments is inauthenticity. Being authentic means keeping both the letter and the spirit of your commitments. Authenticity means acting with sincerity and full capacity to accomplish your commitment.

Another way to understand the three aspects of authenticity is: 1) Being true to yourself, 2) being true towards others, and 3) being true to the expectations of others. Keeping your commitments with authenticity applies to your inner dialogue (your inner commitments to yourself), your commitments to other people, and the expectations of others *even if you had no obvious commitment with them.* This last idea may seem strange, but it is also necessary. Sometimes the expectations that others have of you are higher than your own expectations of yourself and beyond your existing relationships towards others. This is a way for you to grow, so those expectations cannot be ignored. You need to fulfill the highest expectations of you in all three ways.

Your word needs to be your bond, and it needs to be sincere and authentic. Otherwise, people will realize you are not sincere and they will not trust you. You will also not trust yourself. You know that you are lying to yourself. It can even become an unconscious habit to the point that you don't even realize you're lying to yourself. Then you're really in trouble!

When you can't trust yourself to be sincere and authentic, once again your life falls apart. The Universe knows your status. In reality, you never get away with anything. Be careful with your agreements. Don't make them lightly. Watch your thoughts. Before you agree to do something, think about what it really means. What is the level of commitment? What's going to be required of you? Are you really going to do it? If so, then go ahead and make the commitment and follow through. Also, be aware of the unspoken commitments and the expectations that life has of you. None of us exist in a vacuum. We are connected to all of life and we need to respond to life with authenticity, our sincere best.

Noble Principle #3 - Responsibility

Responsibility means not only being responsible for your own thoughts and actions, and everything happening within you, but also being responsible for the thoughts and actions of people in your life, for their behavior, and also for all the happenings around you. At first, this may seem completely unworkable and unfair. How can we be responsible for the thoughts and actions of others or for the events happening around us? Let's look at the bigger picture.

You may have heard the phrase, "You create your own reality." Everything that happens in your life, happens because somehow you attracted it, you created it. You may not know how you did it. It may have been unconscious, but everything that happens in your life happens because you positioned yourself to make it happen. You put yourself in certain situations. You were at the wrong place at the wrong time. You trusted someone you should not have trusted. You made a decision that went against your intuition. You harbored the wrong thoughts and emotions.

There are innumerable things that caused you to end up where you are now. Generally, the whole thing has been an unconscious process. You have not been aware. And because you were not aware, you THINK you were not responsible. But you ARE responsible. If you take responsibility for everything in your life, then you can exercise control over it and you can change it, heal it. If you think that life just happens randomly, then you lose control, lose direction, and lose your power. Nothing happens by accident. All effects have causes. When the causes are unconscious, the effects are usually undesirable. But if you take responsibility, you can change everything. The extent to which this can be taken, is amazing.

Example: This example comes from an ancient Hawaiian healing practice known as Ho'oponopono®, revived and adapted by the late Hawaiian sage Morrnah Nalamaku Simeona. It's derived from more ancient knowledge from the East. The principles are universal and have been used since time immemorial. It's based upon: 1) acknowledgment of responsibility, 2) recompense, and 3) forgiveness as a way to heal ourselves and others.

Here is a true story. A clinical psychologist, Dr. Hew Len, a student of the teachings, took a position at an asylum for the criminally insane. It was a hellish institution. Inmates were utterly insane and aggressive, and the staff was overwhelmed, depressed, defeated, and ineffectual.

The psychologist chose to take responsibility for the situation as his own creation and applied the four parts of Ho'oponopono. He took action as a recompense for his creation, as a means to heal himself, and in the process, to heal others.

First Part: "I'm Sorry." If you create something that you don't want, then surely you can be sorry for that creation and then do something to make recompense. Here, the psychologist realized that he had created these people, he had created this hellhole, and took responsibility for this undesirable creation. To make recompense, the psychologist simply reviewed the records of the inmates daily. He saw only a name, the history of the inmate, and perhaps a photograph. He never clinically met them or interacted with them. He only sat in his office and said within himself, while feeling the pain of the inmate he was reviewing: "I'm sorry." He was genuinely sorry for creating them in the hellish way they existed. Whatever pain he could feel in them he could sense in himself. Of course, this required self healing. He knew that because they were in his life, they were his creation. So he set about healing himself and his creation.

Second Part: "Please Forgive Me." If you have done something undesirable, then it makes sense to ask for forgiveness. You want to set things right. Asking for, receiving, and offering forgiveness is a powerful process for healing. Mentally, the psychologist simply asked for forgiveness and truly forgave himself for his creation. Asking for forgiveness is addressed to that oneness which connects him to the inmate. Asking, receiving, and offering forgiveness – all of it – comes from the one consciousness that pervades all that exists.

Third Part: "Thank You." If you ask for, or offer forgiveness with others, a "thank you" is warranted, since you no longer have to bear the burden of your mistake, or else you release others of the burden. In either case, there is an opportunity for both of you to grow, and so you offer your "thank you." Still, if you have created an undesirable situation, you should do whatever is in your power to make recompense in a practical way. The psychiatrist then mentally thanked the divine oneness for the opportunity to set things right, to make recompense.

Fourth Part: "I Love You." Love is the most powerful healing force. Love means genuinely caring about the welfare of others and yourself. It is not only a sentiment, it's a powerful radiating force. You have the opportunity to love all aspects of this creation, because at a very deep level, they are really aspects of your own self. You do not live in isolation. At a subtle level, we are all one. When you love others, you are loving yourself. The psychologist mentally affirmed this truth and sent out a sincere wave of love.

These four parts of Ho'oponopono can be used in any order. They can be used to heal yourself and the world around you.

What happened from Dr. Len doing this work was unbelievable, really astounding. Little by little everyone improved. Even the staff completely changed. Over the course of four years, all of the inmates, except two, were healed and released from the institution. In the end, the institution was closed with the last two inmates relocated. This all took place because one person took responsibility for the creation he experienced in his life and set about healing himself of his own creation. Whether you look at it as healing yourself to heal others, or healing others to heal yourself, it is the same thing, because we are all interconnected at the level of the oneness of consciousness.

The important thing to note is that this is something each of us can do when we are affected by the tragedies around us. Whether you are looking at the victims or the perpetrators, you can take responsibility and practice this methodology with all of them. It is a way to clear the misperceptions and energies that cause undesirable conditions. You may not have political or economic power to bring about changes, but even without such resources, you have love that you can radiate into any situation.

I'm sorry, please forgive me, thank you, I love you.

This Hawaiian system is one way of taking responsibility, but there are many other ways. First you take responsibility for yourself and do your inner work. Then take responsibility for conditions in the outer world, which is a reflection of yourself. Essentially, that means working with people – helping people to awaken to their true possibilities. Enriching people, helpin to fulfill their highest desires.

Taking responsibility means you are responsible for everything in the world. If you take responsibility, you can change it. If you don't take responsibility, you feel powerless. If you want the world to be a better place, then take responsibility whenever and wherever you can. We are all responsible for our leaders' greed, ineptitude, irresponsibility, and lack of care. We are responsible for corporate greed and abuse. We are responsible for the environment, for all the pollution and nuclear radiation. We are responsible for all the wars and starvation. We are responsible for the unnecessary pain and slaughter of billions of innocent animals eaten for food. We are each responsible for everything. At the deepest level of existence, you ARE everything, so you ARE responsible. This understanding of our true existence as consciousness, and our connection to it as unique individuals, will be explored in the next chapter.

It should be noted that the psychologist did not do this work alone. He taught others at the institution about the process and they used it as well. This reinforces the idea that when more people take responsibility, more powerful effects can be created. It should also be noted that it could have been accomplished much faster.

I mention this method by name because it became an Internet sensation. Yet, if other elements of the Extraordinary Healthcare system had been used, perhaps the prison ward could've been emptied in weeks or months instead of years. If you just use one good method such as Ho'oponopono and then live on hamburgers, ignoring other important realities, you won't accomplish nearly as much, nor as quickly. Everything matters.

Rapid Mental and Emotional Healing through Diet

The Hawaiian prison example showed how healing could be accomplished through Ho'oponopono, a psychological-spiritual intervention. It addressed one level or approach to mental healthcare, but it didn't include physical causes. The typical hospital-prison diet, itself, contains so much violence along with low-quality, low-nutrition foods. It is tainted with all manner of unnatural additives. If the physical, nutritional aspect of natural healthcare had been included, the results could have been dramatically accelerated. For example:

In Appleton, Wisconsin, at the Central Alternative High School, a study was conducted that resulted in a massive reduction in violence. It was accomplished in only weeks by radically changing the diet to a more natural diet, free of additives and junk foods. The dropout rate at the school was 90%. The halls were filled with altercations, dangers, and weapons. After the new diet was introduced, virtually all violence ceased and dropouts were reduced to zero. Drugs, weapons, and suicides were also reduced to zero. Learn more – http://www.feingold.org/PF/wisconsin1.html The primary change was to a healthier, more natural diet that included more fresh foods. Even though the results are dramatic, and took place in only weeks, it also does not represent the totality of what can be accomplished. Even more can be done. Dramatic healing can happen in only days. For example:

In India, Kiran Bedi, as Inspector-General of Prisons, accomplished an extraordinary transformation in an Indian prison in only 10 days through a sattvik (pure) vegetarian diet and an extensive program of vipassana meditation. A movie was made, documenting the process entitled, "Doing Time, Doing Vipassana". The knowledge now exists to completely transform our society and the world. It appears to be entirely possible to virtually empty all of our hospitals and prisons by healing the people through the techniques of Extraordinary Healthcare.

The key element in all of these efforts is taking responsibility. Various methods were used to bring about transformations in mental healthcare, some of which were more effective than others. The more methods you can include, the more rapid the results will be. Combined methods create combined power.

Noble Principle #4 - Enrichment

Your primary purpose in life must necessarily be to enrich the lives of others, as well as your own life. Why? Everything you have comes from your interaction with people. Your food, your home, your clothes, all your possessions, your ability to earn a living, your education, everything you can think of comes because of your contact with people, with nature, and with all aspects of life on earth. The more you can enrich the lives of other people, and improve the environment to support life, the more your own life is enriched.

Life is always expanding in every way possible. There are some people in the world who believe the world is overpopulated, that we need to get rid of this huge population. This concept is invalid. The only reason our large population is a burden is because of wrong education. If everyone had the education to unfold their infinite potential, including these four noble principles, we would very rapidly create a golden age. The more people, the better. The extraordinary capability and creativity of fully awakened people can solve all the world's problems, no matter the population.

Your primary purpose on earth is to enrich people, and to enrich all life around you. If all you do is take and never give in return, you are a thief. Taking and not giving to others is just selfishness. It leads to misery, because soon, no one will want to give you anything. The whole universe will work against you. Everyone needs to find some way to contribute to the lives of others and to life as a whole. Every time you interact with someone, they should come away from that interaction enriched, better off than before.

The world is in desperate need of a cultural transformation. One of the most powerful ways to heal yourself and to heal the world is to teach these four noble principles: Integrity, Authenticity, Responsibility, and Enrichment. They should be gently and wisely taught to everyone in your life – leaders, bosses, subordinates, friends, and family. They should be taught and practiced everywhere. A cultural transformation is the only way a Golden Age can become a reality.

The Four Extraordinary Powers

We all have supernormal powers. There are four of these powers. You may not think of them as supernormal powers, but they have the capability to create supernormal transformations.

The Power of Words

The words you speak can transform the listener. Think of the "I have a dream" speech by Martin Luther King. Words have the power to uplift and inspire us to new levels of accomplishment. In this case it created a whole movement for the transformation of a society. Words can affect our friendships and our business relations. A wrong word can end a relationship and create an enemy. Words have tremendous power. They can inspire a person to become a saint or to train a terrorist. Adolf Hitler also used the power of words. We have to recognize the power of words and how they can be used for good or evil. Just as you need to watch your thoughts carefully, also watch your words, watch your speech.

The Power of Thoughts

The power of thoughts is the power of ideas. Ideas are what transform people and civilizations. The thoughts that you think can be a useless collection of random chaos or they can be focused and creative plans to help uplift your life and the community around you. To have control over your mind, to culture powerful and creative thought, is one of the greatest powers and assets in your life. Ideas are a great power. They are really a super power. They are responsible for all the advancement of humanity. When you learn to harness the power of your own mind, then you become a powerful, creative force in the world.

The Power of Feeling

The power of feeling is also a super power. When you can feel the pain that others are going through, you can have compassion. Feelings provide the power for your motivation. You can never do anything unless you have the power of feeling behind it. The ultimate power of feeling is loving compassion. It's worthwhile to cultivate a feeling of love for all people and for all life. Your purpose for coming to planet Earth is to become a being of love. This is not something you want to miss. Do everything in your power to cultivate devotion to all of humanity. Only when you sincerely care about fulfilling the needs and wants of others will the Universe come to support you.

The Power of Action

All the words, all the thoughts and plans, and all the love will not have much impact unless they are put into action. You have to live it. The power of action means living and radiating your highest state of consciousness, and taking powerful action to accomplish something worthwhile, something that will enrich all life around you. Any job, even an ordinary clerical job, or a checkout job at the supermarket, can be an opportunity for you to express the power of action and living from your highest awareness.

How many people you can help depends upon your sphere of influence. You can work at any level and make a contribution. You can always make a difference no matter where you are. But if you can develop your skills and expand your sphere of influence, you can help many more people. All the great teachers have said that you don't really know your power until you begin to use it and do your best. When the Universe sees you doing your best, it comes to carry you to heights that you could not have imagined. Just begin. Continue to expand and develop your skills so that you can help at a higher level. Helping to enrich the lives of others is what gives life satisfaction, and your life rewards will be a million times more than you give.

Never feel powerless. You always have these four extraordinary powers to draw upon. Wherever you are, whoever you are with, you can use your four extraordinary powers. Combine your four extraordinary powers with the four noble principles and you have a winning combination.

Visualization and Verbal Suggestion - Using Your Mind Correctly

We all think in both pictures and words. They both represent ideas that are independent of either the picture or the word. The idea is the same in any language and many pictures can represent the same idea. When you want to use your mind to accomplish something, generally you are working with ideas expressed either as language or pictures. The deeper these ideas can operate within your system, the more powerful they can be.

In the section on energy healing, I introduced the idea of building bio-energy in your system through deep breathing. I also suggested other methods of collecting energy through intention. Then that energy was directed through intention and attention. Attention means localizing your conscious awareness on a particular place or thing. Intention means focusing energy with a particular intent or idea.

Intentions and ideas are expressed as pictures (visualization) or language, words, either mentally or verbally. Both can work, but visualization is far more powerful. There are techniques that use only language, such as autosuggestion and affirmation. There are techniques that use visualization to impress the suggestion. There are also techniques that use sound without reference to any meaning or idea – just the quality of sound itself. How to use your mind, how to culture your most valuable qualities of heart, how to expand consciousness – these are the most critical subjects for the life of all human beings. Let's look at some of these techniques.

Visualization vs. Suggestion

If you say you're going to do something, but you see yourself doing something else, which one do you think will win out? It turns out that what you say is not as powerful as what you see. If you cannot see yourself doing it, it won't happen. Likewise, if you see yourself doing something that you know you should NOT do, again the visualization usually wins out. It's more powerful. I talked about watching your thoughts earlier. What this means is 1) listen carefully to your inner verbal dialogue, 2) carefully watch your inner movies. If they are not what you want then cancel the existing thought and replace it with something worthwhile. Cancel verbal dialogue verbally. Cancel pictures and movies by visually shattering them and replacing them with better pictures and movies.

Visualization is more dominant, because visuals represent a richer set of information. What determines your action is a combination of the ideas that you hold, both verbally and visually, plus the force of emotion behind them, the support you give them, the responsibility you take for them. When ideas, as language and visualization, combine with the energy of emotions, such as enthusiasm and compassion, you take action. We all act more on feeling than logic. Thoughts, as language or visualization, give the direction, but emotion is the driving force. The most powerful way to change your behavior is to unify what you say, what you see, what you feel, and, of course, what you do.

Say-See-Feel-Do

If you want to guide your life in a particular direction then you can apply the formula, *say-see-feel-do*. Say to yourself what you want to do. See yourself doing it in pictures and movies. Feel how it feels to be doing your planned activity. Feel the inspiration or joy. Then do it. If you combine all of these, then you won't be conflicted inside. Otherwise, you will be at odds with yourself, and you won't be able to sustain yourself in any particular direction without tripping yourself up. As you plan your day each morning, use this formula. *"Say-See-Feel-Do"*

Your Self Image

It's virtually impossible to manifest anything that conflicts with your self image. Your self image is the overarching controller of your life. The most important thing you can do is to build a strong and beautiful self image. You should see yourself as a great being, a saint, a genius, a creative artist, a leader. You are really much more than that, but we have been trained to disparage ourselves. Self-criticism, putting yourself down, not recognizing your worth, is false humility, useless. It is as useless as being egoistic, seeing yourself as superior to others. In truth, you are unique, you are not in competition with anyone. You should see yourself as nothing less than a divine being, then you will be able to accomplish great things.

Rebuild your self image by carefully watching your inner dialogue. Cancel negative thoughts, then replace them with something extraordinary. It's a developmental process over time.

Another powerful methodology to transform your self image is to dissociate from your patterns. When your self image is associated with failures, negative patterns, incompletions, or any other limiting conception of yourself, it pulls you down. Disconnect from what you think of as your identity, with all its limitations.

One powerful way to disconnect from a limited identity is to associate with an infinite identity. Expand what you think of as you to include the whole universe. This technique will be covered in more detail in the chapter on consciousness.

Likewise, what you project into the outer world, to other people, should inspire them to greatness. Help others build a higher self image of themselves. Always listen to others with sincerity and be willing to accept feedback gracefully from others on how you can become a more ideal being. Offer suggestions to others from a place of love, if they are receptive.

Culturing Successful Behavior

The main obstacles to using your mind successfully and changing behavior are: 1) the backlog of conditioning, 2) bad mental habits, 3) emotionally charged events, and 4) the emphasis on logic throughout our educational system. I've already introduced some techniques to help. Let's look at mind and behavior more deeply.

There are three types of behavior. The lowest level is reactive behavior. Reactive behavior is based purely on past conditioning. If someone says something to you that you don't like, you react without thinking. You may even start a fight. Most of our culture, our business models, our competitive sports, even the idea of competition itself exploits this kind of behavior. It says, "I am separate from you, and I am going to win. You are going to lose." Reactive behavior is often intensified by hormone imbalances that can create highly aberrant, even heinous behavior. It can lead to the destruction of families, societies, even countries.

The next level of behavior is logical behavior. Instead of reacting, you try to sort out a better solution logically, so that both of you can win. You explore good logical reasons for your choices. This kind of behavior is based on intellect and it operates at a higher level than instinctive or reactive behavior. You try to be reasonable, logical. You search for agreement and solutions.

Logic can only compute a limited number of variables and can only predict consequences based on a limited set of data. It can only operate on already known facts and can't function in novel or unknown situations. It's far better to be logical than to be reactive. When you are logical, at least you use the right reasons to change your behavior. But logical instruction alone is not enough. It's necessary to understand the reasons why you are doing something or why you choose not to. The next level of behavior, beyond logical behavior, is intuitive behavior.

Intuition is connected to the whole. It can compute everything at once, without logic. It is knowingness. You know without knowing how you know, but you know with an inner certainty. It has no negativity, separatism, or egotism connected with it. It is pure, light, energetic, and wise. This kind of behavior comes with inspiration and eliminates the drudgery of constant calculation. This is where you want to be.

A new science is developing about how to set a desire or intention within yourself that will accomplish your goals without having to know the process or the details. Usually, the logical or thinking mind always wants to know "how," but those "how-to" details are rarely available. There's a better way. All you really have to know is "what" you want. If you can program that desire into the right place, which is the central brain, then your connection to the Universe works out the details.

It turns out that we can bypass the logical mind with all its conditioning, expectations, limitations, confusions, and other drawbacks. The way to bypass both the reactive and logical mind is to bypass the logical circuits of the brain, the cortex. The real power of the brain is in the center of the brain, the midbrain. If we program this part of the brain with visualization rather than verbalization, then we can accomplish our desires far easier – because that part of the brain is the most connected and most powerful. We can use *say-see-feel-do* at the location of the central brain. To do that, let's understand the brain.

Understanding the Brain

The human brain is a miracle. We may never fully understand it, but there are a few things you should know in order to best use it. The brain has different layers or sections devoted to different purposes. Without going into any great detail, let's look at three basic areas. 1) The brainstem and the cerebellum, the lower part of the brain, connects to the body and controls basic metabolic functions and coordination. 2) The central brain includes the master endocrine glands and many specialized structures. 3) The outer brain includes the prefrontal cortex, the cortex, and the various outer lobes of the brain. The educational system, plus family and social conditioning are what program the outer brain. This outer brain is responsible for producing reactive and logical thoughts and behavior. The chaos of our mind is due to the faulty programming of the outer brain.

However, the real power of the brain is the central brain. This area of the brain contains all the magical, mystical, truly amazing components of the brain. Some examples are: the pineal gland, the thalamus, the hypothalamus, the pituitary, the amygdala, hippocampus, and other esoteric structures. This region of the brain can bypass the need for logic and overcome the chaos of the outer brain. You don't have to know what all these structures do. Probably no ordinary human does at this point. All you have to know is that it's possible to set an intention in this part of the brain and that intention will manifest itself in outer reality. We just need to know how to program the brain.

Properly Programming Your Brain

According to the yogis and masters in India, the way to program your brain for success is to visualize what you want at the sixth chakra and take it into the center of the brain, the midbrain. This is like giving an instruction to the whole cosmos, placing an order for what you want in your life. Again, be very careful how you use your thoughts. Only see what you want, rather than trying to avoid what you don't want. See exactly what you want without any negative conditions or conflict between what you say, see, feel, and are willing to do.

Say it, see it, and feel it. Take responsibility for it. Support it willingly. Then, because you are universally connected to the underlying consciousness behind everything, circumstances will then begin to operate in your favor. You only have to allow the Universe to support you and not react in opposition when the things that you really want start coming your way. Decide what you want and then live with trust that the universe knows how to bring it to you. Seize opportunities as they arise and work with sincerity to make them happen. Follow your intuition. According to the ancient teachings, this formula can truly work miracles. You can use it for business success, personal success, relationships, anything that you want to manifest in your life.

Sound and Healing

I've talked about thoughts as language and thoughts as visualization. Another option is the use of sound to create a change in the structure of the brain and mind. Vibration is a science that the Western world is just beginning to grasp. Techniques of using sound to bring about a purification or enhancement to the brain/mind were developed thousands of years ago by yogis and siddhas, perfected beings living in the high reaches of the Himalayas and in the Kevari River region of India. This science is not generally available, but I want you to know that it exists.

I'll present some of these discoveries and give you a few practical tools that you can use in the next chapter. Working with the mind constructively is more powerful if you can develop a higher state of consciousness. In the next chapter, I'll explain how consciousness is realized and how you can accelerate healing by expanding consciousness.

Summary of Mental Healing

Review this chapter and select the methods that you want to use. Schedule these in your calendar and daily to-do list so you get them done. The ones you cannot do immediately, put into your reminder system to jog your memory later.

Be more aware. Listen to your verbal language both as thoughts and speech, observe your inner pictures and movies. Get yourself into a state of completion with your past. Weed out the thoughts and patterns that no longer serve you. Decide which thoughts and patterns from the past you want to fulfill and which ones you want to cancel. Set high goals. Program your central brain with these goals. Recognize opportunities as they arise and take spontaneous action: make phone calls, send emails, develop plans, etc. Learn and practice *The Four Noble Principles*. Heal yourself by seeing your life creation as a reflection of yourself and take responsibility for it. Use the Hawaiian method Ho'oponopono if you like. Find a way to make amends to others for your past lack of integrity and inauthenticity. Practice forgiveness and keep yourself in a continuous state of gratitude. Use your four super powers. The power of words, thoughts, feelings, and action – radiating and living it.

The unenlightened mind always tries to keep you in a state of drama – pursuing illusions, fantasies, and false happiness. This drama is based on past incompletions. Realize you can never find relief from problems or find lasting happiness through anything outside of yourself. Both the pursuit of pleasure and ignoring pain, can never bring lasting happiness. This includes all possessions, relationships, wealth, success, fame, or any other pursuit. It isn't that you can't have those things, but when you believe they will bring you happiness, you get into trouble. Of course, the opposite is also true. Poverty, conflicts, failure, and ignominy will not bring happiness either.

When you live in the state of incompletion, filled with suppressed emotions such as self hatred, every decision you make will bring misery. When you find yourself being dragged down, STOP EVERYTHING. Do completion with the current incident and the previous events that were precursors for the emotion you are caught up in. Clear your past of all incompletions as much as possible on a daily basis. Then your natural enthusiasm and love of life returns. Only when you clear all of your past incompletions and replace self-doubt with trust, self-hatred with love, and self-denial with self-affirmation, will your life have power, bliss, wisdom, and joy. You restore the willingness and openness to embrace life, and to contribute to life. Then, whether you have relationships like marriage or not, whether you have wealth, fame, and success, or not, you will live in a state of fulfillment beyond anything money or success can buy.

There are two kinds of happiness. One kind is temporary and is based on external circumstances such as success, pleasure, and getting what you want. Happiness derived this way always has an end and we are always fighting to prevent that loss. The other kind of happiness is causeless happiness. It is derived from your inner state of consciousness. Once fully gained, it can never be lost. It is a state beyond the mind. It's the subject of the next chapter on Healthcare and Consciousness. It is the state of ultimate healing. The ideal is to have both inner happiness and outer success, but sacrificing the inner to achieve the outer is an inconceivable loss.

To achieve both inner and outer success, first clear your inner mental space of everything that has dragged you down. Then reprogram your inner space, change your self image. See yourself in the highest possible light. Say it, see it, feel it, then take action to become it. You will then achieve success in the inner world and outer world.

You now have extremely powerful and practical ways to accomplish your mental healthcare. You can take your power back, you can heal your mental space, and you can be in control of your life. As you will see in the next chapter, the control you are activating is from a higher level of yourself, not your ego self. Take the time you need to heal. Work consistently with yourself. Do NOT berate yourself. Your self talk is VERY significant and it should always be constructive. It should never make you feel powerless, but should reinforce your natural power. Stay far away from guilt and shame. They do not serve you. Whenever you collapse into powerlessness, you are on the wrong path.

Schedule a regular time each day to consciously reprogram your biocomputer. The half hour or more before sleep is a good time to clear your inner space of all incompletions and patterns. Use the time to upgrade your mental healthcare.

Use your mental talk and imagery to create the conditions you desire. Do NOT use it to see yourself with problems. Seeing yourself with problems creates problems. Thought directs energy and creates realities. Create the reality you want by changing the focus and content of your thoughts.

program your self image, which is the basis of all success. Below is an action plan with the essentials from this chapter that you can post to your reminder system.

Action Plan - Chapter 11, Mental Healing

1. Understand garbage in, garbage out. Choose your experiences carefully. Disconnect the TV. Eliminate the garbage, introduce sublime experiences.
2. Nurture your mind with the best this world has to offer: the wisest mentors, the best books, and the most inspiring media.
3. Watch your thoughts like a hawk. Know what you are thinking, why you are thinking it, and the expected result.
4. Slow your mind by slowing your breath. Breathe in and out 4-5 seconds, up to 8-10 seconds.
5. Overcome conditioning by 1) Not feeding it, 2) Recognizing/canceling useless thoughts, 3) Programming useful thoughts and a new self image. (Details below)
6. Begin recognizing where you are caught by fantasies of greed and fear. Observe the play and recognize how it can never lead to fulfillment. Recognize how it keeps you in a constant state of dissatisfaction and unhappiness as you keep trying to seek pleasure and avoid pain.
7. Choose to not resist reality as it is. Non-resistance should be your first response to any life event. Then decide whether to 1) intelligently oppose, 2) creatively change, or 3) accept the reality. When you see things as they are, solutions become self evident. Your logic and intuition will guide you. Your best option is almost always to change things through your creativity, imagination, courage, inspiration, and productive work.
8. Reality is in the present moment, fantasies are always misguided projections about the past or future. Continuously bring yourself back to recognizing your living presence existing in this present moment. Fantasy is different from constructive imagination.
9. Use imagination, creativity, and visualization to transform your current reality into a better future – in practical ways, not just fantasizing.
10. Forget "positive thinking." Do not fight with negativity. Examine your negative programming. Positivity is your natural state and returns when your negative programs have been purged from your system. That process is the process of completion: 1) Bring your highly charged negative thoughts to the surface, 2) Scan your life history and find the event and the decision you made to adopt the negative mental pattern 3) Relive the event consciously, from a place of objectivity, disassociation, non-identity until the incident no longer produces an emotional reaction, until the charge on it is gone 4) Understand the pattern, the decision you made back then, and recognize it is not serving you. Understand the wrong interpretations and

assumptions you made about reality 5) Decide you are no longer going to fulfill this decision. It was a mistake. As you choose your new reality, other negative, controlling incidents may show up 6) Again, process each past incident until its emotional aspect dissipates and the charge is gone. Correct your decisions and interpretations associated with the event. Be complete with it. 7) When your slate is clean, program in what you really want. Create your new future with Mental Healthcare sessions.

11. Understand the 4 choices: 1) Feels good, is good, 2) Feels good, is bad, 3) Feels bad, is good, 4) Feels bad, is bad. When you make choices, what category does it fall into? Examine your past and upcoming choices.

12. Constantly live the Four Noble Principles: 1) Integrity, 2) Authenticity, 3) Responsibility, 4) Enrich yourself and others. Use Ho'oponopono.

13. Observe your thoughts, your words, your pictures, your movies, and your feelings. Use your four super powers: Words, Thoughts, Feelings, and Action – radiate a high state of consciousness, take action. Be powerful.

14. To be without inner conflict, make what you say, see, feel, and do agree. "Say-See-Feel-Do". Say it (affirm it in language), See it (visualize it in pictures and movies), Feel it in your heart, and Do it (take action).

15. To use your mind successfully, remove these obstacles: 1) Past conditioning, 2) Bad mental habits, 3) Emotionally charged past events, 4) Excessive emphasis on logic and linear thinking. Mental Healthcare sessions make this possible.

16. Recognize the three levels of behavior: 1) Reactive, 2) Logical, and 3) Intuitive. Understand how you are behaving at any time.

17. Upgrade your self image. Program the central brain through visualization at the 6th chakra - what you Say, See, Feel, and are willing to Do.

18. Build a strong and beautiful self image. See yourself as a great being, a saint, genius, creative artist, and leader.

19. Offer inspiration to others to rebuild their self image. Be a sincere listener and accept feedback from others gracefully.

Chapter 12
Healthcare and Consciousness

Consciousness Is the Ultimate Healer

A Guide to Expanding Your Consciousness

What to Expect

Consciousness is one of the great mysteries of life. When you wake up in the morning, you know you are conscious, you know that you exist. Yet consciousness varies greatly from barely conscious to superconscious. The more conscious you are, the easier it is to comprehend everything. Consciousness illuminates mind, intellect, heart, body, and senses. Just as a light illuminates a room, consciousness lights up everything about you. Without that light, you cannot exist. The brain does not create consciousness, consciousness creates the brain... and everything else. When you expand consciousness, you expand every facet of life.

Degrees and States of Consciousness

You probably remember in school that some students learned everything easily. They made straight A's without trying very hard, while most of the class struggled to understand. What was the difference? Did you notice that "A" students were not only better at academics, but often excelled at practically everything. The difference is not just IQ, it's consciousness. What is consciousness? Let's look at an example.

When you wake up in the morning and you're groggy, you can't function well, you operate at a minimal level. When you wake up a little more, all your faculties improve. That's the difference between lower consciousness and higher consciousness. Now, what if you could keep waking up?

At higher levels of consciousness, all your abilities rise – your ability to know and understand, your IQ, your ability to develop new talents, your ability to enjoy life, your ability to love, and your ability to heal. The quality and intensity of your life depends upon consciousness.

Can you increase consciousness? The answer is a resounding "Yes!" This is the most important fact on planet Earth. When you expand your consciousness, your life expands. The quality of your life is directly related to your level of consciousness.

We can understand degrees or levels of consciousness by the common experience of waking up barely conscious, then waking up to our normal waking state. But there are also entirely different *states* of consciousness. For instance – deep sleep, dreaming, and waking are all completely different from each other. What is possible while dreaming seems completely different from what is possible in the waking state. In deep sleep, nothing is possible. We are all aware of these three states, but could there be others? Again, the answer is "Yes." There is a fourth state of consciousness. Later, we'll explore the 5th, 6th, and 7th states of consciousness. First, let's look at this matrix to discover the fourth state:

	Thoughts	No Thoughts
Self Aware	Waking State	??
Unaware	Dream State	Deep Sleep

In the waking state you are aware that you exist, and you have thoughts. In the dream state, you have thoughts, but you are unaware of your existence. Only a fantasy world of thoughts exists. You have no control over them because the self-aware "you" is not present. The awareness of self-existence is missing. When you become self-aware, you wake up out of the dreaming state into the waking state. In deep sleep, you are unaware that you exist, and you have no thoughts. There is a fourth category. To be aware, to be conscious, but with no sensory or mental activity, no thoughts, only pure consciousness, pure self-existence.

It is this fourth category that is vitally important. It is pure awareness or consciousness by itself, unalloyed, uncontaminated by anything else. The key to expanding consciousness is to repeatedly immerse yourself in this fourth state.

Pure consciousness is the stuff that illumines all of our experiences and it is always available. It is the watcher, the observer. It is that which sees the eyes seeing, hears the ears hearing, watches thoughts come and go, feels emotions come and go. It is a separate field that observes all the changes without ever changing itself.

For instance, you can remember being a child. When you had a child's body and a child's mind, you were completely different from how you are today. But something is not different. That something is the essential you, the consciousness that experienced the child's body and child's mind. When you were a teenager, you thought and acted like a teenager. You were different from the child. But something was not different. That something is the consciousness that was observing when you were a teenager. From the time you were born to becoming a child, then a teenager, then an adult, everything about you – your body, mind, and emotions all changed – but the aspect of you that was observing is unchanged. This is what gives stability and continuity of you being the same person. It has never changed and it will never change in the future. This aspect of you always exists. Consciousness is beyond the body, senses, mind, and emotions. It is the pure observer of everything. It is your essential Self.

At any moment, you can shift your focus from the outer world to recognize that there is an inner aspect of you that is observing. When you do that, the observer becomes more dominant. Notice right now that there is something inside you observing this text, observing your mind's reaction to it. Notice how it becomes more dominant when you do that.

But you can never observe the observer itself, because it is the observer that observes. If there were a separate observer to observe the observer, it would lead to infinite regression. So you can never observe it, but you can BE it. You can recognize that it exists at your inner core. You can allow it to become more dominant by shifting your awareness towards it, by shifting away from both the outer world of objects and the inner world of thoughts and sensations, to be the observer. You simply shift your attention deeper into inner space to arrive at the Self-referral state of the observer. This inner core, the observer within you, is pure consciousness, the fourth state of consciousness. It never changes, it is constant, pure.

Awakening Consciousness

Repeatedly recognizing pure consciousness at your inner core, awakens and expands consciousness in the waking, dreaming, and pure sleep states. There are a thousand ways to do it. Most of them involve shifting away from (or minimizing) outer sensory and mental experience, and settling into recognizing and being the observer. It's easy to do, but unfortunately, it's rarely taught in any part of the world.

Essentially, I'm talking about different methods of meditation that allow you to recede from the outer world and allow the inner world of consciousness to become more dominant. As it is, the outer world is most dominant. That's why most people have so little control. It's like the driver of a car who doesn't realize he is behind the wheel. The car is out of control and he doesn't realize he could control it.

251

Another example is going to the movies, that I mentioned earlier. Let's review that example in terms of consciousness. You remember attending a particularly exciting movie. When you first sat down in the theater, you realized that you were in the theater. As the movie progressed and became more exciting, you forgot where you were. You became hypnotized by the images in front of you and you became the hero, the character on the screen in the movie. When the hero goes over the cliff, you go over the cliff with him and your heart starts pounding and racing.

You are now dominated, hypnotized by the movie and you don't realize that you exist, that you are sitting in a comfortable theater. You are in an un-self-aware condition. It's more like a dream. You are in a temporary state of hypnotic amnesia about who you are, a conditioned state of chaos and drama from the movie. You are, in fact, being programmed with the full force of this violence within the movie because of your un-self-aware consciousness. This is a very dangerous thing. Only when the lights come on at the end of the movie, do you realize that you are safe, you are okay, that you exist separate from the movie. The problem is, due to your unconscious state, you have now been infected by the violence. It leaves an indelible scar.

Likewise, your daily experience is just like a movie, and you are the watcher. When your life gets too much drama, like with the movie, you get caught up in it. You are hypnotized by the images coming in through your senses. You get completely lost, overshadowed by events. If you stop to realize that at your essential core you are the observer, then the movie of life does not overshadow you anymore. If you can come back to the silent, stable place within yourself, you can realize that you are okay, safe, at peace just like at the end of the movie when the lights came on. Then you are no longer a victim of the life-movie and can decide how you want to respond.

As with the car example, you realize that you are the one behind the wheel. You can take control of the car and drive differently. The more you COME BACK to the inner state of recognizing that there is an observer, a silent observer, within you that is never affected by any of the drama, then the more awake you become. You are then able to take your power back and become the powerful, loving, conscious being you were meant to be.

Methods to Awaken Consciousness

It's easy to achieve the fourth state of consciousness and awaken higher states of consciousness. All you need to do is minimize sensory and mental activity. Allow it to subside. Shift the emphasis of your awareness from the outer world (and mental world), to the place of the observer, and allow it to be more dominant. Practically speaking, you need to begin by using techniques. For most of us, the mind is too chaotic, too full of thoughts. We don't realize we could drop easily into the silence of consciousness that is behind it all. So we have to do some technique to start.

Slow Your Breath to Slow Your Mind

Most people can't simply turn off their mind, so we use techniques. It turns out that the mind closely parallels the breath. When you're excited you breathe more and faster. When you're peaceful you breathe much slower. It works the other way around, also. If you slow your breath, your mind slows down and you regain control of it by restoring your connection to consciousness, Self.

Start with Breathing Deeply

As I mentioned in an earlier chapter, you always start with deep breathing. Substantial breathing before meditation really helps to clear out the "cobwebs." All you have to do is breathe deeply and rapidly. Continue until you begin to feel a little lightheaded, then keep yourself in that highly charged state for a little while, perhaps a few minutes.

In the yoga system, breathing methods are called pranayama. Two deep breathing methods are kapalabhati and bhastrika. Kapalabhati pranayama is a deep, rapid breathing technique that uses forceful exhalation in which you quickly lift the abdomen up and pull inward toward the spine. You rapidly, forcefully expel air, about twice per second. For inhalation, you just relax the abdomen and inhalation takes care of itself. Bhastrika pranayama is also deep and rapid, but gives equal weight to the in-breath and out-breath. You can use either, but kapalabhati massages the abdominal organs more, which has greater health benefits. Try them now to experience the difference.

Next, Ultra Slow or Sigh Breathing

Ultra slow breathing and sigh breathing were taught in the bio-energy and mental healing chapters. They are a great next step after oxygenation with either kapalabhati or bhastrika pranayamas. Try it now. Start breathing to a count of five-seconds in and five-seconds out. After a few minutes, increase the timing to 10 seconds. How did it feel? Did you notice how soothing and quieting it was for your whole system? Long, ultra-slow breathing really helps to take you into a meditative state. Forget about counting once you get a sense of the timing.

You could also use sigh breathing before or after ultra-slow breathing. When you breathe out, just give a big, long sigh. Within a few minutes, you will regain a deep peace and calm.

Meditation by Observing Your Breath

This is a classic meditation derived from the ancient Yoga or Vedic tradition, from thousands of years ago. All you do is breathe in and out slowly and place your attention at your nostrils. Observe your breath at your nostrils as it goes in and out. If your attention goes somewhere else, which it does, simply come back.

It seems like a simple technique, and actually it is, but we tend to make things so complicated as our mind races around. All you do is gently return to observing the breath at the nostrils – observe it as it comes in, feel it enter your body, and finally observe it going out. As you do this, you will notice how much calmer you feel. Don't try to keep your mind from wavering and losing focus on the breath. Forcing or suppressing your mind by effort never works. You are just allowing your attention to be at the nostrils and gently returning when you realize it's not there. There is no force or effort and no resistance. If you practice this technique for a few weeks, for 20 to 30 minutes twice a day, it will have quite a profound effect.

Watching the Gaps Between Breaths

Watching the breath is a very powerful technique to get deep into meditation. Once you are familiar with watching the in-breath and the out-breath, you can refine the technique. When you breathe, air is not always moving. At the end of the in-breath, before you breathe out again, your breath is perfectly still. The same is true when you breathe out and before you breathe in again. Your breath at the turnaround is perfectly still. These two still points are longer than we realize. The next step in the breath meditation is to watch these gaps between in-breathing and out-breathing. At those two points, the mind is not active.

When your mind is not active, it's easier to recognize the place inside you that is observing. What you are doing is allowing your attention to settle deeper, away from the outer world and into the observer space that is watching, observing. That pure space is always there, always has been there, always will be there. It can be recognized and allowed to become more familiar, more dominant at any time. You just shift your frame of reference from outer to inner and allow the inner observer to be more dominant. That inner consciousness is your own presence. It is your pure existence, beyond the body, mind, and senses. It is the basis of and the watcher of all three.

Observe Your Thoughts

Just as watching your breath slows the thinking process and brings you into the present moment, so does observing your thoughts. Ordinarily, you have a stream of thoughts going on all the time. It's often referred to as a *stream of consciousness*, but really, it's a stream of unconsciousness. You are not really present and your mind is running by itself, uncontrolled, chaotic. When you bring your awareness, your presence, to observe the thinking process itself, then your thinking is automatically controlled without effort. You don't have to control your mind. In fact, trying to suppress or control your mind by effort doesn't work.

When you watch your thoughts, you can be aware that there are thoughts and also something that is observing. That observer is consciousness itself, your presence. In every experience there are always three things: 1) the object, 2) the process of observing, through the senses or mind, and 3) the observer.

You can shift the focus of your awareness from "objects," such as the breath or thoughts, towards the presence that is watching, which is your innermost Self. This shifting of your focus from the objects of awareness, towards recognizing the presence that is watching (awareness itself), awakens and strengthens consciousness/awareness/presence.

Your Presence is Realized More in the No-Mind State

Just as there is a gap between breaths, there is also a gap between thoughts. It's easier to recognize the observer as having its own status, its own separate existence, in the gaps between thoughts. In that space, the mind is not thinking. It's in the no-mind state, the silent-mind state, the state when your awareness, your presence exists by itself. This gives a greater opportunity to recognize your presence, pure existence, pure Self. When this is practiced repeatedly, continuously, consciousness progressively awakens to higher levels.

Meditating 24 Hours a Day

Since that space of the observer, your presence, is always there and always available (even during sleep), you can at any point allow yourself to shift your dominant awareness to that of the observer, your own inner presence. You can constantly withdraw your attention back into itself. This means you don't always have to meditate with eyes closed. Whatever you are doing, you can do while established in recognition of the presence of the observer. It takes a little practice only because it is unfamiliar, because you have generally been drawn into the outer world of senses and objects. It's just the opposite of allowing yourself to be drawn excessively outward, dominated by the drama of the senses and the mind. It's best to practice when you are doing simple things, safe tasks, not while driving.

Generally, it's easier to begin meditation with eyes closed because there is less distraction. Once you understand it and have some familiarity with the observer, you can instantly shift that direction anytime, anywhere.

You always have the option to put your attention on anything you want to. In this case, no matter what you're doing, you can come back to the state of recognizing your own presence as fundamental to the process of experiencing. It is always there. That continuous Self referral experience strengthens pure consciousness, the presence inside you, the presence that IS you. As you regain a stronger sense of Self awareness you can begin to use it.

Using Self-Awareness for Conscious Healthcare

At the deepest level, it is awareness, consciousness that heals. Bio-energy healing uses this awareness to heal. Consciousness has four primary aspects to it: energy, bliss, intelligence, and compassion. Consciousness, your presence, IS life energy. It is the stuff of life itself. It is pure intelligence, pure compassion, pure bliss, and pure life energy. That's why when you direct your attention, your presence, onto some part of the body, it has such a profound influence. The intensified, localized presence of awareness does the healing work. You can enhance the quality of healing through intention, by infusing your desired outcome into the process. This is related to the process of what is called samyama in the ancient Vedic tradition. Though we associate consciousness with energy, bliss, intelligence, and compassion, it is really at the deepest reality, featureless, pure, beyond all qualities. As it becomes expressed, these beautiful qualities come forth. We can use consciousness to bring forth qualities and realities through the ancient technique of *samyama*.

Samyama - Using Self-Awareness to Cause Desired Outcomes

The Vedic tradition includes the yoga and siddha traditions that are thousands of years old. The process of samyama is detailed in the Yoga Sutras of Patanjali. The sages of India discovered it many thousands of years ago as they explored all aspects of consciousness and the human condition.

I talked about suggestion and visualization in an earlier chapter, now I would like to introduce a deeper methodology. Consciousness is like fertile soil. Whatever you plant in it will grow. All you have to do is decide what you want to plant. Here's how it works. If you entertain an idea, represented either by language or by visualization, and then drop that idea into consciousness, it will manifest. Suppose for instance you have a stiff neck. If you 1) localize your awareness on your neck, 2) think the idea "be healed," 3) allow that idea to settle deeper and deeper towards your own consciousness, your own presence, then that idea gains power and becomes manifest. Your neck will be healed, though it may take repeated application. Initially, the full force of the method is not generally available because of 1) your inexperience, and 2) your embedded stress that prevents you from settling into your innermost consciousness. Yet, it still happens every time, at least partially, and the impediments are released as you practice. Let's look at it in more detail. It's a very subtle but powerful process.

Samyama has three parts: Choosing an idea, allowing that idea to settle deeper and deeper towards your own consciousness, then it merges with consciousness – which strengthens the idea and causes it to manifest. The process is really simple, but it requires a little practice to experience how it works. Choose an idea, shift awareness from the idea to subtler, quieter, more abstract levels – towards your inner presence, Self awareness, consciousness. As you approach consciousness itself, the idea becomes subtle, hardly differentiated from consciousness. Finally, it becomes one with Self-consciousness as you enter the Self referral state of pure consciousness. Essentially, you choose an idea, then pause for a few seconds and allow yourself to settle deeper into silence. The idea comes with you as you settle into and become one with your own presence.

Samyama is working with ideas taken to the level of pure consciousness. You can represent ideas with words and pictures. It may also include feelings. But the idea is different from language. If you spoke a different language your words would be different, but the idea is the same. Likewise, the same idea can be represented with different pictures. Feelings are also part of the idea "package." But the idea is subtler and is independent of the language, visualization, or feeling used to recall it. When you return to the idea during samyama, it is the idea you are returning to, the remembrance, not the language you first used to express it. It is essentially, "Say, See, Feel, *Be* instead of Do." It is the non-doing complement of "Say, See, Feel, Do." Samyama helps you to take control of your mind in a completely new way.

Your mind likes to play tricks on you and it will do anything to protect its ego even if it is destructive. Either you are the controller of your mind, or your mind takes control of you and messes with you. Your mind can be your worst enemy or your best friend. You have to watch your thoughts like a hawk. Don't feed what you don't want. Only feed what you do want. As you continue to feed what you want, and avoid feeding what is not useful, you train your mind to be responsive to your true desires. Then your mind becomes your best friend. Samyama is a new way to feed your mind.

You can quickly transform your inner mental and emotional state through the technique of samyama. The method is to choose an idea and drop that idea into the absolute stillness of your pure presence. For example, choose "compassion," "joy," or "bliss." Then go inward, toward the part of you that observes. That idea begins to powerfully manifest and the emotional quality that you have chosen is boosted. You feel more compassionate, joyful, or blissful. It only takes a few seconds.

Try it. Think the word "bliss," then pause for a few seconds as you sink deeper into pure Self. Shift the dominance of your awareness from the idea to the observer. It may be 5, 10, even 15 seconds as you sink deeper. Then the result wells up inside you momentarily. Repeat again. Think the idea and then let go and drop into the silence, be the observer. The result wells up in you more powerfully each time. Repeat over and over again. Soon you will notice your inner space change and you will feel blissful. Bliss will grow tremendously as you repeat the process. The resulting lightness will begin operating on your endocrine system, causing it to produce new healing chemicals. Keep creating this joy and bliss over and over again. You could do this for several minutes at a time, a few times a day.

As you return to the idea of bliss, you will find that you don't need to pronounce the word at all, you will be able to return to the idea as an idea without a mental pronunciation. So when you come back to it, it doesn't need to be a clear pronunciation just a recognition of the idea and then again dropping into silence, into the no-mind, silent-mind state. One way to return to the silent-mind state easily is to recall the idea and then breathe out a deep sigh. At the end of the sigh there is no mental activity. Think the word or the idea and then give a deep sigh and remain in that space for a few seconds. With experience, you can just shift, you won't need to use the sigh.

When you first begin, it may not happen instantly. It's a skill and an art that develops as you practice. Read these instructions many times until you understand them. Practice a lot until you can keep yourself in an uplifted state, a state of power, loving compassion, joy, bliss, enthusiasm, or any other beautiful quality you want.

The whole process only takes a few seconds. It's a subtle process but a very powerful one. You shift the focus of your awareness from a chosen idea to the observer. Choose an idea you want to manifest and drop into pure consciousness, the Self, the inner observer. In that process, the idea merges with consciousness and then manifests. How powerfully and how quickly it manifests depends upon how expanded your consciousness is and how artfully you can merge the idea with consciousness. It also depends upon how many blocks are in the way.

Often, the first thing that happens is a reaction as your system tries to break through any blockages or conditionings that are keeping the idea from manifesting. Note that when any blocks are purged from your system there will usually be a physiological and psychological expression of that release. As with all such phenomenon, do not be concerned. Such releases come and go. Whenever you have an intense release, simply observe it from the place of being the innermost observer. Settle back into your deepest inner space and simply observe it disappear.

When the impediments have been released, there is a clear path for the idea to manifest. The idea doesn't have to be an emotion. It could be anything you want – any ability, any quality, perfect health, a new car, a house, anything. Just be aware and ask for only good things. Here, we are interested in healthcare. The advantage of using this technique for healing should be obvious. The whole power of consciousness, life energy itself, can be brought to bear in the healing process.

An example: I was once with a friend who, while working in the kitchen, badly sliced his finger with a knife. We took him to the hospital to get stitches. But as usual, the emergency room was slow to act. He was in a lot of pain and we were keeping the bleeding stopped by compression. In a few minutes, I taught him this technique. In order to reduce the pain, we used the word "anesthesia." He just focused on his finger, mentally introduced the concept "anesthesia" and then dropped back into Self-awareness, pure presence. Within a minute or two there was no pain, even later while receiving stitches, there was no pain. The same process could be used to accelerate healing by focusing consciousness on the region to be healed and compassionately sending energy from the hands or heart to the region with the purpose of it being healed – then dropping into pure consciousness to intensify the power of consciousness to manifest healing.

One yogi that I studied with, Ramamurti S. Mishra, MD, a medical doctor, endocrinologist, psychiatrist, and neurosurgeon, claimed that by using samyama to eliminate pain, even open heart surgery could be done without anesthetics. Naturally, you would need to master the technique. It's well worth practicing in order to eliminate pain when necessary.

You can pick any word and use it for samyama: Friendliness, compassion, enthusiasm, peace, joy, etc. Pick any quality you want to manifest in your life, bring the idea to mind, then drop into silence, into the stillness of your pure presence. Repeat every 5-10 seconds. Experiment with it for 5-10 minutes at a time to get a feeling for how it works. Whenever you're in a bad mood, use this method to change your inner state. It only takes a couple of minutes at most. The blockage in your system will be released.

You can use single words, or a short phrase. Examples of suggestions include: I am peace, I am bliss, I am joy, I am intelligence, I am compassion, I am gratitude, I am healed, I am energy, I am life, I am enthusiasm, I am infinite space, I am all that is. You can make up your own suggestions. You can put a visual with it.

How fast the process of samyama works depends upon your state of consciousness, your degree of consciousness, and the purity of your consciousness. The more you have explored and awakened consciousness, the more subtle energies such as kundalini are awakened. Everything great and wonderful comes with the expansion of consciousness. The more consciousness is expressed, the faster and more powerfully samyama works. For an adept, it happens instantly. The third chapter of the Yoga Sutras of Patanjali describes many ways that samyama can be used.

There are thousands of techniques to awaken consciousness. Here are a few more that you can experiment with.

Using Sound To Expand Consciousness

There are primordial sounds that can be used to help expand consciousness. These sounds also arise from the ancient Vedic tradition. These sounds have no translation, but they do have quality, vibration. You can use these sounds to enhance the functioning of your system. Wherever you localize your attention, they will have the most effect. They will have beneficial effects throughout your system, no matter where you use them. These are natural sounds that we have all used anyway. We're just making conscious use of them.

Aah – Whenever we see something beautiful we often express it as ooo's and aah's. When we say the sound aah we feel an expansion. It feels good. It is an expanding sound of creation. You can use these sounds, vocally, out loud, or even better you can use these sounds mentally. They have a wonderful, soothing, expanding effect.

Oooo – This is the sound of the long u or ū. It has a very uplifting, nurturing, sustaining, and healing effect.

Mmmm – Just ordinary humming, using the "m" sound. Like making the sound of a bee. This sound has a transforming effect, a regenerating effect. You've probably noticed that when you feel really bad you tend to make a groaning or humming sound. It helps to heal what's going on and creates a regenerating, transforming effect.

Aaah represents creativity and expansion, ooo represents sustaining fulfillment, and mmm represents transformation. Any of these sounds can be used. One of the most important places to apply these sounds is the central brain. Localize your attention in the central brain and then use the sounds either vocally or mentally.

There is another kind of sound that you may experience inside. It is a causeless, spontaneous sound that arises by itself. It can have many different sounds within it – rolling thunder, a high pitched ringing sound, the sound of the ocean, a flute, ringing bells, a stringed instrument similar to a sitar, the sound of bees, and others. In the East, it is called anahata nadam, the un-struck sound. It is a natural sound that awakens consciousness if you listen to it. Listen to it in the central brain or on the right side. It is often mistaken for tinnitus. It is not a disease or condition, it is an awakening, a natural initiation into higher consciousness provided by nature.

Using Visualization to Expand Consciousness

It has been said that the universe is constructed from sound and light. Just as you can use sound to make a transformation in consciousness, you can use visualization in a number of ways to expand consciousness. Here is a simple but powerful visualization/meditation: Visualize a brilliant light in the center of your head, in the central brain. This is where your most subtle and powerful physiological, psychological, and sensory structures are located: the pineal gland, pituitary, thalamus, hypothalamus, amygdala, and many other extraordinary structures. After visualizing luminous intense light in the central brain, allow the light to enter the whole brain, brain stem, and the spinal cord. Then allow the light to permeate your whole body.

Generally a brilliant white light is used, but other colors have often been used. A sparkling golden light coming into the top of the brain from above has a regenerating, uplifting, and healing effect. Visualize a torrent of golden sparkling light streaming down from above you into the top of your head, filling and energizing your whole body, even surrounding your body. A blue light surrounding your body repels negativity in your space. Also, meditating on the blue sky and bringing that blue expansive sky into your system is a beautiful meditation.

Another powerful visualization technique, which is an all-inclusive technique, is to expand the spatial awareness of your identity. We all have a sense of our personal space surrounding us. We feel it is "us," our space. If somebody comes too close, you feel like they are in your space. Actually, that boundary is an artificial boundary. Your real identity is not limited. If you expand that boundary to include progressively more space, it has an expanding effect on your consciousness.

For instance: Start within your body as being you, which is easy. Then keep spreading your sense of identity to larger and larger spaces. For example: Expand out about 2 feet, then 5-10 feet, 10-20 feet (the size of your room), 50 to 100 feet (the size of the building you're in), the size of your neighborhood, your town, your county, your state, your region, your country, continent, earth, solar system, galaxy, clusters of galaxies, infinite space. One by one, as you expand, feel that everything within that boundary, that space, is you and you are all of that. Ultimately, you are everything. Your real identity is infinite. This is a beautiful way to reconnect with your real identity.

More Meditations and Visualizations

There are potentially hundreds and thousands of meditations and visualizations. Far too many to include here. The essence of all meditations is to make a cognitive shift in your identity, from being only identified with your mind and body to being identified with that presence, that observer, which is constantly witnessing all the activities of your body, mind, senses, and environment. That fundamental identity inside you is the core of what you are seeking. That consciousness contains within it, infinite bliss, intelligence, compassion, and energy. The ultimate healing is to become one with this fundamental identity, which is boundless, infinite.

Superconscious States of Awareness

So far you have understood four states of consciousness: waking, dreaming, deep sleep, and pure consciousness. There are higher states of consciousness. When pure consciousness becomes fully established, it begins to permeate the other three states giving rise to a fifth state of consciousness, often referred to as self-realization, or enlightenment. It's described as being as far above the waking state as the waking state is above dreaming or sleeping. It's the first state where you begin to use your full potential. It's called enlightenment because of the light that is experienced as the mind and body are permeated by higher energies. There is a spiritual energy called kundalini that, when it becomes fully awakened, creates an extraordinary transformation in consciousness. All the founders of religions experienced the superconscious state. That's why they had access to higher knowledge, higher sensory perception, and overflowing compassion. You have the opportunity to experience that superconscious state, but you have to transform yourself enough to recognize that it is already within you.

There are also a sixth and seventh state of consciousness. The sixth state arises as sensory perception becomes subtle enough to experience all the layers of creation, from the gross states of matter to the normally invisible states of subtle energy. You also experience the expansive state of the whole universe to the smallest space within an atom. The seventh state arises when identity recognizes that everything external is also everything internal, made of the same identity, the same stuff – one, non-dual, infinite identity.

Devotional Practices For Natural Healthcare
There is a huge problem in the Western world, actually in most of the world. Through our educational systems, our businesses, and our cultures, we learn language, we learn to read, we learn skills to get a job, but we don't receive any real education for the heart. As a consequence, most people feel emotionally unfulfilled. We don't know how to create a beautiful emotional life. Western culture has extremely high divorce rates and high antidepressant and recreational drug use. We all need to learn how to open and express the beautiful qualities of the heart that are already there, but are going unused.

In some cultures, particularly India, parts of Asia, and the South Pacific, there are daily practices of devotion. In the Western world, we don't understand these practices because most of them are based on what we call idols – what they refer to as gods. Even in the cultures that use these practices, the original concept and purpose behind these practices is often lost.

One of the interesting truths about devotion and expression of the heart is that it doesn't really matter what you are devoted to. It is the act of feeling love, over and over again, toward something higher than yourself that actually matters. It also doesn't matter what you use to represent the object of your devotion. If you were to take a stone, and for you that stone represents the highest divinity, it still works. The idols of the East are not being worshiped as an idol, but as a representative of real qualities, real energies, and ancient beings who were once human, but graduated from the human form. It's this ideal, not the idol, that is being worshiped. Ultimately, it is your own higher self, the one consciousness that pervades everything.

It's the practice of love, becoming softer, more compassionate that matters. In ancient cultures, there were many gods, thousands of gods that came to be known over tens of thousands of years. Each of these gods was once a human being who evolved beyond the human level to become superconscious (like the founders of recent religions you are more familiar with). Each of these gods has certain qualities that they exhibited more of – compassion, wisdom, strength, healing power, supernormal abilities, creative power, lightness and joy, and many others.

If you were to make up a list of all the wonderful and best qualities of body, mind, and heart, each of these gods would manifest a superlative combination of certain qualities. These gods, would have a story connected with their life and doings, how they overcame obstacles to reach the superconscious state. These stories in connection with a beautiful depiction of their form, serves as a model, a hero, a mentor that you can learn from today. You can learn to embody those qualities.

What was supposed to happen through devotion is not happening today. That's because devotional practices, as they have been recently taught through many religions, have been to put something or someone on a pedestal, which is fine, but then we put ourselves as lowly, worthless, powerless subjects. Internally, the more everyone praised the one on a pedestal, the less we thought of ourselves with all our conditioned inadequacies, guilt, and failures.

The real purpose of devotional practices was to see the ideal, the god, or object of devotion as a mentor that you, in reality, could mirror. Through identification with the highest qualities embodied in your object of devotion, you rise to embody those same qualities. There was never supposed to be any guilt and self deprecation. We were supposed to rise in dignity and express of all the highest qualities embodied in our beloved. All the so-called bowing down was to represent the dissolution of the ego, the small, confused, distorted self that we all have come to think we are, through our conditioning. As that ego part of you dissolves through identification with the highest ideals of your object of devotion, you are transformed, just as the caterpillar is transformed into a butterfly. Devotion is not for the benefit of any deities or gods, it is for the devotee. Deities don't need anything. It is the practice of loving devotion, sweetness, that transforms you. Once you practice love towards something higher than yourself, any deity or whatever, then you can extend that love to everyone around you. The people you ordinarily meet and interact with are even more in need of your compassion. Devotional activities are a training ground for you to express devotion and compassion everywhere in your daily life.

I recommend everyone make some kind of little altar, and on that altar place a few flowers and make a beautiful platform to practice, learn, and teach by example the practice of devotion towards something higher than yourself. You can talk to that being, that someone, with utmost honesty and sincerity. You can talk about your concerns, your aspirations, and ask that you be guided to unfold your own divinity, to become like the one you adore. Even loving all of nature works. The divine is both with infinite forms and formless. Enjoy it how you want to, in any way that pleases you, but do something to invoke the highest qualities within yourself on a daily basis, not just weekends.

As a practical matter, it's worthwhile to read the stories from all the different religious traditions. The more stories you read, the more resources you have to recognize that you too have divine qualities. Focus on expressing all your divine qualities as you practice being in the presence of your chosen devotional divinity. If we all learn to practice and appreciate devotional practices, we would put an end to all wars. You have complete freedom. Find a practice that appeals to you, but please don't force your practice on others, don't intimidate others. Don't think your practice is the only right one. Everyone should discover their own. You will find that you come to appreciate all traditions. You may even come to prefer another tradition to the first one or two traditions you were introduced to as a child or youth. You have the freedom to explore and grow as you choose, without intimidation, force, coercion, or control from anyone or any institution. You are a free being.

Finding a mentor

Whenever you want to learn something, whether it's a science, an art, a new language, or a new skill, it's easier if you study with someone who already has that knowledge, who has already succeeded. That way, you don't have to learn by making so many mistakes. Even just to drive from one part of a country to another, you need a map, a guide. In order to grow into the person you are capable of being, it's worthwhile to find a guide, a mentor.

There are two categories of mentors. Those at the human level and those at the superconscious level. If you have a choice, it is far wiser to choose a superconscious being as a mentor and guide.

If you don't have access to a superconscious being, or even know how to recognize one, start with books. Start with reading the highest teachings you can find from all the spiritual traditions. Just this intense seeking will start a process of discovery in which you can find a living superconscious being to work with. It's great to read the teachings of those who have passed on. The principles they describe in their teachings are still applicable today, but updated expressions of those teachings for current conditions won't be available. The original founder of those teachings is not here to update them.

It's far better to work with a living superconscious being who can give you real world guidance and update past teachings with new insights relevant to today's world. Ultimately, the same pure consciousness that exists in you, exists in all other people, including all other superconscious beings. It is that pure consciousness that is the foundation and source of everything you seek. Obviously, it is your ultimate guide, but getting access to it with clarity comes much more rapidly through the presence of a living superconscious mentor.

Ultimate Healing Beyond This Life

Everyone knows that this human experience is a temporary state of affairs. At some point, this body must be given up. We don't see anyone who has been living for millions of years. Yet, there is something very curious. You can never remember a time when you did not exist. Also, for some reason, everyone at their core feels like they will live forever. You can remember conditions in your life that no longer exist. The baby that you once were no longer exists. The child that you once were no longer exists. The teenager that you once were no longer exists, yet something about you still exists. The continuity that you experience is your presence, your pure existence which does not change and has never changed. Just as you go to bed at night confident that you will exist in the morning, you will always exist. Your real existence is beyond your body, mind, emotions, and personality. This exposes the reality that you will always exist in some form. The essential you never dies. At the end of your life, if you have attained a deep connection with your inner presence, you can know when you will leave this realm. You can make a graceful easy exit. You will continue with your same high quality of awareness. No worries.

Summary of Chapter 12

The exploration of consciousness is the exploration of life. It's what you came here for and it's the ultimate healing. There are many avenues to choose from. Hundreds and thousands of techniques to expand consciousness. Hundreds and thousands of ideas and truths to explore. Allow yourself to be guided by your deepest intuition. Everyone has a path to explore and your path will change, just as you changed from a child to a teenager to an adult. Avoid getting frozen and stagnant. Keep exploring higher and higher teachings. If you are fortunate, you may even find a living superconscious being to help you. Read all the spiritual literature you can and distill the common principles and ideas embodied in all of them. I wish you the highest success on your journey into consciousness.

Action Plan - Chapter 12, Healing with Consciousness

1. Notice how aware you are at different times of day, notice the states of consciousness, waking, dreaming, and deep sleep.
2. Recognize that there is a fourth state of consciousness, different from the three you know about.
3. Be aware of the observer that observes your thoughts and senses. That observer is the fourth state, consciousness itself.
4. Do breathing techniques: Kapalabhati, Bhastrika, Long Slow Breathing, Sigh Breathing.
5. Meditate on breathing, watch your breath come in at your nostrils, enter your body, and exit at your nostrils. 20-30 min.
6. Observe the breath when it stops – the gaps between breaths – when the breath turns around after the in-breath and again after the out-breath. Your mind also stops and becomes silent at those points.
7. Be aware of your pure presence, your pure existence, the watcher behind all phenomenon.
8. Observe your thoughts. Observe the gaps between your thoughts.
9. Meditate 24 hours a day by recognizing the presence, your pure existence that is always watching everything. Allow the observer to become more dominant than either the outer world or the inner world of your mind.
10. Practice samyama on what you want to manifest in your life.
11. Use sound to transform consciousness 1) Aahhh, 2) Ooo (ū) long U, and 3) Mmmm, humming sound. Practice them at the mid-brain.
12. Use visualization to expand consciousness. Visualize a stream of golden sparkling light coming from high above you into the top of your head, into the mid-brain, whole brain, brain stem, spinal cord, and whole body. Do the expanding-spacial-awareness meditation.
13. Decide to pursue higher states of consciousness and find total healing and fulfillment.

14. Learn about devotion. Be devoted to something higher than yourself. Find a mentor in the highest sense. Make a beautiful altar to express your devotion. Embody all the qualities of your beloved.
15. Explore and find traditions and mentors who add joy and wisdom to your life.

Chapter 13
Putting It All Together

A Day in the Life

A Recommended Daily Life Plan

The most difficult thing in the world for everyone is change. You can make change easier by shifting your attitude. Instead of drudgery or force of willpower, just decide to be adventurous. Be an explorer. You know for certain that if you don't make changes, things will stay the same or get worse. There's always that negative reality to spur you forward. But that approach is not much fun and it doesn't work very well. We always try to stand our ground and resist. We get caught in endless cycles of guilt when we don't follow through. There's a much better way. Just be an adventurer. It's more fun to be an adventurer.

You can either expect it to be difficult and struggle with it, or you can be excited about the adventure. It's like waking up on a cold morning and going out to your car. There's a big difference if you're getting in your car to go to a boring office job or to go on a camping trip. When you're headed for a camping trip, an adventure, you're not fazed by anything. Attitude is really important. Just make everything an adventure. Just decide.

When you're trying to make changes, you can expect that there will be hurdles to jump. You can also expect that as you make changes, life can get incredibly better, which is what you want. Goals can be a motivation, but the process is more important than the multitude of goals or destinations. If this is going to work, you need to enjoy the journey. You enjoy the journey by changing your attitude, changing your perspective, becoming more conscious, and deciding to be more alive and adventurous. It's a simple decision.

Review Your Organizing System

I mentioned early in the book about the importance of creating systems to keep you organized and on track. You have been using your system and adding actions items as you've worked your way through the book. Now is a good time to review and update your organizing system. What's working? What needs improvement? It's difficult to make progress when you get knocked off track. What improvements can you make to stay on track?

A Daily Schedule

Your daily schedule should be designed to maximize joy, inner growth, useful learning, and enrich the lives of yourself and others. For most people today, it's all work and no play. Be sure to schedule time for yourself, time to experience the joys of nature, time to wander, time for peace. Remember, even if you win the rat race, you're still a rat! Try not to live your life like the bulk of humanity does, caught up in unnecessary accumulation with no time for life. Why do things, why support things that you don't believe in? Choose the things that truly add value to your life and to the lives of others.

Here's a simple schedule:

Morning Routine
- Rise early with the sun, or even before sunrise
- Drink water to rehydrate
- Answer the calls of nature
- Bath or shower
- Skin nourishment and protection
- Dental care
- Exercises: yoga, aerobic exercise, lymphatic exercise, strength exercise, acupressure and reflexology, or other physical conditioning. If you do heavy morning workouts, have your bath or shower afterwards.
- Breathing exercises
- Morning meditation and devotions
- Breakfast, if you eat breakfast

Productive Morning Work
- Work to enrich yourself and others
- Add to your skills and knowledge

Enjoy Lunch
- Prepare and enjoy lunch, share food with others
- Eat your largest meal when the sun is highest in the sky

Productive Afternoon Work
- Work to enrich yourself and others
- Add to your skills and knowledge

Evening Routine
- Light evening meal, if you eat in the evening. Share food.
- Spend time with friends and family, nourish relationships
- Study the great teachings

Weekends
- Share your gifts
- Enjoy time with friends and family
- Practice your artistic skills
- Be in nature
- Refine and redefine yourself

In general, do things to maximize the quality of your life and the quality of others' lives. Keep things simple. Spend more time accumulating wisdom and experiences than accumulating things. The more you enrich others, the more you are enriched.

Notes on Creating a Daily Schedule

Arise early, preferably without an alarm (or use a gentle alarm). Look at a clock and suggest to yourself before sleep when you would like to awaken. If you practice, your mind will awaken you at the appointed time. You can always set a backup alarm. When you first wake up, breathe deeply 10-20 times to energize your system.

Upon Rising: Do a morning cleanse. Scrape the white coating off of your tongue and rinse your mouth with warm water. Then drink a glass or two of water to rehydrate. Use the toilet, then shower and shave. Apply skin protection lotion.

For dental care, Ayurveda recommends that you first swish your teeth with a small amount of sesame oil for 5-10 minutes to kill bacteria and build healthy gums. You can even do this while in the shower. Don't swallow. Spit it out. Then brush and floss your teeth. It's actually much more pleasant than you expect once you get use to it. It really helps your gums and teeth.

Do some morning exercise. Yoga, or other light exercise. Some people like to do running or aerobic exercise before morning shower.

Meditate for at least 1/2-1 hour if possible (start with 20 minutes) 1-2 hours of meditation per day is not unreasonable for advanced practitioners. Or practice living in the meditative state continuously.

Work at something the feels right for you and improves the life of others as well.

Your activities during the day should be filled with purpose, power, and sharing your life with others. Avoid wasting your life through mindless habits, mindless media, and wasted time. Meals should be a time to nourish yourself with the best quality materials the world has to offer. Eat in the happy presence of others and do what you can to enrich everyone. Avoid complaining. Take creative action on the things you believe in.

Also do an evening meditation for a half hour, or more if you like. This will refresh you so you can enjoy your evening activities.

Spend evening hours increasing your skills, reading the best inspiring materials you can find, or in some way advancing yourself and your family.

The evening cleanse, can be like morning, then sleep.

Chapter 14
Natural Healthcare Resources

How to Use These Resources

Too Much!

When looking at all the changes that need to be made to create a natural health lifestyle, it can appear be *too much!* If you don't use some kind of system and take it step-by-step, it can be difficult to make the changes. You may feel overwhelmed and give up. If you use a system, it will be easy. Just take it one step at a time.

This chapter is a practical and useful chapter. It contains the resources you need. From time to time, it's also worthwhile to review the action steps at the end of each chapter. Turn to the beginning of any chapter, then back up one page to see the action items for the previous chapter. Put new reminders in your organizer to keep yourself on track. Keep your organizer system current, otherwise you can be overwhelmed. This chapter is not just a reference and resource chapter. It should be read through at least once so you know what is here, so you can find it when you need it.

This chapter includes suggestions for:

1) Classical Natural Cures: How serious conditions have been healed

2) Shopping Lists: Foods to avoid, foods to purchase, herbs and spices

3) List of packaged spices to save time

4) List of edible flowers

5) Recipe formulas, meal planning ideas

6) Links to physical exercise charts, healing charts, and more

Review of Basic Concepts in Natural Healthcare

Natural healthcare is unlike the conventional allopathic healthcare system. Natural healthcare recognizes that there are very few conditions created by a single cause. Virtually all problems arise out of weakness, and weakness has multiple causes on all five levels. The methodology in allopathic medicine is generally to prescribe one drug, one magic bullet, to address a problem. It is very rarely effective, even in the short term, and often causes multiple problems and side effects that lead to more drugs and more problems. Ultimately, allopathic medical intervention is the third leading cause of death. It is largely a failed system, yet there is some hope that the field of regenerative medicine will reverse this trend.

The new natural healthcare approach is entirely different. It is not "medicine" at all. Instead, it changes the ecology of your body, mind, emotions, and consciousness and the ecology of your living environment to promote greater strength on all levels. No single therapy is used for any condition, rather a variety of life enhancing modalities are combined together, each of which adds healing power. Layering multiple natural techniques together brings extraordinary results and is the foundation of Extraordinary Healthcare. The choice of modalities to combine can be approached logically, intuitively, or by studying past successful best practices. This constructive, regenerative approach is synergistic. Any single technique, modality, or therapy may contribute only 5-10% towards the solution, but several methods collectively often combine into a powerful 100% solution. In fact, natural healthcare doesn't actually treat diseases. It simply builds strength in your body, mind, heart, and consciousness. This enables your body to heal itself with it's own extraordinary capabilities. Natural solutions are gentler, so they must generally be applied more frequently and over a longer timespan. The advantage is that they truly heal the underlying causes.

First let's review the universal methods that apply to all healing, then in the listings below, I'll provide some particulars that apply to specific conditions. As with all knowledge, review the recommendations, use your intuition for guidance, and check with experts that you trust.

Short Summary of Extraordinary Healthcare

Physical Healthcare: Change the pH of the body, remove congestion, remove toxicity, provide high enzyme nutrition, provide complete mineral nutrition, remove parasites, increase oxygenation, provide adequate hydration, remove toxic exposures, cleanse and heal the digestive tract, fast to purify the body, avoid high glycemic foods, get all five kinds of exercise.

Bio-Energetic Healthcare: Massively increase bio-energy in your body. Focus your attention and intention where you feel discomfort to direct the energy there. Clear the meridians and acupressure points. Clear the aura. Utilize the healing power of nature. Practice yogic breathing techniques.

Emotional Healthcare: Heal emotions by flooding areas of physical imbalance and areas of pain with compassionate loving attention. Relive painful incidents while dissociated until the incidents have no emotional charge. Tap acupressure points. Replace destructive emotional thoughts. Shift attitudes. Learn the lessons revealed through your emotions. Use light and sound therapies. Use music constructively. Observe the symbols in your life. Forgive yourself and others. Practice nonresistance. Eliminate exposures to negative emotional media. Keep a gratitude journal Practice cathartic meditations. Understand how emotions are created.

Mental Healthcare: Understand how your mind has been programmed. Carefully choose your exposures to all media. Watch your thoughts carefully. Always know what you are thinking – why you are thinking it – what the expected result will be. Slow your mind by slowing your breath. Heal your mental patterns by consciously reliving past incidents while remaining dissociated. Recognize and cancel past decisions and interpretations of reality that no longer serve you. Affirm new constructive choices. Understand your motivations that come from greed and fear. Understand the four kinds of choices. Live the four noble principles. Stay out of conflict by ensuring "say-see-feel-do" are all in agreement. Re-create a new self image. Use the primordial sounds. Practice meditation. Realize that you have extraordinary powers: The power of spoken words, the power to think creatively, the power to feel compassionately, and the power to act, to radiate and live totally.

Consciousness and Healthcare: Understand degrees and states of consciousness. Connect with your pure consciousness that is beyond mind. Practice breathing and meditation techniques. Observe the gaps between breaths and between thoughts. Reside in your pure being, in your essential presence. Learn and practice samyama to create the life you want. Use primordial sounds to expand consciousness. Use visualizations to expand consciousness. Understand and use devotional practices. Study the highest teachings of all spiritual traditions. Find an enlightened mentor to help you.

Classical Solutions for Serious Conditions

Listed below are a few of the major health conditions in America (and other countries adopting the Western lifestyle). A short list of classical natural solutions follows each listing. In the natural approach to healthcare, the solution to all degenerative conditions is to create regenerative effects in the mind, heart, and body and minimize destructive forces. All the knowledge and methods described throughout the book apply. The classic solutions listed below are just a short list of suggestions.

Heart Disease – Dissolve circulatory system deposits using the universal solvent – ordinary water. Extensive experience of Dr. Batmanghelidj, M.D.

confirms that drinking half your body weight in ounces of water daily, with a pinch of sea salt in each glass, will dissolve and remove the deposits that cause congestive heart disease. Also, go for daily gentle walks. Heart and blood vessel congestion simply dissolve. The pinch of natural sea salt in each 8 oz glass prevents electrolyte loss and provides trace minerals. Balance your pH. Live on the natural diet to build healthy tissues. Schedule uplifting events in your life so you don't have a "heavy heart." Minimize stress in your life through meditation and breathing techniques, so your heart is not trying of keep up with an impossible lifestyle. Use bio-energy healing.

Cancer – Please be aware of misinformation and disinformation when it comes to the treatment of any disease, especially cancer. There are vested interests at play. Always ask, "Who is benefitting? Who gets the money?" If the recommendation comes from years of experience and costs nothing to implement, it may actually have more creditability. For instance, a 12 year, peer reviewed study published in the Journal of Clinical Oncology concluded that chemotherapy, was a 97% failure in the treatment of all adult cancers. It is a very expensive therapy with extremely poor results, yet it is highly promoted by the American Cancer Society and the medical profession generally. It is promoted because they have no other expensive chemical protocol to offer. Doctors and hospitals get huge financial kickbacks for prescribing it. Science has been politicized to a great degree and no longer follows scientific protocols. The scientific medical establishment has largely become morally bankrupt.

Independent researchers and those who found self cures for cancer can provide testimonials, but cannot afford expensive clinical trials research. The established mainstream cancer industry always points out that there is little or no clinical research or peer reviewed scientific studies to back up the claims of alternative therapies. How could there be? Such studies would cost millions of dollars and there is no financial incentive to study free, un-patentable treatments.

According to the experience of cancer survivors and alternative cancer researchers, cancer does not like high alkaline, high oxygen, high enzyme, high antioxidant, high mineral, high life-force energy environments. Many alternative practitioners feel that cancer is actually very easy to cure, and even easier to prevent. Here are the general recommendations:

Balance the pH of your body, raise your pH to about 7.6. Live on a high enzyme, low glycemic index diet. 100% raw foods and juices are ideal – many people have cured themselves of cancer through diet alone. There are even reports of people curing stage IV cancer by juicing and drinking 5 pounds of carrots per day. Remove pathogens – viruses, bacteria, fungi, and yeasts – from your system with the various pathogen cleanses. Use colloidal silver for cancers instigated by viruses. Practice meditation and uplifting emotional practices to lift yourself out of depression and into joy. Practice deep yogic breathing – pranayamas. Practice lymphatic exercises to clean the lymphatic system. Enrich the lives of other people as much as you can to shift the focus and purpose of your life. Stay in gratitude. Use bio-energy healing.

Use alkalizing therapies. Use ordinary baking soda, and/or other sodium, potassium, calcium, and magnesium minerals (4 major alkaline minerals in the body). Supply adequate minor minerals such as selenium. Supply trace minerals. Many diseases are invited by mineral deficiencies.

One popular free therapy is the use of baking soda. The protocol is available for free (http://www.cancertutor.com/Cancer02/Simoncini.html). Many people have had success with his protocol. Use alkalizing herbs. One popular and successful regimen is Essiac Tea.

Essiac Tea to Cure Cancer and Auto Immune Diseases
(Approved in China as a valid cancer therapy)

Essiac tea was used successfully by Rene Caisse, RN to cure many people of cancer. It includes four healing herbs that were given to her by the Canadian Ojibwa Indians. Later, she worked with her research partner, a medical doctor, to expand the formula to eight herbs. The four herb formula is: 1) Burdock Root, 2) Turkey Rhubarb Root, 3) Sheep Sorrel (the whole plant including the root) 4) Slippery Elm Bark

Additional herbs added later are: 5) Blessed Thistle, 6) Kelp, 7) Red Clover, and 8) Watercress. Both the 4 and 8 herb versions are original. The expanded 8 herb formula is considered more effective.

I have not used this therapy but many people endorse it. Even if you had the formula percentages by weight, which are not disclosed precisely by anyone, it would be time consuming and difficult to reproduce due to the varying nature of herbs in how they are grown, when they are picked, and how they are prepared. The organization with the best knowledge of the formula is http://www.discount-essiac-tea.com

They are willing to provide the herb mix for free to anyone in need. They appear to be ethical and can provide instructions. I have avoided recommending herbal approaches for healthcare because of the knowledge required to harvest, assess, and use them well. But that doesn't mean they are not a powerful regimen. They can have remarkable healing power. There are many ways to reverse cancer and this could be an asset for those who would like to pursue it.

Diabetes – Same approach as cancer. Change the nutritional landscape of the body through high alkaline, high oxygen, high enzyme, high antioxidant, high mineral, high life-force energy environments. This is true for all degenerative diseases. Many people have cured diabetes in 30 days or less just through dietary change – 100% raw foods, especially vegetable juices. Also use bio-energy healing.

Obesity – Live primarily on raw vegetable juices. Begin a modest exercise program, especially lymphatic exercise. Live exclusively on raw foods that are low on the glycemic index – juices, raw soups, salads, slaw, and smoothies, especially green smoothies. Watch the movie "Fat, Sick, and Nearly Dead." Eliminate pathogens, especially yeasts. Find new ways to approach emotional fulfillment, especially develop a new self image. Practice meditation.

Infectious Diseases – Do a pathogen cleanse. Raise your pH to normal levels. Live on the natural diet. Get sufficient rest. Practice meditation. Avoid destructive foods and habits. Use bio-energy healing. Use colloidal silver, essential oils, and herbal cleanses.

Lung Conditions – Same as infectious disease. Extensive lymphatic exercise. Eliminate pulmonary infections using inhaled atomized essential oils such as lavender oil (get expert recommendations for other essential oils for internal use) and/or use atomized, misted, colloidal silver which requires no special precautions. Use bio-energy healing.

Depression – Use continuous tone light therapy (yellow light). Practice meditation. Develop a new self-image. Live on the natural diet. Eliminate toxic substances and environments. Heal your relationships. Use bio-energy healing. Quit any job that supports or promotes the death of humans or animals. Work only in a life supporting vocation. Start a gratitude journal. Shift your focus to enriching the lives of others.

Scoliosis – Scoliosis is a lateral curvature of the spine. Often there is a rotation of the rib cage. It's a common condition with about 3% (6-9 million people) affected in the United States. Medically, the cause is not understood for most cases. I'm aware of two primary causes: Mercury toxicity and trauma. Physical and emotional trauma are primary causes in my experience. When a person is traumatized, they react by tightening their muscles and psychologically and physiologically recoiling.

The induced tension in the muscles is not released and continues to pull and distort the body. When the trauma is released, the muscles relax, and the body assumes its normal alignment. I have been able to reverse mild conditions in one hour using bio energy healing (See photos on my website). Most cases take longer. I have developed protocols that people can use at home to reverse the condition over time. When someone is traumatized, it not only affects muscles and physiology, but body chemistry, the energy fields of the body, the meridians, and acupressure points.

All Other Conditions – Use your intuition to select modalities on all five levels from throughout the book. Remember it's easy for the body to heal itself when it has the right resources and high life force energy.

Food Shopping, Transportation, and Storage

Natural healthcare begins by rejuvenating your body with the best nutrition. By now you have located the best shopping resources suggested in chapter 4 under the heading, Wise Shopping. If not, review that chapter and find the best products and sources available in your area.

You can keep your produce fresher after purchasing by transporting and storing it properly. If you have a long drive between shopping and home, it's worthwhile to put your produce in an ice chest with reusable frozen cooler packs, gel packs, or reusable ice cubes. When you store vegetables in the refrigerator, especially greens, you can make them last twice as long by putting them inside a linen bag and put the linen bag inside a plastic bag. This prevents them from becoming mushy and from drying out. Linen and hemp fabrics do not rot or disintegrate when wet.

Shopping Lists and Recipes

The single most important decision for health is healthy food. Below is a shopping list for items to avoid and items worth buying. I also include herb and spice blends, which often have medicinal value, and make meals delicious. Basic recipe formulas are included to get you started.

Foods To Avoid and the Reasons Why

For most rapid healing you must cleanse your system. To do that, it's better not to consume ANY of the following "foods" or other items listed below in ANY amount. Your body can do a better job without them. As a life-style change, it would be best to avoid these non-foods permanently.

When you overload your body with damaging "foods," healing is more difficult or impossible.

1. Meat — Causes putrefaction, poisons the body, contains pesticides, antibiotics, and other toxins. Meat (animal carcass) is a totally unnatural food for humans. No one would ever live and eat like a carnivore does. The renowned China Study found no safe lower limit for meat consumption in the causation of cancer. Seafood is measurably contaminated by the Japanese nuclear plant meltdowns. You may want to monitor the severity. Avoid foods from the ocean anyway. They are unnatural for humans.

2. Eggs — Same as meat, when cooked, proteins turn into a coagulated, rubber-like substance that is not healthy. Many people are allergic to eggs.

3. Dairy products — NO pasteurized, homogenized milk. For other dairy products such as butter or cheese, there can be exceptions depending upon your body type. A small amount of cultured milk products, such as yogurt, kefir, buttermilk, or sour cream (some brands) can be useful to re-establish intestinal flora (even better, use sauerkraut or biological supplements). Vata constitutions (thin, lightweight body type) can sometimes tolerate pure dairy products such as butter, ghee, and cheeses. Many people, especially those of Asian or African descent, are allergic to most dairy products, which often cause skin eruptions.

4. Sugar, brown sugar, and corn syrup — Avoid all white sugar, sugar products, corn syrup, and all products made with corn syrup, which includes practically all packaged foods. White sugar and corn syrup are both known to increase the incidence of cancer and diabetes. Virtually all corn syrup is from genetically engineered corn, which has been shown in French studies to cause cancer. Also, many white sugar products have been processed through bone char and are not vegetarian. A large proportion of white sugar comes from genetically engineered beets, and so should be avoided. Brown sugar is the same as white sugar, but with molasses added. Practically all processed foods contain these sugars, which leads to the recommendation to eat no processed or packaged foods. Occasional use of whole sugar, (whole, evaporated cane juice such as Sucanat, Demerara, etc.), gur or jaggery (from Indian food stores), or whole natural syrups such as honey, blackstrap molasses, or sorghum (non-GMO), are acceptable. NO sugars, fruits, fruit juices, or sweet foods at all if you have candida yeast or any other yeast infestations. Avoid pasteurized fruit juices (virtually all commercial fruit juices are pasteurized). It's far better to eat the whole fresh fruit.

5. White table salt – Ordinary white salt is pure sodium chloride, stripped of all useful minerals. It usually has non-food additives. Use whole sea salt, it supplies trace minerals and rare earth minerals. Soy sauce and tamari, which have been used for centuries, are a reasonable substitute if made

with sea salt. Soy products must come from organic, non-GMO sources, (which may be difficult to find).

6. All white flour and white flour products, without exception. All so-called "vitamin enriched" products. "Enriched" means all the good stuff has been taken out to feed animals and a few synthetic substitutes have been tossed in.

7. Alcohol – None of any kind, in any amount. It's the red grapes, not the wine, that has nutritional value. Alcoholic beverages have no human value.

8. Nicotine – NO smoking whatsoever, no chewing tobacco.

9. Caffeine – NO coffee, colas, chocolate, or black tea – depletes adrenals, creates caffeine headaches. Eat an orange for a pick-me-up. Natural chocolate powder is healthy and high in antioxidants, but candy "chocolates" are flavored, sugary, hydrogenated, unhealthy fats, and are not useful in human nutrition.

10. NO soft drinks, without exception, even diet varieties – The only beverage worse than acidic sugar water is alcoholic acidic sugar water. It causes mineral imbalances and destroy enzymes. Sugar and synthetic sugar substitutes are both suspected of causing cancer.

11. NO frozen foods – They are devitalized. Dried foods are a better substitute, if dried at low temperatures. Frozen foods are acceptable if there is no choice.

12. NO microwaved foods or water (devitalizes, denatures, and distorts energies). Creates chemical changes in foods.

13. NO hydrogenated oils (denatures the oils) – Use raw olive, coconut, or hemp oil, (some safflower, sunflower, sesame, flax or walnut oil is OK). Eat foods that have natural oils in them. Organic ghee is usually tolerated.

14. NO additives such as artificial flavors, artificial colors, artificial sweeteners, or preservatives

15. NO tap water. Drink pH balanced spring water, well water, or properly filtered tap water. Also, bathe in filtered water if possible. Tap water has been tainted by mindless city regulations with fluoride and chlorine compounds and is not healthy. Better to avoid it. Bottled water is usually just filtered tap water. You have to check whether it comes from uncontaminated wells or safe reservoirs. Many countries now protect their water supply from bacteria using oxygen instead of chlorine. A huge improvement.

Super Nutrition

If you have any condition that needs healing, eat at least 3/4 of your foods fresh and uncooked, preferably 100%. Ideally, use organic foods grown on mineral-rich soils. Conventional commercial foods can have nutritional content many times less than organic foods – for trace minerals, even hundreds of times less (depending upon the soils). Include some super foods in your diet: Kelp or other seaweeds for trace minerals (if collected before or far away from nuclear wastes contamination), nutritional yeast, omega-3 essential fatty acids (raw vegetables, flax oil, walnut oil, chia seeds, hemp oil and seeds), green freeze-dried superfoods (barley or wheat greens, blue-green algae, or spirulina), blackstrap molasses.

What to Eat — The Natural Human Diet

The natural foods for humans are the 3 food groups: 1) vegetables, 2) fruits, and 3) seeds (many varieties). These three can be expanded to 7 food groups: 1) vegetables 2) fruits – from trees & vines, 3) melons, 4) nuts, 5) vegetable & flower seeds such as pumpkin, sunflower, poppy, chia, etc., 6) grains, such as wheat, barley, rice, etc. and 7) legumes (beans) such as lentils, garbanzo beans, etc. Also, there are products derived from these seven foods, such as oils, herbs and spices. A super nutritious healing diet emphasizes green vegetation over other foods. For healing purposes, vegetable foods may be consumed as juices, smoothies, salads, blender soups (uncooked, with fiber), and slaws.

Nuts, seeds, grains, and legumes must be soaked for a few hours until plump, then washed and drained a few times at room temperature for 24 hours to eliminate enzyme inhibitors. Enzyme inhibitors, and other anti-nutrients, protect seeds from decomposing, and are not healthy to eat. To get the most nutrition from any food, make the particle size very small.

You only need a small amount of fermented foods as live cultures. Grains and legumes, the primary source of carbohydrates for most cultures can be cooked. Essene breads from sprouted grains are unfermented, unleavened, and uncooked. They are simply dehydrated wafers.

Nuts and seeds can be prepared in a variety of ways. You can chop them for use as a garnish. For sauces and dressings, finely blend them with liquid and a small amount of oil and spices. Make nut and seed milks by blending with water. Make spreads, patés, loafs, crackers, and numerous entrées. Study raw food and vegan recipes online for a wealth of ideas. There are hundreds of Internet sites with recipes. Also, see our Food Formulas later in this chapter, so that you can create your own recipes spontaneously from what you have on hand. This new approach to diet can be wonderfully delicious.

Basic Menu Ideas

Breakfast

Green Smoothie: In cold weather, drink warm herbal teas to warm up. If there are no healing or weight-loss requirements, natural muesli or even cooked grains, like oatmeal, are okay. If you need healing, avoid cooked foods for at least a few weeks.

Lunch

Vegetable Meal: Large salads with soaked nut/seed dressing, Greens/ Veggie/Fruit Smoothie, Raw Soups, Soaked Nuts/Seeds, Sprouted Grains and Legumes. Favor legumes over grains if you need to lose weight. Cooked grains are high in starches and quickly convert to sugars and are not recommended for losing weight or if you have any health condition. Substitute legumes instead, particularly sprouted lentils and garbanzo beans. If there are no strong healing or weight loss requirements, enjoy cooked vegetables, whole grains, and legumes. As long as your pH remains above 7.4, and you don't have strong healing requirements, you can eat 20-30% cooked foods.

Fruit Meal: Fruit salad with 2-3 pieces of fruit or melon. Fruits go well with raw soaked nuts and seeds, but not so well with cooked foods. Wonderful soaked nut and seed toppings and dressings with herbs and spices can be used for added nutrition.

Dinner

Same as breakfast or lunch, but lesser in quantity.

Your Food Shopping List

Vegetables

The primary food for high nutrition is vegetables. The best vegetables of all are dark leafy greens, but any vegetable high in chlorophyll is good. Greens can be eaten in salads, blended into raw soups, or used in cooked vegetable dishes. Vegetables fall into several categories: 1) Salad greens, 2) vegetables that can be enjoyed raw, and 3) vegetables that are too bitter, tough, or difficult to eat raw and are better marinated or cooked. Marinating with lemon (or vinegar), oil, and salt helps break down tough vegetables, increases bioavailability of nutrients, and improves digestibility.

Salad Greens & Green Veggies

Tender Salad Greens	Nutritious Greens	Green Veggies
Lettuce: (Romaine, Bib, Boston, Red Leaf), Mache, Spinach, Chard & Collards (when young), Tatsoi, Bokchoy, Parsley, Cilantro, many other Chinese greens (Mizuna, etc.)	*Cooked or Raw:* Cabbage, Chard, Kale, Collards, Mustard Greens, *Use Sparingly Raw:* Endive, Escarole, Arugula, Radicchio, Frisée, Watercress	Asparagus, Broccoli, Cabbage, Celery, Peas, Green Beans, Sugar Snap Peas, Snow Peas, Yard Long Beans, All Sprouts

Raw, Cooked, and High Calorie Veggies

Raw Veggies	Cooking Veggies	High Calorie Veggies
Beets (grated), Bok Choy, Other Chinese Greens, Broccoli, Cabbage, Carrots, Cauliflower, Celery, Corn (organic, freshly picked) Cucumbers, Jerusalem Artichoke (Sunchoke), Jicama, Peppers, Radish, Spinach, Swiss Chard, Sugar Snap Peas, Snow Peas, Tomatillo, Tomato, Squash, Water Chestnut, Zucchini	Artichokes, Asparagus, Bamboo Shoots, Beets, Bok Choy, Broccoli, Brussel Sprouts, Cabbage, Carrots, Cauliflower, Corn (Non-GMO only), Eggplant, Green Beans, Greens (Collards, Mustard, & Turnip Greens), Kale, Kohlrabi, Okra, Peppers, String Beans, Spinach, Swiss Chard, Tomato, Zucchini	Carrots, Corn, Sweet Potatoes, White Potatoes, Butternut Squash, Acorn Squash, Winter Squash, Chestnuts, Parsnips, Rutabagas, Turnips, Yams, Pumpkins

Greens and many other vegetables, although high in nutrition, are not high in calories and won't provide the energy you need for daily life. But they are perfect if you want to lose weight. You can eat large quantities of high-nutrition, low-starch vegetables. You can even juice them. You will never be hungry and you will get all the nutrition you need. Weight will simply melt off. Once your weight is down to normal, then you can enjoy other foods in greater quantities. High calorie vegetables are for energy once you are at normal weight.

Explore the variety of vegetables in asian and international markets. They include: Yu choy, sher li hon, a choy, gai lan (Chinese broccoli), choy sum, ta ku choy, sweet bok choy, amaranth greens, red shen choy, tong ho, gongura leaf, methileaf, calaloo, verdolaga, cactus pear, cactus leaf (nopal), jicama, chayote squash, tomatillo, lotus root, gobo (root), nagaimo, Korean radish, and many more.

Fruits

Fruits	Berries	Caloric Fruits & Melons
Apple, Apricot, Cherry, Fig, Grapefruit, Grapes, Guava, Kiwis, Kumquat, Lemon, Lime, Mango, Nectarine, Orange, Paw Paw, Peach, Pear, Persimmon, Pineapple, Plum, Pomegranate, Tangerine	Blackberry, Blueberry, Boysenberry, Elderberry, Gooseberry, Loganberry, Marionberry, Raspberry, Strawberry	Avocado, Banana, Coconut *Dried Fruits:* Apricots, Cranberries, Currants, Dates, Figs, Prunes, Raisins *Melons* (high glycemic index/low calorie): Cantaloupe, Casaba, Honeydew, Muskmelon, Sharlyn, Santa Claus Melon, Watermelon

All fresh fruits and veggies can be blended together to form a variety of smoothies, salads, and soups. Fruits are perhaps our most natural food. Although sweet, the kind of sugars they contain are much slower to convert to energy or fat in your body. Whole fruits are not a problem. Papaya is omitted from the list because most of it is now genetically engineered.

Nuts & Seeds

Nuts	Seeds
Almonds, Brazil Nuts, Cashews, Macadamia, Hazelnuts, Pecans, Pine Nuts, Pistachios, Walnuts	Chia, Flax, Hemp, Poppy, Pumpkin, Sesame, Sunflower

Soaking nuts and seeds until plump, draining/washing, and letting stand for 24 hours is necessary to eliminate enzyme inhibitors, which are bad for digestion. It also makes these hard-to-chew products more assimilable. Nuts and seeds are best blended into toppings, sauces, and dressings.

Grains

Flaked (rolled) Grains	Grains
Barley, Oats, Rye, Wheat	Amaranth, Barley, Cornmeal (non GMO), Buckwheat, Kamut, Millet, Oats, Popcorn, Quinoa, Rice (brown, wild, many other colors & varieties), Rye, Spelt, Teff, Triticale, Wheat

Soaking grains until plump, draining/washing, and letting stand for 24 hours improves nutrition significantly. It also shortens cooking time. Grains can be allowed to sprout fully over several days, then blended and used in many ways. Grains are starchy foods and not recommended for losing weight, use legumes instead for long-term energy.

Legumes (Beans)

Legumes (Beans)	
Anasazi Beans	Kidney Beans
Appaloosa Bean	Lima Bean (baby & large)
Azuki Beans	Mung Beans
Lentils (Black, Green, Red, Yellow, French)	Navy Beans
	Peanuts
Black Turtle Beans	Pinto Beans
Chickpeas/Garbanzo Beans (black or tan)	Red Beans
	Scarlet Runner Beans
Bolita Beans	Soybeans
Channa Dal	Split or Whole Peas (green, yellow)
Cranberry Beans	Urad Dal
Dhal	
Great Northern Beans	

There are literally hundreds of legume varieties around the world. This is a small list of the most common varieties available. Two of the most important legumes are lentils and garbanzo beans. Cooked properly and seasoned with herbs and spices, they can provide long-term energy and are high in nutrition. Lentils and chickpeas can easily be sprouted and eaten raw (delicious when properly seasoned).

Herbs and Spices

Herbs and Spices

There is a reason Columbus was trying to reach India and the Spice Islands (Indonesia). Herbs and spices add incredible flavors to foods. They also have healing properties. Here's a list of the most common herbs and spices. When you shop for herbs and spices, start by looking at prepared blends from different ethnic groups: Mexican, Italian, Thai, Indian, Chinese, etc. Note the combination of herbs and spices used and their order listed on the package – the order is from most to least used in the blend. This will give you a great head start in making your own blends.

The herbs and spices below can be used individually or in blends. Herbs and spices should be added to virtually every preparation to improve health values. They can also be used in dressings, sauces, toppings, icings, spreads, milks, etc.

I have omitted onions and garlic because of their steroidal properties and their tendency to produce aggressive behavior. They do have medicinal properties, which have short term value.

Agar-agar - Gelling agent made from seaweed.
Allspice - Aromatic, used in baked goods.
Arrowroot - Used to thicken.
Asafoetida/Hing - Very strong, use only a pinch. A substitute for onions if used in cooking, not for raw dishes.
Basil - Spicy, good in almost any savory dish.
Bay Leaves - Robust. Use whole leaf, remove from dish after cooking. One dry leaf placed on top protects stored dried beans, grains, and flours.
Black Salt - Salty and pungent. Has a slight sulfur taste to it. Excellent on apples and apple sauce.
Caraway Seed - Pungent.
Cardamom, Seed/Ground - Aromatic. Delicious in east Indian and sweet dishes.
Cayenne Pepper - Hot, use sparingly.
Chervil - Green tasting. good in salad dressings, Italian style dishes, and soups.
Chili Powder - Spicy, use in ethnic dishes, especially Mexican. Most chili powders sold in stores have garlic in them. If you want just chilies, powder your own.
Chinese Five Spice - A blend of spices especially nice for sweet foods and desserts.

Cinnamon, Stick/Ground - Spicy/aromatic. Good in baked goods and most winter squash.

Cloves, Whole/Ground - Spicy/aromatic. Use just a little, good in baked goods and most winter squash.

Coriander, Seed/Ground - Slightly bitter. Takes gas out of beans if combined with cumin. Good in east Indian savory dishes, and many others.

Cream of Tartar - Used in baking.

Cumin, Seed/Ground - Slightly bitter. Removes gas from beans. Good in salads (whole seeds).

Curry Powder - Spicy and hot. Excellent with most vegetables, grains, and beans. Many blends are available.

Dill Seed, Dill Weed - Seed is sourish, weed is very green tasting and slightly sour. Excellent in salad dressings and breads.

Fennel - Sweet/aromatic. Excellent in east Indian stir-fries, salads, dressings, and winter squash.

Garam masala - Sweet, spicy, slightly hot. Good with most vegetables, especially stir-fries.

Ginger, Fresh/Powdered - Hot/spicy/pungent. Excellent for digestion, good in dressings, stir-fry dishes, and desserts.

Marjoram - Aromatic/slightly sweet. Used in Italian dishes and dressings.

Mustard, Black or yellow - Use whole seed or ground - Spicy/pungent. Good in dressing and east Indian curries.

Nutmeg - Spicy. Excellent in baked goods and winter squash.

Oregano - Aromatic, slightly bitter. Used in Italian and Mediterranean dishes.

Paprika - Spicy/sweet. Good in sauces, dressing, and to garnish mashed potatoes.

Pepper - Hot/spicy. Use sparingly in sauces, dressings, and as a condiment.

Peppermint - Sweet/spicy. Excellent tea for digestion, very soothing. Use in dressings, salads, and smoothies.

Rosemary - Aromatic. Good on almost anything that isn't sweet, especially breads, potatoes, dressings, and sauces.

Sage - Aromatic. Used in stuffing. Try in dressings, stir-fries, and breads.

Salt - Flavor enhancer, use moderately.

Sesame Seeds - Nutty flavor. Delicious base for sauces.

Spearmint - Sweet/spicy. Excellent tea for digestion, very soothing. Use in dressings, salads, and smoothies.

Tamari/Soy Sauce - Salty. Use in place of salt in oriental dishes. Has a distinct flavor that can be used in any dish as a substitute for salt.

Tarragon - Sweet/pungent, slight licorice taste. Used predominantly in Italian and Mediterranean dishes, salads, dressings, and sauces. Too much will create a soapy flavor.

Thyme - Bitter. Used in Italian and Mediterranean dishes, breads, and salad
   dressings.
Turmeric - Bitter. Ingredient in curry and mustards, can be used by itself.
   Use sparingly. Good in east Indian dishes. A major ingredient in mustard.
Vanilla Bean - powder or liquid, for vanilla flavor.

Packaged Indian-Ayurvedic Herbs and Spices / Typical Ingredients

Packaged Herbs and Spices	Typical Ingredients
Companies: Shan, MDH, Sakthi *Package Names:* Pav Bhaji Chana Chaat Chunky Chat Sambar Chaat Masala Dahi Bara Chaat Fruit Chaat Dry Mango Powder	Red Chili, Paprika, Coriander, Cumin Seed, Green Cardamom, Brown Cardamom, Ginger, Cinnamon, Green Mango, Dry Mango Powder, Clove, Mace, Fenugreek Seed, Anise Seed, Nutmeg, Fennel, Carom (Ajwain, Bishop's Weed), Bay Leaf, Citric Acid, Musk Melon, Black Pepper, Pomegranate Seeds, Mint Leaves, Caraway, Asafoetida, Curry Leaf, Turmeric, Long Black Pepper, Salt

For other spice blends, search the Internet for recipes. For instance,
search "ethnic spice blends." Typical ingredients for European and
Mediterranean spice blends (omitting onion and garlic): Salt, Basil, Cumin,
Coriander, Parsley, Sage, Rosemary, Thyme, Marjoram, Oregano, Fennel,
Dill Weed, Toasted Sesame, Celery Seed, Paprika, Chervil, Savory, Tarragon,
Black Pepper, Cayenne Pepper.

Thai and Chinese spices often include the Indian and European spices
along with Mint, Ginger, Coconut, Lemongrass, Mustard Seed, Lime Zest
(or other citric zest).

As you can see, when you switch to a healthy diet you are really switching
to the most flavorful, gourmet diet possible. It is also extremely healthy
because these herbs and spices have many health benefits. You learn how to
spice foods by experimenting. Your tastes will change as you become more
adjusted to a lighter more nutritious diet. Your spicing will change as you
change. The only big mistake you can make is to use too much of a very
strong spice or herb, such as cayenne pepper, asafoetida, clove, or tarragon.
Don't be afraid to use a variety of herbs and spices. It's not unusual to use
1-3 tablespoons in a dish for 2 to 3 people.

Edible Flowers

Edible Flowers
Anise Hyssop, Apple, Arugula, Bachelor's Buttons, Bee balm, Calendulas, Carnation (all dianthus), Chamomile, Chervil, Chicory, Chrysanthemums, Clematis, Daisies, Dandelion, Daylilies, Dill, Elderberry, English Daisy, Fennel, Fuchsia, Geranium, Hollyhocks, Impatiens, Iris, Japanese Honeysuckle, Lavender, Lilac, Linden, Lovage, Marigold (Tagets Signata & Tagets Tenuifolia), Nasturtium, Okra, Passion Flower, Pansies, Petunia, Pineapple Sage, Primrose, Redbud, Red Clover, Rosemary, Roses, Safflower, Sage, Scarlet Runner Bean, Scented Geraniums, Snapdragon, Squash Blossoms, Sunflower, Sweet Violet - all varieties (leaves too), Sweet Woodruff, Thyme, Tulips, Violas. Most herb flowers. Never eat commercial flowers.

Edible flowers can be added to salads for beauty, color, and fun. Some flowers have a spicy flavor. Most flowers taste like they smell. This list has been checked for safety. If you are unsure about identification, then it's better not to eat them. Never use commercial flowers. They are usually treated with various chemicals and often grown with pesticides! Use only organically grown flowers from your own garden or from an organic grower you know and trust.

Foods from your own garden always taste better than commercial produce, because they're so much fresher. Expand your gardening knowledge and share gardens with friends. Here are some resources.

Your Gardening Knowledge Base
Indian System
http://palekarzerobudgetspiritualfarming.org
Bhutan System (Includes Indian systems)
Training Manual on Low Cost Organic Agriculture (pdf)
Includes conventional organic practices (that are of lesser value) but also Indian microbial methods...
http://www.snvworld.org/es/publications/training-manual-on-low-cost-organic-agriculture
Korean System
http://gilcarandang.com/recipes/
Search the Internet: "indigenous microorganisms IMO" and "beneficial indigenous microorganisms"
Japanese System
http://en.wikipedia.org/wiki/Natural_farming
http://en.wikipedia.org/wiki/Masanobu_Fukuoka

Permaculture System
http://en.wikipedia.org/wiki/Permaculture

Community Agriculture
Research the terms *Agroforestry*, *Forest Gardens*, *Permaculture*, and *Edible Landscaping* for systems of sustainable food security for larger communities and for regional food planning.

Natural Seed Sources for North America
For other areas of the world, search for "open pollinated seeds" and "heirloom seeds." Talk with local organic gardeners and seed saver exchanges. These are the seed sources we use most often:

Seed Sources:
Baker Creek Heirloom Seeds, www.rareseeds.com/
Pinetree Gardens, www.superseeds.com
Territorial Seed Company, www.territorialseed.com
Botanical Interest, botanicalinterests.com
Johnny's Selected Seeds, johnnyseeds.com
Renee's Garden, www.reneesgarden.com (interesting flower seeds)

Other Resources:
Native Seed/SEARCH, www.nativeseeds.org
Seed Savers Exchange, www.seedsavers.org

There are a lot of good smaller companies out there, too. Local seed sources will have seeds that are acclimated to your local environment and soils. Be sure to check that they've signed the Safe Seed Pledge. If they haven't, their seeds may contain GMO seeds, or they support companies that produce GMO seeds. Avoid potentially dangerous GMO seeds.

Saving your own seed is a good option, too. There are many good books. Two books I can recommend are:
Seed to Seed by Suzanne Ashworth and *Saving Seeds* by Marc Rogers.

Recipe Formulas
There are now so many recipes on the Internet that there's little value in putting recipes here. Instead, I'll suggest a few recipe *formulas* that will allow you to build your own recipes using the ingredients that you have on hand. I rarely use recipes anymore, except for occasional baked goods. One of the problems with recipes from books is that you often don't have all the ingredients. These recipe formulas allow you to make generic recipes, using what you have on hand. You may want to put your recipes into an app on your portable device, so you can have them readily available.

Green Smoothie Formula

2-3 fruits (one citrus)

1 C liquid (water, juice)

80% Mild Tender Greens (like spinach)

20% Dark Nutritious Greens (like Kale or Chard)

Nuts, &/or Seeds, if desired (2-3 tsp, soaked)

Pinch of Salt

1 tsp Cinnamon or Chinese 5 Spice if desired

Raw Soup Formula

1-2 cups of liquid (Nut milk, water, etc.)

2-3 Veggies, (tomatoes work well)

Greens - (not too much, or too bitter)

Avocado - (if desired, makes a creamy soup)

Nuts, &/or Seeds (2-3 tsp, soaked)

1/2 Lemon (or vinegar) to taste

2 tsp Sweetener (or a few dates/raisins, or fruit)

2 tsp Salt

2 tsp Herbs & Spices

Raw Soup Example

2 Cups Water

2 Cups Roma tomatoes, chopped

1/2 Cup sun-dried tomatoes, soaked in water

1 Cup Celery, chopped

1/4 Cup Red Pepper, chopped

1/4 Cup Fresh Basil, chopped (or 1 T dried)

3 Dates, soaked

1/8 tsp Cayenne Pepper (if desired)

Salt to taste

Blend in a blender or high-speed blender

Nut & Seed Dressing or Topping Formula

3 Tbsp Soaked Nuts & Seeds

1-2 Tbsp Herbs & Spices,

Water or Nut Milk,

A little oil or avocado (if desired),

Lemon or other citrus, or vinegar,

Salt to taste

Sweetener to taste

For fruit toppings, use sweet spices and only a pinch of salt.

Use a small jar and blender to blend into a creamy dressing or topping.

With less liquid, it can even be an icing for a sweet treat.

Chunky Salad Formula

Sliced Tomatoes

Chopped Jicama

Chunks of Avocado

Nut and/or Seed Dressing

Salad Formula

75% Mild Tender Greens

25% Dark Nutritious & Spicy Greens

2-3 Vegetables Chopped or Shredded

1-2 Dried or Chopped Fresh Fruits

Nuts & Seed Dressing

Thin Wraps (Similar to Dosas, Burritos, Crepes, Tortillas, etc.)

(I call these "Dosaritos" a contraction of Dosas and Burritos)

2/3 to 3/4 Whole Wheat Flour

1/3 to 1/4 Bean Flour (i.e. Garbanzo or Lentil Flour)

Salt to taste

Spice blends to taste

If you like a lighter, less dense wrap use baking powder & baking soda, 2:1, as you would with pancakes, otherwise no leavening is needed.

Add water to make the consistency of a very thin pancake-type batter.

Pour onto a lightly oiled pancake skillet at medium heat, cook both sides.

Fill with shredded vegetables, lettuce, and savory nut/seed dressings. You can also fill with bananas, fruits, sweet nut/seed toppings, and sweet spices such as cinnamon or cardamom for a dessert.

Omega-3 Drink Formula

Omega-3 Nutrient-Dense Milk

3 Tbsp soaked blend of Seeds & Nuts: Flax, Chia, Sunflower, Walnuts

1-2 C Almond Milk or water

Sweetener to Taste

Pinch of Salt

If desired, 1 Tsp of Rosewater or 1/4 tsp Cinnamon powder

Fermented Foods

Sauerkraut

To make sauerkraut, shred cabbage in a food processor. Make some of it smaller and smash it with a large wooden dowel or plunger to make a little cabbage juice. Add a teaspoon of sea salt per cabbage and only enough water to cover when pressed down. Compress tightly into a large crock pot. Use a plate, smaller crockpot, or a casserole dish that fits snugly inside the large crockpot to compress the cabbage. Keep it pressed down with a weight. I use a casserole dish that fits nicely inside of my crockpot. Let it sit at normal room temperatures of 70-85°F for 3-7 days. Check every day or two for sour taste. When done, salt to taste and eat. Keep sauerkraut juice away from furniture as it can ruin the finish.

Fermented Dosas / Dosaritos

This is our fermented non-traditional formula version.

To make a thin *fermented* batter, use water, grain flour, and legume flour (2/3 to 3/4 grains, 1/3 to 1/4 legumes). For grain flour, you can use rice, wheat, barley, rye or any grain. If you don't have flour you can put grains in a blender and blend on high speed. It won't be as fine as flour, but it works. Combine this with garbanzo, lentil, urad dal, or any legume flour. Blend legumes to turn them into a coarse flour if you don't have flour.

Add grain and legume flour to an open container of warm water, cover with a towel. Put in a warm place overnight. During the winter, I use a heating pad set on low and put the container on two chopsticks, so it doesn't touch the pad. Cover with the towel. By morning it will become fermented and smell like sourdough bread. Make thin "pancakes" or crêpes (dosaritos) and fill the wraps with savory veggies or fruit fillings. If you didn't use flour but used coarse blended grains, blend into a smooth liquid before using it.

Bokashi Formula

The Fermented Dosa formula is also our bokashi inoculant formula. The lactobacillus bacteria can be multiplied afterward by adding brown sugar or molasses. You can also mix it with yogurt or milk to create greater volumes of friendly bacteria. Do not keep it sealed tightly since high pressures can build up. Allow room at the top to prevent overflow.

Marinated Foods

An alternative to fermenting or cooking is marinades. It's another way to break down tough vegetables to make them more palatable. They will have more nutritional value than cooking. To marinate vegetables, coat or soak them in vinegar (or citric acids such as orange or lemon), salt, olive oil, and herbs and spices. To preserve food values, marinate in the refrigerator in a closed container. This is rather similar to soaking them in salad dressing. Tough plant tissues are softened by the action of salt and acids.

Skin Care Formulas
All skin care formulas can be made in a blender jar. Any 1/2 pint or pint jar will fit on an Oster blender and perhaps on others. Some blenders have their own small blending jars available. Check your blender for options.

General Skin Care
Skin Rejuvenation (Makes ~ 5-10% vitamin C solution)
Skin Rejuvenation Ingredients:
1/2 to 1 part powdered vitamin C
10 parts of water
2 parts vegetable-source glycerin
Splash it on after a shower or bath. A spray bottle also works. Keep out of eyes.

Natural Cold Cream
Useful for removing makeup. Simple natural formula.
Ingredients:
1/2 Tbsp of bee pollen - optional
1 Tbsp of rosewater (available at Indian groceries)
1/4 cup vegetable glycerin
1/4 cup grated beeswax
1/2 cup almond or sunflower or other vegetable oil

Directions:
Blend the bee pollen and rosewater, set aside.
Mix glycerin, beeswax, and oil and heat just until melted
Blend the oil, then add water and blend again until fully blended

Skin Moisturizer
Lightly coat your skin with a moisturizer after a shower or bath, especially in winter.
Skin Moisturizer Ingredients:
4 parts oil – olive or coconut oil is best, but any vegetable oil is good
4 parts water – add some rosewater for a nice scent
1 part bee's wax or shea butter (these make a more solid creamy lotion)
1 Vitamin E capsule, if available, protects from spoiling and helps your skin.
Warm oils and waxes before blending, then blend in warm water, add vitamin E.

Fruit Facial Peel
This is a low-cost treatment to replace expensive spa treatments.
A fruit facial peel removes dead cells from the outer layers of your skin. There are hundreds of formulas. They all use natural fruit acids and enzymes. Papaya has

lots of enzymes, pineapple also has enzymes but more acid. All fruits have acid and enzymes in various measures. Unripe fruits are more acidic. The mix of ingredients can vary widely. Use a more acidic mix for a stronger peel, more papaya, honey, and aloe for a gentler peel. You can also add yogurt, or milk.

Facial Peel Ingredients:
10-15 parts papaya pieces
1 part pineapple pieces
1 part orange juice
1 part honey
1 part aloe vera gel if available
1 part chamomile tea if available

Directions:
Blend the ingredients in a blender jar
Start with a clean warm wet face using a warm wet towel to soften the skin. Massage onto your face and neck. Let sit for 5-10 minutes. Rinse with warm, then cool water. Peels can be drying. Use a moisturizer to protect your skin. Do this peel no more than twice a week. Search the Internet for "papaya fruit facial peel" for lots of ideas. Many other fruits also work. Strawberries are often used. Test first if you are sensitive.

Skin Exfoliating Body Scrub

Many formulas for body scrubs use some mild abrasive and oil. The abrasive is usually salt or sugar, but oatmeal and various flours have also been used. Coffee grounds help to reduce cellulite.

Ingredients:
3/4 cup coffee grounds, oatmeal, and/or flour, etc.
1/4 cup sugar and/or coarse sea salt, (2/3 salt to 1/3 sugar works well)
Coconut and olive oil, just enough to cover. Stir to mix well.

Directions
Mix all ingredients thoroughly. After you've washed your body, massage the scrub onto wet skin. Cover your body, and rinse with warm water. You can expect this to take a several minutes. Do this treatment in the tub or shower so you don't make a mess of your bathroom or house.

Hair Conditioning Treatment

There are many natural hair treatments that use natural ingredients from the kitchen: apple cider vinegar, olive oil, almond oil, yogurt, honey, avocado, banana, etc. Here's a simple formula. You can find more on the net with a quick search.
Ingredients:
1/2 cup plain yogurt
1/2 cup honey

Directions

Mix ingredients together and massage into your hair. Let sit for 20 minutes. Rinse with warm water followed by cool water to seal the process.

Natural Toothpaste
Make your own natural toothpaste:
2 tsp clay powder – either bentonite or kaolin clay (natural food store)
1/2 tsp natural salt
1 drop of peppermint or spearmint essential oil

Mix in sufficient water to make a paste, double or triple the recipe to make more. It only takes a minute to two to make this up, so you can make it weekly or bi-weekly. Be careful not to add more than a drop or two of essential oil. The oils are very potent. If you add too much, you can dilute with more clay, salt, and water.

Make Your Shaving Razor Last for Months (Even a Year or More)
After shaving, take a few seconds to dry your razor by swishing side to side across a towel, moving backwards to avoid cutting the pile. Then stroke your razor backwards on your thigh for 10-20 strokes. It works the same way old-time barbers sharpened straight razors with a leather strap. Your thigh, or any expanse of skin, is the "leather." Your savings will pay for this book several times over! Plus, you'll always have a sharp razor!

Resources, Charts, Links, and Other Goodies
pH Paper - Micro Essential Laboratory Cat. # MF-1606

Iridology and Reflexology charts - Innerlightresources.com

Dr. Bernard Jensen books on iridology and bowel cleansing.

Additional resources that I could not include in the book because of large format requirements, color graphics, videos, and more will be available from my website. This is the place to go for the latest updated information. http://ExtraordinaryHealthcare.com

Downloadable Charts:
- Dynamic Tension-Resistance Exercises for Strength
- Classic Yoga Exercises
- Classic Pilates Exercises
- Reflexology Chart
- Iridology Chart

Speaking Engagements, Seminars, and Workshops
For speaking engagements for your organization please contact me through my website.

I also offer seminars and workshops for people who want a more in-depth experience. Be sure to sign up on the website if you would like to be notified.

Personal consultations are available for individual "house calls" anywhere in the world via telephone or two-way Internet video conference. See the web site for more information.

Programs for Businesses

Companies and organizations may want special presentations and programs for staff and employees to provide optimal wellness and natural healthcare for their employees and to reduce healthcare costs for the business. I offer wellness and natural healthcare programs for businesses, especially the Extraordinary Healthcare™ Program.

Visit http://ExtraordinaryHealthcare.com

29456566R00173

Made in the USA
Charleston, SC
13 May 2014